Nursing
Delegation and
Management
of Patient Care

Second

Nursing **Delegation** and **Management** of Patient Care

Second Edition

Kathleen Motacki, MSN, RN, BC
Clinical Professor Saint Peter's
   University School of Nursing
Jersey City, New Jersey
Secretary, New Jersey Consortium of
   Chapters
Sigma Theta Tau International Honor
   Society of Nursing

Kathleen Burke, PhD, RN
Assistant Dean in Charge of Nursing
   Programs
Professor of Nursing
   Adler Center for Nursing Excellence
   Ramapo College of New Jersey
Mahwah, New Jersey

ELSEVIER

ELSEVIER

3251 Riverport Lane
St. Louis, Missouri 63043

NURSING DELEGATION AND MANAGEMENT OF PATIENT CARE,
SECOND EDITION

ISBN: 978-0-323-32109-9

Notices

Knowledge and best practice in this field are constantly changing. As new research and experience broaden our understanding, changes in research methods, professional practices, or medical treatment may become necessary.

Practitioners and researchers must always rely on their own experience and knowledge in evaluating and using any information, methods, compounds, or experiments described herein. In using such information or methods they should be mindful of their own safety and the safety of others, including parties for whom they have a professional responsibility.

With respect to any drug or pharmaceutical products identified, readers are advised to check the most current information provided (i) on procedures featured or (ii) by the manufacturer of each product to be administered, to verify the recommended dose or formula, the method and duration of administration, and contraindications. It is the responsibility of practitioners, relying on their own experience and knowledge of their patients, to make diagnoses, to determine dosages and the best treatment for each individual patient, and to take all appropriate safety precautions.

To the fullest extent of the law, neither the Publisher nor the authors, contributors, or editors, assume any liability for any injury and/or damage to persons or property as a matter of products liability, negligence or otherwise, or from any use or operation of any methods, products, instructions, or ideas contained in the material herein.

Previous edition copyrighted 2011.

Library of Congress Cataloging-in-Publication Data
Motacki, Kathleen, author. | Burke, Kathleen, 1952-, author.
Nursing delegation and management of patient care / Kathleen Motacki,
    Kathleen Burke.
2nd edition. | St. Louis, Missouri : Elsevier, [2017]
LCCN 2015045932 | ISBN 9780323321099
| MESH: Nursing Care | Nursing Care--organization & administration
    | Leadership
LCC RT89 | NLM WY 100.1 | DDC 362.17/3068--dc23 LC record
available at http://lccn.loc.gov/2015045932

Content Strategist: Yvonne Alexopoulous
Content Development Manager: Jean Fornango
Content Development Specialist: Danielle M. Frazier
Publishing Services Manager: Jeff Patterson
Project Manager: Lisa A. P. Bushey
Design Direction: Teresa McBryan
Senior Book Designer: Maggie Reid

Printed in the U.S.A.

Last digit is the print number: 9 8 7 6 5 4 3 2 1

Dedication
Robert E. Motacki, Jr.
November 9, 1984, to November 17, 2013
Kathleen Motacki
Kathleen Burke

KATHLEEN MOTACKI, MSN, RN, BC

A Clinical Professor at Saint Peter's University School of Nursing, Jersey City, New Jersey, Kathleen Motacki has more than 39 years of experience in nursing, 12 years as a Professor of Nursing, and currently teaches 4-year traditional nursing courses and in the RN-to-BSN progam at the Jesuit College of New Jersey. Her areas of clinical and classroom expertise include pediatric nursing, leadership, and community health. She has taught pediatric NCLEX® review sessions. She holds board certification in pediatric nursing from the American Nurses Credentialing Center (ANCC). She was on the ANCC examination-standard-setting committee and on the content expert panel for the new pediatric credentialing examination. She was the lead investigator for the American Nurses Association School of Nursing Curriculum Study on Safe Patient Handling and Movement. She received the 2008 National Occupational Research Agenda (NORA) Partnering Award for the American Nurses Association Safe Patient Handling and Movement Training Program for her role in the Schools of Nursing research project. She also received the Daisy Award and the Marianne Rooney Award for nursing excellence from the New Jersey Consortium of Chapters, Sigma Theta Tau International Nursing Honor Society. She is past president of the Epsilon Rho Chapter and the Mu Theta Chapter At Large and currently serves as the Secretary for the New Jersey Consortium of Chapters, Sigma Theta Tau International Nursing Honor Society. Professor Motacki obtained her BSN and MSN in transcultural nursing administration from Kean University, Union, New Jersey. She has published a continuing nursing education series for contact hours, "Safe Patient Handling in Pediatrics," in the *Journal of Pediatric Nursing*. She has published two books with Springer Publishing: *The Illustrated Guide to Safe Patient Handling and Movement* and *The Illustrated Guide to Infection Control*. She has presented at conferences throughout the country on safe patient handling and movement, as well as on peer-reviewed nursing publications.

KATHLEEN BURKE, RN, PhD

Kathleen Burke presently serves as the Assistant Dean in Charge of Nursing at Ramapo College of New Jersey, the state's public liberal arts college. In this position, she is the chief administrator of a 550-student program with prelicensure and RN-to-BSN and -MSN programs. She has been in this position since 2007. In this role she has created academic/clinical partnerships between the college and The Valley Hospital, Ridgewood, New Jersey; The University of Sierra Leone in West Africa; and Kwame Nkrumah University of Science and Technology in Kumasi, Ghana. Additionally, she has served as research advisor to three large Magnet Hospitals in New Jersey and is presently working with St. Joseph's Regional Medical Center (a four-time Magnet-recognized organization). Before that, she was the Assistant Dean of the UMDNJ (the state's health sciences university) School of Nursing, in charge of the Northern Region.

She has extensive clinical nursing experience, having started as a staff nurse in the Veterans Administration system, then moving to local community hospitals and up the professional ladder to supervisory roles, Director of Performance Improvement, Director of Clinical Education, and Senior Vice President of Nursing.

Kathleen has served as a member of Quality New Jersey as an examiner, trainer, senior examiner, and Member of The Board of Judges from 1995–2003. She was a 10-year member of the Baldrige Board of Examiners. She has also facilitated training and served on writing panels and scorebook review panels. She has participated in and led numerous site visits on both a state and national level. She led the first of the new Baldrige Collaborative Assessment Teams.

She is a consultant to the National League of Nursing Centers of Nursing Excellence Program. Kathleen is presently serving on the Board of Trustees of The Valley Home Care System in Ridgewood, New Jersey. She previously served on the Board of The Mountainside Hospital in Glen Ridge, New Jersey. She is the sole academic representative to the New Jersey Council of

Magnet Organizations and the Northern New Jersey Council of Magnet Organizations.

She holds a Bachelor's Degree from Rutgers, The State University of New Jersey, College of Nursing. Her Master of Arts degree is from New York University, Division of Nursing, and she holds a PhD in Nursing Theory and Research from New York University. She was an AACN/Wharton Leadership Fellow in 2014. She is a member of the American Nurses Association, the National League for Nursing, New Jersey Organization of Nurse Executives, Sigma Theta Tau International, and the New Jersey Council of Magnet Organizations.

CONTRIBUTORS

Mary Jo Assi, DNP, RN, NEA-BC, FNP-BC
Director of Nursing Practice and Work Environment
American Nurses Association
Silver Spring, Maryland

Una M. Doddy, RN, MPH, MBA
Clinical Instructor of Nursing
Ramapo College of New Jersey
Mahwah, New Jersey

Gina M. Dovi, MSN, RN, CPHON
Clinical Level III Staff Nurse
Pediatric Hematology/Oncology/BMT
Hackensack University Medical Center
Hackensack, New Jersey

Kathy Faber, RN, MSN, CNL
Clinical Nurse Leader in Neonatology
St. Joseph's Regional Healthcare System
Paterson, New Jersey

Donna Grotheer, MSN, RN
Director of Organizational Education
Hackensack University Medical Center at
    Pascack Valley
Westwood, New Jersey

Catherine Herrmann, BSN, RN, CCRN
Registered Nurse
Hackensack University Medical Center
Hackensack, New Jersey

Sandra D. Horvat, MSN, APN-BC, CPN
Clinical Assistant Professor
Saint Peter's University
School of Nursing
Jersey City, New Jersey

MaryAnn Hozak, MSN, RN, NEA-BC
Director
Innovative Nursing Practice & Quality Outcomes
St. Joseph's Regional Medical Center
Paterson, New Jersey

**Beverly S. Karas-Irwin, DNP, RN, NP-C, HNB-BC,
    NEA-BC**
Director of Nursing Magnet Programs
Center for Professional Nursing Practice
New York, New York

Judith Kutzleb, DNP, RN, CCRN, CCA, NP-C
Vice President, Advanced Practice Professionals;
Primary Care Provider–Adult Primary Care
Excelcare Physician Network
Holy Name Medical Center;
Assistant Professor/Coordinator MSN
Adult–Gerontology Graduate Program
Fairleigh Dickinson University
Teaneck, New Jersey;
Adjunct Faculty
Touro College of Osteopathic Medicine
New York, New York

Beth McGovern, MSN, RNC-OB, CHSECH
Clinical Practice Specialist
Women and Children's Services
The Valley Hospital
Ridgewood, New Jersey

Bonnie Michaels, RN, MA, NES-BC, FACHE
Northvale, New Jersey

Lauren E. O'Hare, EdD, RN
Dean, School of Nursing
Saint Peter's University
Jersey City, New Jersey

Joan Orseck, RN
Human Resources Business Partner
Holy Name Medical Center
Teaneck, New Jersey

Cristina Perez, PhD, RN
Assistant Professor, Nursing
Ramapo College of New Jersey
Mahwah, New Jersey

Eddie A. Perez, RN, MHA, NE-BC
Director of Nursing
Medical Surgical Services
St. Joseph's Regional Medical Center
Paterson, New Jersey

Eleanor Schiavo, MS, RD
Registered Dietician
St. Joseph's Regional Medical Center
Paterson, New Jersey

Theresa Szucs, MSN, RN, CPHQ
Corp. Director of Quality & Performance Improvement
St. Joseph's Healthcare System
Paterson, New Jersey

Shirley Bennett Thompson, RN, BSN, BSBA, MSHA, FACHE
Consultant and Health Care Executive
Shirley Bennett Thompson Consulting, LLC
Jackson, Florida

Judy Urgo, MSN, RN
Staff Nurse
Hackensack University Medical Center
Hackensack, New Jersey

Tina Vacante, MSN, RN
Registered Nurse
Hackensack University Medical Center
Hackensack, New Jersey

Maureen Washburn, RN, ND, CPHQ, FACHE
Chief Clinical Officer
DNV GL–Healthcare, Inc.
Milford, Ohio

REVIEWERS

Michelle Beckford, DMH, RN
Associate Professor of Nursing
Saint Peter's University
Jersey City, New Jersey

Corinne Ellis, DNP, ANP, RN, BC
Assistant Professor
Felician College
Lodi, New Jersey

Janis McMillan, RN, MSN, CNE
Nursing Faculty
Coconino Community College
Flagstaff, Arizona

Cheryl Perna, MSN, RN
Lecturer/Clinical Instructor
University of Nevada Las Vegas
Las Vegas, Nevada

Darlene Sredl, RN, PhD
Teaching Professor of Nursing
University of Missouri, St. Louis
St. Louis, Missouri

Linda D. Wagner, EdD, MSN, RN
Professor, Department of Nursing
Central Connecticut State University
New Britain, Connecticut

Nursing Delegation and Management of Patient Care, Second Edition, is designed to assist nursing students and novice nurses to begin developing an understanding of the myriad issues facing them as managers of care and the potential nursing leaders of tomorrow. This is only a beginning; the concepts of management and leadership are changing daily. Health care is moving at an unprecedented speed, and it is imperative that we all attempt to keep up. The important lesson here is that we as nurses need to keep current, questioning and focusing on what is "best" for our patients and practice.

There is massive information, in both the scholarly and commercial literature, that focuses on what makes a good manager or leader. It is important that nurses keep in touch with this literature, but they need to be able to differentiate between what is "best evidence" and what is best-selling fiction. As you move into practice, your professional organizations, your health care library/librarian, and your own engagement in the profession will be your best allies. Keep in touch with the current literature, and continually strive to improve the care that you deliver to patients and families. Remember. Continuous improvement is continuous!

This book is divided into five sections, four of which deal with the components of the Magnet Model; the final section deals with issues of importance to new graduate nurses. The Magnet-focused sections deal with the following:

Transformational leadership

Structural empowerment

Exemplary professional practice

New knowledge, innovations, and improvements

The last section deals with issues of importance to newly graduated nurses.

Integrated throughout these components are the delineated areas of competence for the nurse manager (AONE). These areas of competence include the following:

- Financial management
- Human resource management
- Performance improvement
- Technology
- Strategic management
- Clinical practice based on current evidence

Other competencies are necessary for the art of managing health care. This is leading the people of health care. These competencies include the following:

- Human resource skills
- Relationship management and influencing behaviors
- Diversity
- Shared decision making

And lastly, there are competencies for creating the leader in yourself:

- Personal and professional accountability
- Career planning
- Personal journey disciplines
- Optimizing the leader within

FEATURES

The text is organized according to these competencies of nurse leaders and managers. Each chapter includes a Clinical Corner box written by a nurse leader who shares a current practice that is used in practice. Additionally, there is an evidence-based discussion from a current piece of literature that reviews current research and/or best practice. It is our hope that the reader gleans some ideas from these sections to spark their own practice. Each chapter concludes with some NCLEX®-exam style questions that may prove helpful in reviewing the content.

ANCILLARIES

Evolve Resources for Nursing Delegation and Management of Patient Care, Second Edition, is available at http://evolve.elsevier.com/Motacki/delegation/ to enhance student instruction. This online resource is organized by chapter and includes the following:

For instructors:
- NEW! TEACH for Nurses
- Test Bank Questions
- PowerPoint Slides
- Image Collection

For students:
- NCLEX®-exam–style practice

PREFACE TO THE STUDENTS

Nursing Delegation and Management of Patient Care, Second Edition, is designed to assist you as you prepare to become the nursing leaders of tomorrow. To help you make the most of your learning experience, here are the key features that you will find in this text:

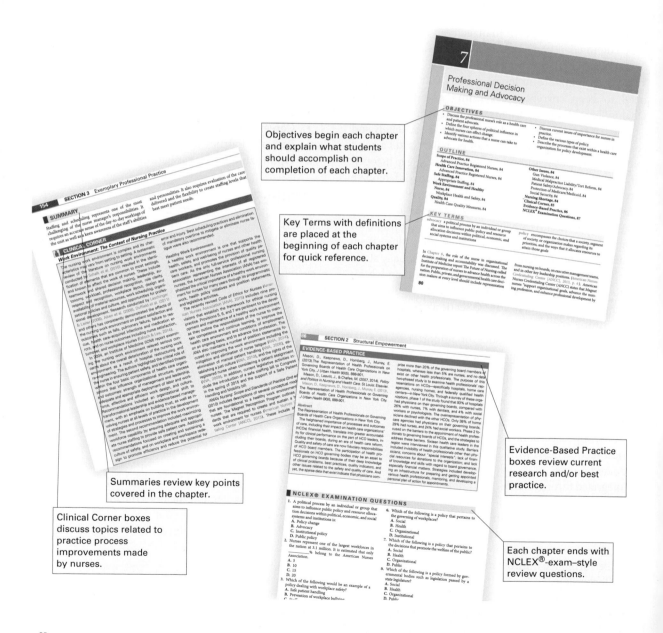

Objectives begin each chapter and explain what students should accomplish on completion of each chapter.

Key Terms with definitions are placed at the beginning of each chapter for quick reference.

Summaries review key points covered in the chapter.

Clinical Corner boxes discuss topics related to practice process improvements made by nurses.

Evidence-Based Practice boxes review current research and/or best practice.

Each chapter ends with NCLEX®-exam–style review questions.

ACKNOWLEDGMENTS

Thank you to Dr. Kathleen Burke, who agreed to take on this project with me. Her knowledge and expertise have made this book an excellent and exceptional resource for senior-level students and new graduate nurses. She was key in making the second edition even better than the first. She is truly a visionary and is an exemplary leader in nursing education. Her lead on the clinical corners and the evidence-based practice boxes makes this book unique. Thank you to the contributors and reviewers for their expertise and input. Thank you to senior acquisitions editor Yvonne Alexopoulos, senior developmental editor Danielle Frazier, and project manager Lisa Bushey for their unending patience with this project. Finally, thank you to my loving family for always being supportive in my nursing endeavors, my husband Robert, my lovely daughter Lisa, my baby John, my brother-in-law Brian, and to my new family, Mirza David Ashraf, my son-in-law, and his mother, Dr. Elizabeth Ashraf. To my family members who have gone before us, Irene and Edward Motacki, Ted Tatarek, and my loving son, Robert, Jr; may they rest in peace. They are always in my heart and prayers.

Kathleen Motacki

Thank you to Kathleen Motacki for asking me to assist her in this project. Also to Jean Kenworthy of Elsevier, who suggested my name to Kathleen. Thank you to the contributors and reviewers for their expertise and input. Thank you to senior acquisitions editor Yvonne Alexopoulos, senior developmental editor Danielle Frazier, and project manager Lisa Bushey for their unending patience with this project. I would also like to thank my many colleagues who assisted with the evidence-based practice boxes and clinical corners. Their names are listed under Contributors. Thanks also to all of the marvelous nurses I have worked with over the years ... and to Elaine, Peggy, Kathleen, Cristina, Asha, Diane, Maisha, Julie, Pat, Donna, Andrea, Joan, Debi and Ulysses at Ramapo, in addition to the nurses of the New Jersey Magnet Consortium of Magnet Organizations, who have extended the reach of professional nurses throughout the state.

Kathleen Burke

CONTENTS

Transformational Leadership

SECTION OUTLINE

Transformational leaders are those who stimulate and inspire followers to achieve extraordinary outcomes and in the process develop their own leadership potential. They inspire, motivate, stimulate, and attend to each individual's concerns and needs (American Nurses Credentialing Center [ANCC], 2013). They also evolve the organization through strategic planning to meet current and future needs and strategic challenges.

The strategic planning of the organization occurs at all levels and must align with the organizational priorities to continually improve the levels of performance across the organization. Wherever nursing is practiced, the nursing leadership must develop structures, processes, and expectations for clinical nurse input and involvement across the organization (ANCC, 2013).

This section deals with the leadership structure within health care organizations: the structures and processes, underlying strategic planning, regulatory environments, and financial management.

1

Leadership and Management

OBJECTIVES

- Identify the various leadership theories.
- Differentiate between leadership and management.
- Discuss the role of the manager.
- Review the different management levels in nursing.
- Identify differences between a nurse manager and a nurse executive.
- Differentiate between the various types of competencies of patient care managers.

- Compare the nursing process and the management process.
- Discuss activities used by the nurse manager to support the nursing and management processes.
- Identify the day-to-day activities of the care manager.

OUTLINE

KEY TERMS

first-level manager manager responsible for supervising nonmanagerial personnel and day-to-day activities of specific work units

leadership ability to influence people to work toward the meeting of stated goals

management act of planning, organizing, staffing, directing, and controlling for the present; process of coordinating actions and allocating resources to achieve organizational goals

middle-level manager manager who supervises first-level managers within a specified area and is responsible for the people and activities within those areas; generally acts as liaison between first-level and upper-level management

upper-level manager top level to whom middle manager reports; primarily responsible for establishing organizational goals and strategic plans for entire division of nursing

LEADERSHIP VERSUS MANAGEMENT

Just because someone is in a leadership position, it does not automatically follow that this person is a leader. Some people have false assumptions about leaders and leadership. Many people believe that the position and title are the same as true leadership. Having the title of chief nurse does not necessarily mean that the person in that position is a leader, while being a staff nurse does not mean that person is not a leader. New nurse managers often make the mistake of believing that along with the new title comes the mantle of leadership. Leadership takes a tremendous amount of effort, time, and energy. **Leadership** can be defined as the use of individual traits and personal power to influence and guide strategy development. Leaders need to "do the right thing," be future oriented, be visionary, focus on purposes, and empower others to set and achieve organizational goals. According to Porter-O'Grady and Mallach (2015, p. 20) the major tasks of the twenty-first century health care leader are:

- Deconstructing the barriers and structures of the twentieth century.
- Alerting staff about the implications of changing what they do.
- Establishing safety around taking risks and experimenting.
- Embracing new technologies as a way of doing work.
- Reading the signposts along the road to the future.
- Translating the emerging reality of health reform into language the staff can use.
- Demonstrating personal engagement with health reform.
- Helping others adapt to the demands of a value-driven health system.
- Creating a safe milieu for the struggles and pain of changing practice and service.
- Enumerating small successes as a basis for supporting staff.
- Celebrating the journey and all progress made.

Management is the act of planning, organizing, staffing, directing, and controlling for the present. Management can be taught, whereas leadership is usually a reflection of personal experience.

As shown in Figure 1-1, leaders show the way, although managers labor to produce the day-to-day

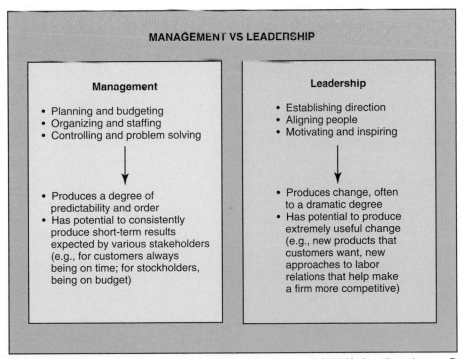

FIGURE 1-1 Management versus leadership. (Data from Kotter, J. [1996]. *Leading change*. Boston: Harvard Business School.)

TABLE 1-1   Comparison of Leadership and Management

	Leadership	Management
Motto	Do the right thing	Do things right
Challenge	Change	Continuity
Focus	Purposes	Structures and procedures
Time frame	Future	Present
Methods	Strategy	Schedule
Questions	Why?	Who, what, when, where, how?
Outcomes	Journeys	Destinations
Human	Potential	Performance

Bennis, W., & Nanus, B. (1997). *Leaders: The strategies for taking charge.* New York: Harper and Row.

outcomes. Leaders focus on effectiveness, and managers deal with efficiencies (Figure1-1).

COMPARISON OF LEADERSHIP AND MANAGEMENT

A further review of leadership and management focuses on the major themes of each role (Table 1-1). The nurse, as manager, works collaboratively to achieve the desired outcomes of quality care, fiscal responsibility, and customer satisfaction by coordinating the care of individuals, families, groups, or populations through the effective use of technology, resources, information, and systems. Some health care agencies will differentiate between the level of academic preparation of the nurse and the expected competency of the manager (Table 1-2).

TABLE 1-2   Competencies of Associate Degree in Nursing (ADN) and Bachelor of Science in Nursing (BSN) Nurses

Skill	Associate Degree in Nursing	Bachelor of Science in Nursing
Management of care	Coordinates, organizes, prioritizes and modifies care provided for the individual, family or group. Assigns and delegates care appropriately.	Coordinates, organizes, prioritizes, and modifies care provided for the individual, family, group, or population. Assigns and delegates care appropriately. Develops, implements, and evaluates population-based health care programs.
Management and leadership concepts	Applies management and leadership concepts. Uses effective communication and conflict management skills in promoting a positive milieu.	Analyzes the management process and leadership concepts for implementation. Uses, and coaches others to use, effective communication and conflict management skills in creating a positive milieu.
Professional development	Contributes to the professional development of health care providers.	Promotes and evaluates professional development of health care providers.
Nursing care delivery systems	Participates in implementing and evaluating traditional and alternative nursing care delivery systems.	Develops and evaluates traditional and alternative nursing care delivery systems.
Management goals	Identifies and participates in influencing management goals.	Demonstrates a beginning leadership role in establishing and influencing management goals.
Standards of care	Participates in evaluation and development of standards of nursing care.	Develops and evaluates standards of nursing care.
Change	Demonstrates flexibility and effectively influences the change process.	Evaluates the need for change and demonstrates flexibility in promoting planned change.

THEORIES OF LEADERSHIP

There are numerous theories of leadership. How the leader approaches leadership is often very dependent on their personal experiences. Leadership also relies on the organizational structure and culture of the health care facility. Four of the more common leadership theories have evolved over time: trait theory, behavioral theory, contingency theory, and contemporary theory.

Trait Theory

Leaders are presumed to possess certain traits that are leadership specific. Leadership traits include drive, persistence, creative problem solving, initiative, self-confidence, ability to influence others, and intelligence. The thought is that these traits when put into practice will result in positive outcomes.

Behavioral Theory

The focus of behavioral theory is not what leaders do, but how they behave. Behaviorists characterize leaders by their style of practice:

- Autocratic leaders change behaviors within the organization through the use of coercion, authority, punishment, and power.
- Democratic leaders influence change within the organization through participation, involvement of staff in goal setting, and collaboration.
- Permissive or laissez faire leaders assume that people are able to make their own decisions and complete their work without any facilitation of the leader.
- Bureaucratic leaders influence the behavior of the organization through organizational policies and rules.

Contingency Theory

Often leaders use different leadership styles in different situations. A leader may use an autocratic style in a disaster management situation, but a democratic style in strategic planning. This ability to adjust one's approach to the situation is called situational leadership or contingency theory.

Newer concepts of leadership are a combination of prior work in the field and include such descriptors as charismatic, connective, shared, and servant leadership. A charismatic leader has the ability to engage others because of their powerful personality. Connective leadership draws on the leader's ability to bring others together to effect change. Shared leadership acknowledges that no one person can accomplish the work of the organization. Self-directed work teams and shared governance epitomize this philosophy. Servant leadership puts other people and their needs before the leader's self-interest.

Two leadership theories prevalent within health care today are transactional leadership and transformational leadership. In transactional leadership, there is an exchange between the leader and the employee. The needs of the employees are identified, and the leader provides rewards to meet those needs in exchange for performance. This type of leadership usually occurs in a hierarchical organization, that is, one in which decision making occurs at the top of the structure and is communicated to the employees. Transformational leadership is more consultative and collaborative. Kouzes and Posner (2002) identify five basic practices in transformational leadership:

1. Challenging the process, questioning the ways that things have always been done, and creatively thinking of new ways of doing things.
2. Motivating and inspiring shared vision or bringing everyone together, moving toward the shared goal.
3. Empowering others to act.
4. Modeling the change.
5. Praising the employee for the work done.

Transformational leaders behave in ways to achieve superior results by employing one or more of the four core components of transformational leadership (the four Is):

Idealized Influence (II): Leaders serve as a role model for followers: they exhibit high ethical behavior, instill pride, and gain respect and trust. Followers tend to identify with their leaders and desire to emulate them; leaders are perceived by their followers as having extraordinary capabilities, persistence, and determination.

Inspirational Motivation (IM): The degree to which the leader articulates a vision that is appealing, motivating, and inspiring to followers. Leaders with inspirational motivation communicate optimism about future goals, provide meaning for the task at hand, and challenge followers with high standards. The visionary aspects of leadership are supported by communication skills that make the vision understandable, precise, powerful, and engaging. The followers are willing to invest more effort in their tasks because they are encouraged and optimistic about the shared vision and goals.

Intellectual Stimulation (IS): The degree to which leaders challenge assumptions, take risks, and stimulate and solicit followers' ideas. Transformational leaders encourage followers to be innovative and creative by questioning assumptions, by reframing problems, and by challenging them to approach old situations in new ways.

Individualized Consideration (IC): The degree to which the leader attends to each follower's need for achievement and growth, acts as a mentor or coach to the follower, and listens to the follower's concerns and needs. The leader provides empathy and support, keeps communication open, and places challenges before the followers. IC also encompasses the need for respect and celebrates the individual contribution that each follower makes to the team (Bass & Riggio, 2006, cited in ANCC 2013 2014 Magnet Application Manual, p. 75).

One form of governance often used by transformational leaders is shared governance. This is a democratic, dynamic process resulting from shared decision making and accountability (Porter-O'Grady, 2001). In shared governance there is the creation of organizational structures that allow nursing staff the autonomy to govern their practice (Batson, 2004). Shared governance is a key principle in the ANCC's (*American Nurses Credentialing Center*) Magnet Recognition Program. ANCC shared leadership/participative decision-making is a model in which nurses are formally organized to make decisions about clinical practice standards, quality improvement, staff and professional development, and research (*American Nurses Credentialing Center* [ANCC], 2013, p. 74).

LEADER VERSUS MANAGER

As you advance in your nursing proficiency, you will eventually take over some managerial tasks. You may even be asked to become a nurse manager. However, just because you take on some managerial tasks does not necessarily make you a nurse manager. Also, just because you are an excellent clinical nurse does not mean that you will become an excellent manager. In some organizations the only promotion opportunities occur through progression to management. If you do not see yourself in such a role, it will be important for you to work in an organization that also has promotion opportunities for nurses who remain at the bedside. The competencies of a nurse manager need to be developed,

and the process of manager development occurs through education, mentorship, and professional growth. As discussed earlier, management is not synonymous with leadership, although management is a part of leadership.

Management and leadership are different (Bennis, 1994, p. 45):

- The manager administers; the leader innovates.
- The manager maintains; the leader develops.
- The manager focuses on systems and structure; the leader focuses on people.
- The manager relies on control; the leader inspires trust.
- The manager has a short-range view; the leader has a long-range perspective.
- The manager asks how and when; the leader asks what and why.
- The manager has their eye on the bottom line; the leader has their eye on the horizon.
- The manager imitates; the leader originates.
- The manager accepts the status quo; the leader challenges it.
- The manager is the classic good soldier; the leader is their own person.
- The manager does things right; the leader does the right thing.

In addition, the leader needs to be able to operate under the evidence-based management tenets identified in the Institute of Medicine (2004) report on work environment. These five tenets are (1) balancing efficiency and patient safety; (2) promoting trust; (3) creating and managing change; (4) implementing shared decision making around work design and flow; and (5) establishing a learning environment.

Management is a complex process of coordinating and directing the actions of others to accomplish an organization's objectives. It also involves the assignment of resources to these groups so that the objectives can be met. It is achieved through six functions: planning, staffing, organizing, directing, controlling, and decision making (Carroll, 2006).

Planning determines what needs to be done. This may refer to what needs to be done for a single shift or for a longer period, such as the year. Staffing refers to the selection and assignment of specific people to accomplish the tasks (see Chapter 13 for discussion on delegation). Organizing is the process of coordinating all resources to meet the goals. It is a fluid activity requiring knowledge of the organization and people and having the ability to alter the plan, staffing, and organization if the goals are not being met. Directing deals with the skills necessary to motivate the staff to accomplish the assigned tasks. In this function, you need to be able to provide the proper resources, set clear goals, and foster a work environment that encourages goal achievement. Controlling is accomplished through the setting of professional standards, compliance with standards of performance, and the ability to lead a staff to excellence. Finally, decision making is the result of these five actions. According to Sullivan and Decker (2001), the key steps of decision making are (1) identification of the problem, (2) establishment of criteria that can evaluate potential solutions to the problem, (3) seeking alternative solutions, and (4) selection of the best option based on the organizational mission, vision, strategic objectives, and available resources.

COMPARING THE NURSING PROCESS WITH THE MANAGEMENT PROCESS

The nursing process focuses on assessing, analyzing, planning, implementing, and evaluating. The management process is used to meet patient needs in an efficient and effective manner with available resources. The management process consists of five phases: identification of needs, identification of resources, planning, organizing and direction, and controlling.

LEVELS OF MANAGEMENT

Cipriani (2011) states that nurse managers "at all levels work together to address emerging trends, adopt innovative ideas, and work toward the shared goals of quality, efficiency, and excellence in practice. They guide and lead frontline nurses while contributing to an organization's success." There are levels of patient care management in most institutions. The organizational structure of the organization will determine the titles and the span of authority of the various levels of patient care management (Box 1-1).

First Level

The first-level manager, also known as a first-line manager, nurse manager, or head nurse, is responsible for supervising the work of nonmanagerial personnel and the day-to-day activities of a specific work unit or units (Box 1-2). This manager is responsible for the

---

> **BOX 1-1** **Three Levels of Management Are Used in Nursing**
>
> | | |
> |---|---|
> | First | Nurse manager |
> | Middle | Director |
> | Upper | Executive |

From Sullivan, E. J., & Decker, P. J. (2005). *Effective leadership and management in nursing* (6th ed.). Upper Saddle River, NJ: Pearson/Prentice Hall. pp. 60-61.

> **BOX 1-2** **First-Level Manager Responsibilities**
>
> - Clinical nursing practice.
> - Patient care delivery.
> - Use of human, fiscal, and other resources.
> - Personnel development.
> - Compliance with regulatory and professional standards.
> - Fostering interdisciplinary, collaborative relationships.
> - Strategic planning.

From American Organization of Nurse Executives. (1992). The role and functions of the hospital nurse manager. In *American Hospital Association advisory*. Chicago: American Hospital Association.

---

units on a 24-hours-a-day/7-days-a-week basis. The first level manager straddles the worlds of staff and upper management, ensuring a two-way flow of information (Cipriani, 2011).

Key tasks for a first-line nurse manager may include the following (adapted from Carroll, 2006, p. 32):

- Preparing orientation schedule in collaboration with nursing education department.
- Submitting time schedules for nursing shifts.
- Assigning staff for patient care during shifts.
- Making budget recommendations to the middle and upper levels of management. These budget needs are made based on unit needs and patient acuity (see Chapter 4).
- Calculating the amount of staff needed per shift, per day, etc. This will also include the alteration of staffing plans based on emergencies, sick calls, and changes in patient acuity.
- Making daily patient rounds.
- Conducting staff meetings.
- Conducting employment reviews, including counseling reports and termination.
- Interviewing potential staff members (this is often done in conjunction with middle management).

- Participating in performance improvement and evidence-based practice activities; reviewing of unit performance on National Database of Nursing Quality Indicators (NDNQI) outcome measures, CORE measures, National Patient Safety Goals, infection rates, and other unit-based performance indicators.
- Setting goals with individual staff and for patient-care areas.
- Maintaining current knowledge of the profession and regulatory requirements.

The Scope and Standards from the American Nurses Association (ANA) (2009) for Nurse Administration states that to fulfill the responsibilities, the nurse manager, in collaboration with nursing personnel and members of other disciplines, performs the following:

- Ensuring that care is delivered with respect for individuals' rights and preferences.
- Participating in nursing organizational policy formulation and decision making involving staff.
- Accepting organizational accountability for services provided to recipients.
- Evaluating the quality and appropriateness of health care.
- Coordinating nursing care with other health care disciplines, and assisting in integrating services across the continuum of health care.
- Participating in the recruitment, selection, and retention of personnel, including staff representative of the population diversity.
- Assessing the impact of and planning strategies to address such issues as:
  - ethnic, cultural, and diversity changes in the population
  - political and social influences
  - financial and economic issues
  - the aging of society and demographic trends
  - ethical issues related to health care.
- Assuming responsibility for staffing and scheduling personnel. Assignments to reflect appropriate use of personnel, considering scope of practice, competencies, patient/resident needs, and complexity of care.
- Ensuring appropriate orientation, education, credentialing, and continuing professional development for personnel.
- Providing guidance for and supervision of personnel accountable to the nurse manager.
- Evaluating performance of personnel.

- Developing, implementing, monitoring, and being accountable for the budget for the defined area(s) of responsibility.
- Ensuring evidence-based practice by participating in and involving the nursing staff in evaluative research activities.
- Providing or facilitating educational experiences for nursing and other students.
- Ensuring shared accountability for professional practice.
- Advocating for a work environment that minimizes work-related illness and injury.

Middle Level

The **middle-level manager**, also known as supervisor, director, assistant director or associate director of nursing, supervises a number of first-level managers. These managers usually are within the same specialty or the same geographic location. They may spend more time planning, evaluating, and coordinating and less time with direct patient care supervision than the first-line manager (Box 1-3). They are responsible for the people and activities within the departments they supervise on a 24-hours-a-day/7-days-a-week basis.

Key tasks that the middle-level manager may perform include the following (adapted from Carroll, 2006, p. 33):

- Assessment: Observe whether unit policies and objectives are meeting the needs of the patients and staff. Initiate changes to unit policies based on current evidence.
- Planning: Set short-term and long-term goals for patient care; revise as needed. Align these goals with the goals of the larger patient-care services department.
- Organization: Put plans in action via delegation, committee work, and through shared governance processes.

BOX 1-3 Middle-Level Manager Responsibilities

- Actions of people and activities within the departments they supervise.
- Liaison between upper management and first-level manager.

From American Organization of Nurse Executives. (1992). The role and functions of the hospital nurse manager. In *American Hospital Association advisory.* Chicago: American Hospital Association.

- Control: Analyze results of action plans and evidence-based projects, make changes as necessary, facilitate the growth of staff, and communicate changes and opportunities to upper-level staff and to staff reporting to managers.

Upper Level

The **upper-level manager** or the executive-level manager, is also known as the senior vice president of patient care, vice president for nursing, chief nurse executive, or chief nursing officer (CNO). Middle management reports to the vice president for nursing. According to the American Organization of Nurse Executives (1990), "A nurse executive is a registered nurse who is part of the executive management team and as such is responsible for the management of the nursing organization and the clinical practice of nursing throughout the organization." ANCC defines the chief nursing officer as the highest level nurse with ultimate responsibility for all nursing practice within the organization (ANCC, 2013, p. 64).

The CNO spends the least amount of time in direct supervision. Most of the time is spent planning and working with key stakeholders to move the organization forward. According to the Magnet standards "the CNO is a strategic partner in the organization's decision making" (ANCC, 2013, p. 32). The CNO is responsible for influencing change beyond the scope of nursing to provide for continued excellence (ANCC, 2013, p. 31). They are responsible for establishing organizational goals and strategic plans for the patient care department and driving leadership development and the continued path toward excellence (Box 1-4).

Key tasks that the chief nursing officer may perform include the following (adapted from Carroll, 2006, p. 33):
- Assessment: Understand the organization's internal environment and culture and the external environment (regulatory, technology, community, legislation) in which it functions.
- Planning: Forecast trends in the profession, health care, costs, reimbursement, and regulations, and develop responsive strategic plans.
- Organization: Based on assessment and strategic planning, bring together the appropriate mix of resources, staff, and evidence-based knowledge to assist in the meeting of strategic goals.
- Control: Evaluate nursing policies, programs, services, and performance to ensure that they are consistent with the organization's mission and strategic goals, current evidence, and the profession's standards.

Other managerial roles have evolved over the past few years. To assist the nurse manager or head nurse, the role of charge nurse (patient care manager) has been developed. This expanded staff nurse role grants a staff nurse managerial responsibility on a given shift. This role may be a permanent position or a rotating one. The care manager functions as a liaison between the nurse manager and the activities and staff of the off-shifts.

Key tasks that the care manager may perform include the following (adapted from Carroll, 2006, p. 33):
- Assist in shift coordination.
- Create patient assignments for the shift.
- Deal with personnel issues arising during shift (e.g., sick calls, real-time conflict management).
- Make patient care rounds during shift.
- Trouble-shoot problems that occur during shift.
- Assist staff members with making decisions and prioritizing care.
- Use resources efficiently.
- Perform staff evaluations (this will depend on the organization).
- Serve as liaison between staff of off-shift and first-line management.

COMPETENCIES OF PATIENT CARE MANAGERS

Patient care managers use organizational resources and routines while providing direct patient care. They need

---

BOX 1-4 Upper-Level Manager Responsibilities

- Establishing organizational goals.
- Establishing strategic plans for nursing.
- Integrating work units to achieve the organization's mission.
- Buffering the effects of the external environment on nurses within the organization.

From American Organization of Nurse Executives. (1992). The role and functions of the hospital nurse manager. In *American Hospital Association advisory.* Chicago: American Hospital Association.

to use time productively and collaborate with the inter-disciplinary work group. They use leadership character-istics to manage others within the nursing work group. More specifically, to manage patient care, entry-level nurses perform the following tasks (Wywialowski, 2004, pp. 4–5):

- Identify organizational resources and determine when they are needed.
- Work within various nursing service delivery patterns.
- Use position descriptions to establish the scope and limitations of their own and other nursing work group member practices.
- Manage time purposefully and productively.
- Prioritize patient needs and related care.
- Exhibit flexibility in providing care within available time constraints.
- Show initiative, flexibility, and creativity as leader-ship qualities.
- Think critically to make decisions required to solve patient care problems.
- Collaborate with other health team members.
- Resolve conflicts within the work group.
- Delegate appropriately.

The role of the care manager differs from that of the first-line manager in that the charge nurse or care manager has more limited authority and a limited span of control. The charge nurse may or may not perform staff evaluations; this will depend on the organization. The charge nurse may have more knowledge of staff performance, especially if the position deals with the off-shifts. The typical workday of a care manager or charge nurse is presented in Box 1-5.

Resource nurses are being used in many organiza-tions. The role of resource nurse has developed to role model nurses in areas of clinical decision making and use of resources. The resource nurse is usually a nurse with recognized clinical expertise (clinical ladder posi-tion, certification, and experience) who is able to mentor less experienced nurses as they grow within the profes-sion (St. Luke's Medical Center, 2015). Clinical resource nurses serve as a clinical resource for the identified

---

BOX 1-5 Typical Patient Care Management Routines

7:00–7:30 am: Receive change-of-shift report.

7:30–8:00 am: Complete preliminary assessment of assigned patient needs; complete assigning patient care to coworkers; administer scheduled drugs and treatments before meals or with meals.

8:00–9:30 am: Administer drugs to be given after meals and per agency schedules; complete detailed assess-ments of acutely ill patients and provide comfort and personal hygiene measures; note changes in medical plans and other interdisciplinary diagnostic or treat-ment programs.

9:30–10:00 am: Administer scheduled drugs and detailed assessment of stable patients; provide comfort and personal hygiene measures; implement exercise treatments.

10:00–11:30 am: Obtain feedback from coworkers regarding progress and special needs; provide assis-tance to coworkers, and plan to receive assistance from others for complex procedures; administer drugs before meals; involve patients in routine health education programs.

11:30 am–1:00 pm: Take lunch break and cover for coworkers while they are on break; monitor unstable patients; assist patients with meals; administer scheduled drugs and those to be given with meals.

1:00–2:00 pm: Monitor patient progress; provide com-fort measures; promote patient rest periods; admin-ister drugs to be taken after meals and as scheduled.

2:00–2:45 pm: Monitor unstable patients; seek feed-back from coworkers; complete care plan revisions and documentation not completed earlier; organize data for change-of-shift report; involve patients in health education programs.

2:45–3:30 pm: Give change-of-shift report.

From Wywialowski, E. (2004). *Managing client care.* St. Louis: Mosby.

---

unit/s. They collaborate with nurse leaders, medical staff and nursing staff and provide clinical support to improve patient care and patient outcomes in the unit (Quinn-O'Neill, et al., 2011).

SUMMARY

The role of the manager is very different from that of the nurse. Although nurses need to have strong management skills to deliver patient care, there are additional skills and tasks that are needed to be a nurse manager at any level. Not every nurse will want to be a nurse manager, even through they manage patient care on a daily basis. As a new nurse moves into a managerial role, it is important to realize that a different set of skills and knowledge is required to advance in this role. The American Organization of Nurse Executives has many resources for these roles, and the American Nurses Credentialing Center manages the certification examinations for nurses working in nursing administration.

CLINICAL CORNER

Sustaining Nursing Through Leadership

Leadership exists in nursing as a concept that many have defined, theorized, and characterized, in general and specifically, to the various specialties and roles of the profession. We have a plethora of well-thought and well-intentioned literature that proposes new ideas. We also have theories that are derived from various disciplines, such as business, education, and medicine, and applied to nursing. I have spent many hours reading and gaining insight from others on what leadership in nursing means and what it means to me in my practice. If someone had told me all those years ago, when I was a brand new nurse on an adult medical-surgical floor (trembling with fear at the start of each shift), that I was a leader, I would have laughed. Or I would have fainted from the added feelings of responsibility. Because what I have learned over time about leadership in nursing through practice, reading, and teaching is very simple: to nurse is to lead.

We are all leaders. From the nurse who steps onto a hospital floor or into a patient's home for the first time, to the seasoned practitioner who runs a community-based clinic, to the chief nursing official of a major hospital system — and all of us in between — we lead. People look to us; they need and heed our advice. Being a nurse implies that one is trustworthy, humanistic, and intelligent; a person who is intent on healing and righting the wrongs in life. We naturally accept these implications and take pride in our roles in the community. Every time I answer someone who asks what I do for a living, I know I am changing their perception slightly when I answer, "I am a nurse." The title itself yields a certain amount of respect and dignity that stems from the association of nursing and leadership. Nurses consistently answer to the needs of the public through various roles, and employ traditional leadership characteristics in serving our patient populations. But I often wonder how we are doing in terms of leadership among ourselves. How well are we modeling these traits that we share with the general public to one another? Are we leading each other well as we forge a path through the unstable world of health care today?

I pose the question because of the steady rise in the literature on incivility and horizontal violence in our profession. Much of this has been attributed to work stress, burnout, and high-pressured work environments to which we are commonly exposed. However, these stressful health care environments have and will always exist. In the midst of caring for diverse populations, we forget the diversity among ourselves, which affects how well we work together to preserve nursing as a reputable profession that others will want to join. We forget that we need to lead. The need to embrace horizontal leadership in addressing violence has never been so timely and apparent. We need to bring one another up instead of holding each other down. How do we achieve this? We apply the leadership concept of sustainability, which is critical to this profession.

The term "sustainability" suggests endurance over time without the exhaustion of resources in the interim. A sustainable leader employs characteristics that contribute to the success and longevity of a profession by strengthening its greatest resource: the professionals within. How do we sustain the nursing profession into the future? By committing to lifelong learning, social justice, and succession planning. A sustainable leader knows that the expansion of individual knowledge strengthens the profession when new learning is cycled into practice. New learning is the basis for evaluation and change, which in nursing translates to better outcomes for our patients, our communities, and ourselves. This leader supports the baccalaureate as the entry level for nursing, pursues the advanced degree best suited for their practice, and encourages others to do so. This leader applies this knowledge by participating in evidence-based practice, research, and quality improvement to expand the science of the nursing profession.

Sustainable leadership encompasses the concept of social justice. In terms of patients, this is something that is well understood among most nurses. We take responsibility for our patients, without conviction or judgment. We consider each patient's situation, perspective, and goals as we collaboratively plan care. This is how we directly improve patient outcomes. Do we extend to one another the same considerations: work collaboratively and cooperatively without conviction or judgment to improve our outcomes, either on a smaller or larger scale? A sustainable nurse leader realizes that being just extends beyond patient care, and takes responsibility for the wider environment — on the job and for the profession at large. This includes modeling civil behaviors, embracing diversity within the workplace, and most importantly,

Continued

CLINICAL CORNER—cont'd

Sustaining Nursing Through Leadership

distributing leadership to others. Sustainable leaders remain transparent with their people when it comes to issues that arise and involve them in the decision-making process. This leader knows that more is gained by listening to the group and by trusting that wisdom of a group is greater than any one individual.

As nurses, we are the healers of society. The world will always need nurses, and who replaces us as time passes should matter. Leaving a legacy and influencing those who come after us is another trait of sustainable leadership. It is more accurately defined as succession planning. Although each one of us may not be able to directly select who replaces us, we can place value on those who follow us and lead by example. I am going to use the negative phrase we have used a million times: "nurses eat their young." I do not know when we, as nurses, started being associated with trial by fire at the hands of more experienced colleagues, but we need to change that idea. Our most valuable asset for a strong profession in the future is our young — our new nurses. Give them time, attention, and the right model to follow. Sustainable leaders help to groom the next generation by being authentic. They are true to themselves, accountable for their actions, while maintaining high personal standards and accepting criticism as grounds for personal improvement. We can influence young nurses in many ways — through teaching, precepting, mentoring, and publishing. In other words, leaving your footprint in the sand into which someone else can step. Sustain the profession by embracing and preparing those who come next, who in their turn will guide the next generation of nurses behind them.

I am often reminded of my very first nurse manager when I was a new graduate nurse many years ago. Back then, I did not know enough to put my finger on it, but in hindsight I realize that her goal was to impart lessons to her nurses that would foster individual love and pride for the profession. She had been a nurse for 25 years before she decided to go back to school for her baccalaureate degree in nursing, although it was not a job requirement at the time. She never complained about it and actually seemed to enjoy it so much that she convinced a lot of her nursing staff to go back to college with her. She took time to get to know us individually, learned our personal strengths and talents as nurses, and used us appropriately for unit-based research projects, hospital nursing initiatives, and preparations for accrediting organization visits. If something was happening on or to our unit, we were all informed and we all contributed. When decisions needed to be made, she always sought group input and shared in the process. She observed us with patients and offered advice and suggestions when we struggled.

One time, I remember I came in at 3 PM to start a shift. I had a patient whose status was declining, but I could not identify what was wrong. I was terrified that something was going to happen that I could not control. My manager stayed by my side, talked to me about what I seeing, and helped me care for the patient who was becoming septic. She stayed with me for hours, helped me organize myself enough to care for the rest of my assignment, all the while reminding me that I was a good nurse, learning how to become an excellent one. At that point, so early on in my career, that woman taught me that being a nurse meant so much more than the sets of tasks we do for patients. She led me, without me even realizing it, to expand my education, diversify my thinking, and worry about the future of nursing. She taught me to embrace my role as a contributor to that future, which is what I now try to make my nursing students see: that we are all in this together — that at all levels and positions we must accept the responsibility to lead because we are nurses. It is what we do. And we make greater impacts on health care, the profession, and the world in general when we lead together.

Cristina Perez, PhD, RN
Assistant Professor, Nursing
Ramapo College of NJ

EVIDENCE-BASED PRACTICE

Quinn-O'Neil, B. MEd, RN, NE-BC, Kilgallen, M., MEd, RN, NE-BC, Terlizzi, J., MS, RN, AOCN (2011). Creating a Unit-Based Resource Nurse Program. *A hospital program develops clinical experts to foster best practices on every unit. American Journal of Nursing, 111*(9), 46-51.

Holy Name Medical Center is a 361-bed Magnet-designated community hospital in New Jersey. The nursing care is followed by the principles of Magnet. The norm of this facility is that upper nursing management works closely with all nurses at various levels within the hospital. Upper management respects the expertise of nurses that work at the bedside, directly with the patient. In 2001, nurse leaders realized that not all nurses have expertise in the different areas

EVIDENCE-BASED PRACTICE—cont'd

of nursing. Based on the different needs, the medical center established the resource nurse program. The resource nurse is the clinical leader. The main role of this specialty nurse is to enhance clinical expertise and to provide peer support. Another task of the specialist is to support the nursing staff in problem solving, clinical decision making, and critical thinking. The nurse is also charged with meeting Joint Commission standards and the American Nurses Credentialing Center Magnet requirements. Holy Name initiated its first resource nurse role: pain resource nurse. The next unit-based resource nurse was a skin-care nurse. There is a skin-care resource nurse and a pain resource nurse on each patient unit to meet the needs of the specific unit and the specific shift. There are presently over 80 resource nurses. These nurses help implement evidence-based practice, exemplify the role of the nurse as teacher, and serve as mentors to patients and colleagues. The nurses develop increased expertise in their specialty areas to improve their own practice and mentor their colleagues. Not every staff nurse is chosen to be a resource nurse; nursing management evaluates each staff nurse individually and selects if they feel the nurse is ideal for the position. It is an honor to be chosen to be an expert in the specialty field. The medical center has supported their efforts from the beginning, hence the long-term success of the program. The specialty nurses make walking rounds, develop educational materials, and evaluate outcomes. They are supported to go to conferences

to have the most up-to-date patient-care guidelines for their specific unit.

The result: The quality outcomes have been high, which has led to staff retention and satisfaction. The autonomy and commitment of the nursing staff are key to the program's success. The resource nurse role supports staff RNs in practicing with evidence-based knowledge and skills. Resource nurses provide a foundation for practice, quality improvement initiatives, and nursing research.

The first pain-management resource nurse was charged with an increase of compliance with medication for pain relief. There was a 2-day course that included staff education about pain, teaching skills, and outcome evaluation. The pain resource nurse performed data collection, evaluated the practice, and shared their knowledge with their co-workers. There was also a change in the medication administration sheets, so that was also part of the education provided.

In 2003 the hospital had the prevalence of 10 to 1,000 patient days; this was higher than the national benchmark. Hence the development of the skin-care resource nurse. The program was developed. Nursing administration supported one resource nurse per shift on each unit. The program evaluates types of equipment such as mattresses.

The diabetic resource nurse has also been a success. Patient teaching is key for prevention. Using evidence-based practice, the nurses designed a poster, and provided staff members with new articles.

NCLEX® EXAMINATION QUESTIONS

1. The nurse manager on the labor and delivery unit evaluates that one of the staff nurses has leadership qualities. Which of the following is a basis for this judgment?
   A. The nurse works overtime every week.
   B. The nurse stays long after her shift is over to chart.
   C. The nurse uses a monthly forum to review current knowledge content.
   D. The nurse uses a negative approach when evaluating staff skills.

2. As a nurse, you are aware that one element that is common to the nursing process and the management process is:
   A. Identification of needs
   B. Identification of resources

   C. Planning
   D. Control

3. One main difference between an ideal leader and an organization-focused manager is that an:
   A. Ideal leader maintains the status quo
   B. Organization-focused manager is creative
   C. Ideal leader is a risk-taker
   D. Organization-focused manager is a visionary

4. Which of the following is NOT the middle-level manager's responsibility?
   A. People within the departments they supervise
   B. Liaison between upper management and first-level manager
   C. Establishment of organizational goals
   D. Activities within the departments they supervise

5. The middle-level manager:
   A. Makes hospital-wide decisions
   B. Supervises a number of upper-level managers
   C. Is responsible for the people and activities on a 24-hours-a-day/7-days-a-week basis
   D. Is responsible for their specific shift only

6. You are mentoring a new nurse. You know that which of the following is NOT a mentor's responsibility?
   A. Discuss means to correct chronic tardiness
   B. Offer criticism on nursing skills
   C. Perform a nurse's probation period review
   D. Evaluate the nurse's exact break and lunch times

7. The four skill sets needed by good leaders are:
   A. Self-awareness, self-management, social awareness, and relationship management
   B. Self-awareness, self-management, social control, and relationship management
   C. Self-awareness, self-control, social awareness, and relationship management
   D. Self-awareness, self-management, social awareness, and relationship performance

8. Ruiz (1997) defines the "four agreements" that leaders must make with themselves. They are as follows:
   A. Be impeccable with your word, take nothing personally, make no assumptions, and always do your best, no more and no less
   B. Be impeccable with your actions, take nothing personally, make no assumptions, and always do your best, no more and no less
   C. Be impeccable with your word, take nothing personally, make assumptions, and always do your best, no more and no less
   D. Be impeccable with your word, take nothing personally, make no assumptions, and be appreciative of your staff

9. Leader competencies are a necessary aspect of a leader's role. As a leader, you are aware that the following is needed for this role:
   A. A clear vision and owned purpose
   B. A pessimistic attitude with colleagues
   C. A negative approach with families
   D. A membership with more than three committees

10. The vice president of nursing is responsible for:
    A. Establishing organizational goals and strategic plans for nursing
    B. Developing and maintaining daily assignments
    C. Prioritizing events during disaster plan implementation
    D. Overseeing the mission and vision of the organization

Answers: 1. C   2. C   3. C   4. C   5. C   6. A   7. A   8. A   9. A   10. A

REFERENCES

American Nurses Credentialing Center [ANCC]. (2013). *2014 Magnet application manual*. Silver Spring, MD: Author.

American Nurses Association. (2009). *Scope and standards of practice—Nurse administration*. Silver Spring, MD: Author.

American Organization of Nurse Executives. (1992). The role and functions of the hospital nurse manager. In *American Hospital Association advisory*. Chicago: American Hospital Association.

Bass, B. M., & Riggio, R. E. (2005). *Transformational leadership* (2nd ed.). Mahwah, NJ: Lawrence Erlbaum Associates, Inc.

Batson, V. (2004). Shared governance in an integrated health care network. *AORN*, *80*(3), 493–496 498, 501-504, 506, 509-512.

Bennis, W. (1994). *On becoming a leader*. New York: Addison-Wesley.

Carroll, P. (2006). *Nursing leadership and management: A practical guide*. Clifton Park, NY: Thomson Delmar Learning.

Cipriani, P. (2011). Move up to the role of nurse manager. *American Nurse Today*, March 2011, *6*(3), 61–62.

Institute of Medicine. (2004). *Keeping patients safe*. Washington, DC: National Academies Press.

Kata from Kotter, J. (1996). *Leading change*. Boston, MA: Harvard Business School.

Porter-O'Grady, T., & Mallach, K. (2015). *Quantum leadership. Building better partnerships for sustainable health* (4th ed.). Burlington, MA: Jones & Bartlett.

Porter-O'Grady, T. (2001). Is shared governance still relevant? *Journal of Nursing Administration*, *31*(10), 468–473.

Quinn-O'Neil, B., Kilgallen, M., & Terlizzi, J. (2011). Creating a unit-based resource nurse program. *American Journal of Nursing*, *111*(9), 46–51.

Ruiz, D. M. (1997). *The four agreements: A practical guide to personal freedom (a Toltec wisdom book)*. San Rafael, CA: Amber-Allen.

St. Luke's Medical Center. (2015). *Resource nurse job description*. http://jobs.stlukesmedcenter.com/registered-nurse-clinical-resource-nurse/job/3303764.

Sullivan, E., & Decker, P. (2001). *Effective leadership and management in nursing* (5th ed.). Upper Saddle River, NJ: Prentice Hall.

Wywialowski, E. F. (2004). *Managing client care* (3rd ed.). St. Louis: Mosby.

2

Organizational Structure of Health Care

OBJECTIVES

- Differentiate between a care delivery model and a professional practice model.
- Describe the various organizational structures in health care.
- Identify the management structures of patient care.
- Describe the various modes of patient care delivery systems.
- Discuss the pros and cons of each of the delivery systems.
- Determine the responsibility of the nurse in the various care delivery systems.
- Relate a clinical scenario to each of the delivery models.

OUTLINE

KEY TERMS

care delivery system a system for the delivery of care that delineates the nurse's authority and accountability for clinical decision making and outcomes. The care delivery system is adapted to regulatory considerations and describes the context of care, the manner in which care is delivered, the care competencies required, and the expected outcomes of care (American Nurses Credentialing Center [ANCC], 2013)

case/care management model of care in which the nurse integrates delivery of clinical services across the various transitions of care

functional nursing model of care in which nursing work is allocated according to specific tasks and skills

primary nursing model of care in which one nurse assumes accountability for care delivered by other personnel in a 24-hour period

professional practice model a schematic description of a theory, phenomenon, or system that depicts how nurses practice, collaborate, communicate, and develop professionally to provide the highest level of care (ANCC, 2013)

team nursing model of care in which a group of staff members led by a nurse provides care

total patient care model of care in which the nurse assumes full accountability for care of a group of patients

LEADERSHIP STRUCTURE IN HEALTH CARE

The health care industry is a complex web of patient care facilities and workers with the chief goal of caring for patients in a safe, cost-effective manner. Improving the U.S. health care system requires the pursuit of three aims: improving the experience of care, improving the health of the population, and reducing per capita costs (Berwick, Nolan, & Whittington, 2008). To this end, the organizational structures of most health care organizations tend to focus on oversight, efficiency, and stakeholder satisfaction.

Health care institutions are usually organized according to lines of authority, power, and communication. Structures are defined as centralized or decentralized depending on the degree to which the organization has spread its lines of authority.

Integrative Structures in Health Care

With the dramatic changes that have occurred in health care since 2010, health care systems are now being reorganized to provide for care throughout the various transitions of care. Single acute care institutions have partnered or merged with health care agencies and facilities providing broader care. An example would be a relationship between an acute care hospital with a long-term care facility, a rehabilitation agency, and a home health care organization. These reorganizations also provide increased efficiency and financial stability of services. Organizations may be vertically integrated or horizontally integrated. Vertical integration (affiliation of a particular health care facility with the health maintenance organization) provides for different, but complementary services among the organizations involved. Horizontal integration (shared services or reciprocal services across two or more institutions) allows for shared provision to be made, for instance the provision of maternal/child services by one affiliate and orthopedic surgery services by another.

Organizational Structures

An organizational chart is a visual means of determining the level of centralization or decentralization. A centralized organization is a typical hierarchy that follows a chain of command and is characterized by top-down decision making. The more decision making is "pushed down" through the organizational levels, the more decentralized the organization becomes. A flat organizational structure signifies the removal of hierarchical layers, demonstrating that the authority for action occurs at the point of service (Figure 2-1). In a more decentralized organization, lower-level managers and staff have an increased opportunity for shared governance and often report greater job satisfaction (Rundio & Wilson, 2010).

Functional Structures

Functional structures arrange services and departments according to what they do (Figure 2-2). Departments providing similar functions would all report to a common manager or vice president. In such a structure, nursing units would report to the larger nursing services. Other services in support of patient care, such as respiratory and dietary, might report to a non-nursing manager or VP. This type of structure supports professional expertise but can result in the "silo" effect, in which departments become separate entities with little interaction.

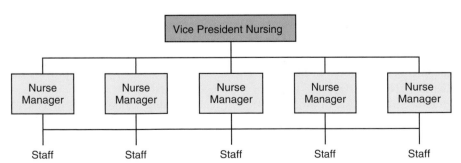

FIGURE 2-1 Organizational structure. (From Yoder-Wise, P. S. [2007]. *Leading and managing in nursing* [4th ed.]. St. Louis: Mosby.)

Product Line Structures

In product line structures, the functions necessary to produce a specific service are brought together into an integrated unit under the control of a single manager (Figure 2-3). For example, the orthopedic service line at a hospital would include all personnel providing services to the orthopedic service population. This might include the orthopedic ambulatory care service, the orthopedic operating rooms, the orthopedic trauma center of the emergency department, and the orthopedic rehabilitation center. Benefits of this model include coordination of all services within the specialty and a similarity of focus. A limitation would be increased expense caused by duplication of services.

Matrix Structures

Matrix structures combine both function and service line in an integrated service structure (Figure 2-4). In a matrix organization, the manager of a unit responsible for a service reports both to a functional manager (vice president for nursing) and a service manager (directors of the services: cardiovascular services, trauma services, surgical services, or women's and children's services). Such a structure requires a collaborative relationship between the service line and functional manager. The nurse is responsible to the nurse manager and vice president of nursing for nursing care and to the program director when working within the matrix.

Integrated Structures

In an integrated health care system (e.g., networks), providers agree to accept the risk of caring for a particular patient segment or population for a pre-established fee. They provide care across the continuum. Preventative care is inherent in this structure, with primary care providers, not the hospital at the center of the structure. Keeping people healthy is the goal of this type of structure, thereby decreasing the need for hospitalization.

In vertically and horizontally integrated structures (health care systems), hospitals, delivery systems, and medical group and health care workers are brought together under one umbrella with shared purpose and unity of control. Potential challenges include relatively high overheads and internal power struggles (Rundio & Wilson, 2010).

In the organizational structure, the nursing department is usually listed on the senior leadership level. The chief nursing officer (senior vice president of patient care, vice president of nursing, chief nursing officer, etc.) is the highest-level reporting nursing officer in an organization. As a new staff nurse, you will report to a unit-based manager. Although you will be ultimately responsible to the chief nursing officer, on a day-to-day basis you might report to a shift charge nurse. This charge nurse (patient care manager) will have the overall responsibility for the patient care delivered during the work shift. There are many delivery systems, and the titles and responsibilities of the nurse and nurse manager vary according to the system used.

MAJOR TYPES OF CARE DELIVERY SYSTEMS

A patient care delivery model is the method used to deliver care to patients. There are multiple care delivery models, and the choice of a model within an organization is dependent on many factors: financial, staffing capability, patient population, organizational mission,

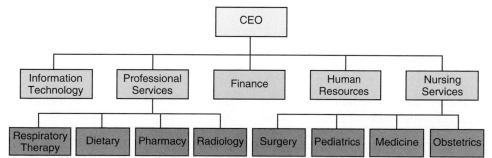

FIGURE 2-2 Functional structure. (From Yoder-Wise, P. S. [2007]. *Leading and managing in nursing* [4th ed.]. St. Louis: Mosby.)

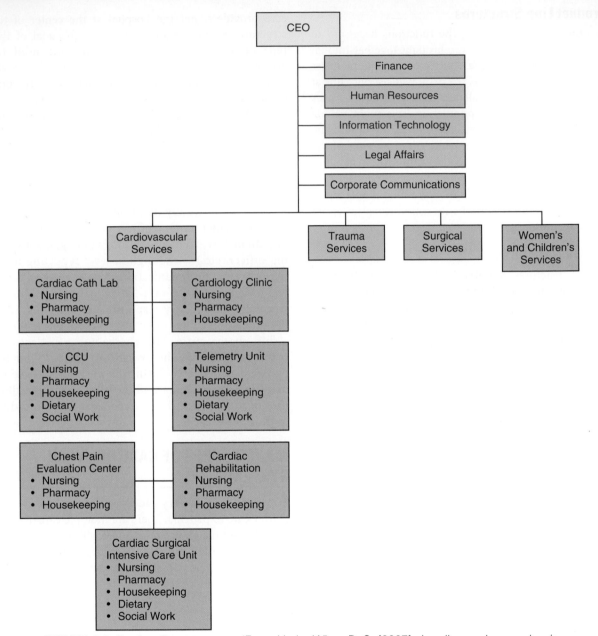

FIGURE 2-3 Product line structure. (From Yoder-Wise, P. S. [2007]. *Leading and managing in nursing* [4th ed.]. St. Louis: Mosby.)

and philosophy. The **care delivery system** delineates the nurses' authority and accountability for clinical decision making and outcomes (ANCC, 2014). It is adapted to regulatory requirements and describes the context of care, the manner in which care is delivered, and the skill set required. The fundamental element of any patient care delivery system (Manthey, 1990) is a combination of the following:

- Clinical decision making
- Work allocation
- Communication
- Management

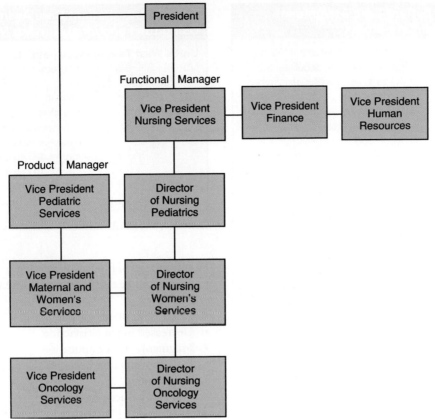

FIGURE 2-4 Matrix structure. (From Yoder-Wise, P. S. [2007]. *Leading and managing in nursing* [4th ed.]. St. Louis: Mosby.)

- Coordination
- Accountability

The following are the models associated with nursing practice:

- Total patient care
- Functional nursing
- Team nursing
- Modular nursing
- Primary nursing
- Case/care management

Total Patient Care

Total patient care is the oldest method of providing care to a patient. It is sometimes called case method (not to be confused with case management). It was the primary care delivery model until the 1930s, and it had a resurgence in the 1990s. In this model one nurse assumes accountability for the complete care of a group of patients. It has been described as a type of primary nursing (Reverby, 1987), but in total patient care the accountability for coordination of care does not extend beyond the assigned shift. This is the type of care seen in private duty nursing and some intensive care units, and was the model of care used by Florence Nightingale.

Advantages of total patient care:

- Quality of care; all care is delivered by a registered nurse
- Continuity of care for a given shift
- High patient satisfaction
- Decreases communication time required between staff
- Reduces the need for supervision
- Allows one person to perform more than one task

Disadvantages of total patient care:

- May not be cost effective because of the number of registered nurses needed to provide care
- Some nurses dislike this model because they believe that some of the patient care activities could be done safely and effectively by others with less skill

TABLE 2-1 Patient Care Assignment Using the Total Care Model

Hester B., RN, MSN	Patient Care Manager 4 West
Joseph Z., RN, BSN	Full patient care, documentation, orders, admissions, discharges: rooms 410 to 414
Maria C., RN	Full patient care, documentation, orders, admissions, discharges: rooms 415 to 417
Joy T., RN, BSN	Full patient care, documentation, orders, admissions, discharges: rooms 418 to 420
Michael Y., RN	Full patient care, documentation, orders, admissions, discharges: rooms 421 and 422
Clarisa T., RN	Full patient care, documentation, orders, admissions, discharges: rooms 423 to 425

TABLE 2-2 Patient Care Assignment Using the Functional Nursing Model

Unit 4 West Telemetry: 30 patients	
Mary L., RN, BSN, charge nurse	All orders, rounds, report
Bob W., telemetry technician	All monitors, rhythm strips Q 4, and chart
Lisa N., RN	Medications rooms 401 to 415, oversee nurse aide Tom R. rooms 401 to 415, charting for rooms 401 to 415, admissions/discharges rooms 401 to 415
Tom R., nurse aide	Hygienic care rooms 401 to 415, feeding, line cart restock

An example of a patient care assignment using the total patient care model is shown in Table 2-1.

Functional Nursing

Functional nursing is a model in which work is allocated according to specific tasks and technical skills. This model was popular from the late 1800s to the end of World War II. In this model the "charge nurse" identifies the tasks/work that need to be completed during the shift. These tasks/work are then divided and assigned to personnel. In this model there would be a "medication nurse," a "dressing nurse," etc. This model of care delivery is oriented to the accomplishment of tasks. It is efficient in times of staff shortages, and you will see patient care units reverting to this delivery mode in times of staff shortage, such as "snow emergencies" when the number of staff is limited. Some institutions with a large variation in the classification of staff (registered nurses, licensed practical nurses, nurse aides, and technicians) to care for patients may also use functional nursing.

Advantages of functional nursing:
- A large number of tasks can be completed in a shift
- The ability to mix staff classifications
- Efficient financially
- Staff members can be trained to master one task

Disadvantages of functional nursing:
- Charge nurse may be the only one with a total view of patient
- Decreased patient satisfaction
- Decreased nurse satisfaction
- Fragmented communication
- Unit coordination becomes the responsibility of the charge nurse
- Fragmented accountability

An example of a patient care assignment using the functional nursing method is shown in Table 2-2. In this assignment, everyone is accountable for a portion of care. The challenge is that all aspects of patient care need to be communicated to the next shift, and the charge nurse must make sure that all pertinent information is known by them and that they are then able to communicate it to the next shift. This can lead to fragmented patient knowledge and a lack of holistic care.

Team Nursing

Team nursing is a delivery approach that uses a group of staff members led by a nurse to provide care. The team is composed of health care workers with a diversity of skills, education, licensure, and ability who work collaboratively to provide care to a group of patients. The registered nurse is the team leader, and she supervises and evaluates the team members delivering care. The team leader can provide care to a patient with complex care needs, but usually does not provide hands-on care. Strong communication skills are essential. This model supports group work and productivity.

TABLE 2-3   Patient Care Assignment Using the Team Nursing Model

Mary B., RN, BSN	Charge nurse Oversight of patients Rooms 410 to 422
Team A	

Betty K., RN	Team leader, Team A
	Rooms 410 to 416
	Documentation, orders admissions/
	    discharges, charting for PCA.
	    Restocks cardiac arrest cart

Maria B., RN	Rooms 410 to 412 patient care Medications Team A
Sara N., LPN	Rooms 413 to 416 Blood sugars, rooms 414, 416
Edith W., PCA	Hygienic care, rooms 410, 412, 414, 415 Assists patients, rooms 411, 413, 416 Vital signs 8a and 12n
Team B	
Tom A., RN	Team leader, Team B Rooms 417 to 422 Documentation, orders admissions/ discharges, charting for PCA
Marci S., RN	Rooms 418, 420 patient care
Michael T., PCA	Rooms 417, 422 hygienic care Vital signs 8a and 12n, Team B Blood sugars rooms 417, 422

Advantages of team nursing:
- Facilitation and overseeing of novice nurses
- Smaller group of patients allows for a higher quality of care than with functional nursing
- Team leader has knowledge of patient needs and can provide coordination of care
- Fixed teams relate to higher quality patient care

Disadvantages of team nursing:
- Increased time needed to communicate within the team
- Expensive because of the increased number of staff needed
- Increased time required to supervise, coordinate, and delegate
- Can lead to omissions in care
- Most educated staff relegated to role of supervision, not direct delivery of care

An example of a patient care assignment using the team nursing model is shown in Table 2-3. In this assignment, care is delivered by a group of staff, all of whom report back to the team leader. It is the team leader who has the decision-making responsibility for the care delivered to the group of patients.

Modular Nursing

A variation of team nursing is modular nursing (Anderson & Hughes, 1993). Modular nursing is based on the physical layout of the unit. Some hospital units were designed to house a number of smaller patient "pods" and as such are structurally divided into smaller patient care areas or substations. Nurses are stationed near the patients. The essential components of modular nursing are as follows:

- A module consists of a group of staff members and a group of patients.
- Patients are grouped by spatial or floor plan clustering.
- Nurse/patient assignment is standardized by cluster.

Advantages of this model center on the physical layout of the assignment and the ease of working in such an environment. Disadvantages center on the need to have consistent numbers of staff members in such a physical environment.

Primary Nursing

Primary nursing is a one-to-one approach to patient care. Each patient is assigned a specific nurse, who assumes 24-hour responsibility for the delivery, implementation, evaluation, and coordination of care. The primary nurse works in conjunction with nurses (associate nurses) on the other shifts to coordinate all care for the patient and family. The primary nurse is responsible for the development and evaluation of the plan of care for the patient. Decision making is decentralized and takes place at the patient's bedside. This is a flexible model and can include a variety of skill mixes. It does not mean that only registered nurses care for patients. The primary nurse plans, coordinates, and evaluates the plan of care, but the care can be delegated to appropriate staff members depending on the patient acuity.

Advantages of primary nursing:
- Improved quality and continuity of care
- Simplified communication
- Increased nurse satisfaction in nurses prepared for the role
- Patients perceive care to be more personalized

Disadvantages of primary nursing:
- Increased number of hours of care per day requires a greater number of registered nurses
- Overall patient satisfaction results are inconclusive
- Can be difficult to implement if patient has multiple unit transfers

An example of a patient care assignment using the primary nursing model is shown in Table 2-4.

Case Management

Case management is a model that mixes both process and care delivery. In hospital nursing it focuses on the achievement of patient outcomes within an effective and appropriate time frame. It is focused on the

TABLE 2-4 Patient Care Assignment Using the Primary Nursing Model

Hester A., RN, MSN	Patient Care Manager 4 West
Joseph T., RN, BSN (primary nurse) 7 to 3 Jody N. (associate nurse) 3 to 11 Evelyn B. (associate nurse) 11 to 7	Full patient care, documentation, orders, admissions, discharges: rooms 410 to 414
Maria C., RN 7 to 3 Cathy C., RN, BSN (primary nurse) 3 to 11 Evelyn L. (associate nurse) 11 to 7	Full patient care, documentation, orders, admissions, discharges: rooms 415 to 417
Joy T., RN, BSN (primary nurse) 7 to 3 Peter U., RN (associate nurse) 3 to 11 Barbara S., RN (associate nurse) 11 to 7	Full patient care, documentation, orders, admissions, discharges: rooms 418 to 420
Michael T., RN, BSN (primary nurse) 7 to 3 Peter B., RN (associate nurse) 3 to 11 Barbara S., RN (associate nurse) 11 to 7	Full patient care, documentation, orders, admissions, discharges: rooms 421 and 422
Clarisa I., RN 7 to 3 Diane O. (associate nurse) 3 to 11 Erline P., RN, BSN (primary nurse) 11 to 7	Full patient care, documentation, orders, admissions, discharges: rooms 422 to 425

entire illness episode and can cross all units in which the patient receives care. It is associated with the use of care pathways/order sets/care maps/protocols/clinical practice guidelines, which are written plans that identify critical and predictable events that must occur throughout a hospitalization and after the hospitalization. The assigned case manager works with the assigned nursing staff to coordinate patient progress through the transition of care pathway. The Case Management Society of America defines case management as "a collaborative process of assessment, planning, facilitation and advocacy for options and services to meet an individual's health needs through communication and available resources to promote cost-effective outcomes" (Case Management Society of America, 2002). The case management model also extends beyond the hospital setting, with case managers working with patients and families in all transitions of care. Some institutions use case managers in partnership with chronically ill patients at high risk for continued hospital readmissions. The case managers work with the patients to coordinate the entire spectrum of care in all settings. Case management has been associated with decreased readmissions for chronically ill patients.

Case managers are often population based, so that one case manager may work with all surgical patients within a hospital, although some institutions do use unit-based case managers. The case manager is assigned to the patient on admission and follows the patient for the entire hospital stay and performs all post-hospital care coordination. Not all case managers are nurses.

Advantages of case management:
- Provides a professional practice model for nurses
- Is cost effective

Disadvantages of case management:
- May lead to fragmented communication
- Needs to be integrated into the care delivery model
- May lead to nurses caring for patients to become more skills focused if the case manager makes all the decisions

Table 2-5 provides an overview of the major types of nursing care delivery models.

The care delivery system delineates the nurses' authority and accountability for practice and outcomes. The care delivery system is integrated with the professional practice model. According to the ANCC (2014), the professional practice model is the "driving force of nursing care" (p. 74). It is a schematic description that depicts how nurses practice, collaborate, communicate, and develop professionally to provide high-quality care for those served by the organization. It is integrated with the care delivery model and promotes continuous, consistent, efficient, and accountable nursing care (p. 64).

Some of the professional practice models that have been embraced by nursing over the past few years include:

Relationship-based care (RBC): Relationships are built with the patient and family. The goal of this model is to work collaboratively with the patient and family to effect positive outcomes.

Transforming care at the bedside: The goal of this model is to empower nurses to improve care processes, delivery, and outcomes at the bedside by identifying initiatives for quality improvement.

Family-centered care: The goal of this model is to care not only for the patient but also for the family by including the family in all aspects of care and decision making as allowed by the patient.

Synergy model of patient care: This model was developed by the American Association of Critical-Care Nurses (AACN). It places the needs of the patient at the core of the model, with a matching of the needs of the patient to the competencies of the nurses. The ideal outcome of this model is the patient moving safely and effectively through the health care delivery system.

TABLE 2-5 Overview of Major Types of Nursing Care Delivery Models

Model	Focus	Clinical Decision Making	Work Allocation	Time Span
Total patient care	Total patient care	Nurse at bedside, charge nurse makes some decisions	Assigning patients	One shift
Functional	Tasks	Charge nurses make most decisions	Assigning tasks	One shift
Team	Group task	Team leader makes most decisions	Assigning tasks	One shift
Primary	Total patient care	Nurse at bedside	Assigning patients	24 hours/7 days a week
Model	**Communication**	**Documentation**	**Outcomes**	**Quality**
Total patient care	Hierarchical: charge nurse gives and receives report	Unknown	May lack continuity of care between caregivers	High: all care delivered by RN
Functional	Hierarchical: charge nurse gives and receives report	Tasks	Fragmented care	Omissions and errors can occur
Team	Hierarchical: charge nurse to charge nurse, or charge nurse to team leaders, or team leaders to team members	Tasks and care plan	Fragmented care	Omissions and errors can occur
Primary	Lateral: caregiver to caregiver	Individualized plan	Continuity of care	Process oriented

From Tiedman, M., & Lookinland, S. (2004). Traditional models of care delivery: What have we learned? *Journal of Nursing Administration, 34*(6), 291-297.

SUMMARY

The manner in which patient care is delivered to patients and families is reflective of the nursing philosophy of the organization. Each model of patient care delivery has advantages and disadvantages for both the patient and the nurse. The role of the nurse in each type of model differs according to the delivery system. It is important to acknowledge your role and responsibilities in the model being used in your institution.

New models of patient care delivery and professional practice are being developed and used across the United States. Some of the newer models combine aspects of the models already in existence. As research and evidence concerning the successes and challenges of the new models evolve, care delivery will change.

CLINICAL CORNER

Transforming Care at the Bedside

Initiated in 2001 in collaboration with the Institute for Healthcare Improvement (IHI) and Robert Wood Johnson Foundation (RWJF), Transforming Care at the Bedside (TCAB) empowered front line staff to drive the health care environment. This nontraditional quality improvement initiative was introduced to health care, specifically medical surgical units, on the heels of the Institute of Medicine (IOM) report that time spent at the bedside by registered nurses was directly tied to overall patient outcomes.

Using a session called a Deep Dive, staff brainstorm on the issues that impact their day-to-day work, common themes are identified after grouping the barriers, and the staff members are challenged to develop "small tests of change." These are developed using the Plan-Do-Study-Act (PDSA) method for performance improvement.

Staff empowerment is driven in the ongoing evaluation of the PDSAs. Staff members are encouraged to initiate change on the smallest scale possible. This enables the staff to adapt, or fine tune, the test of change while working toward a finished product that can be applied on a larger scale. Adapting in this manner leads the process through the necessary cycles until a test of change can be adopted. Adopting a test of change indicates that the staff have reached a process that works and is now a part of the operation of the unit. A significant caveat is the ability to abandon a test of change that does not work. This prevents the staff from wasting time and energy on implementing a process that just does not fit into the operations of the unit.

Successful tests of change are not confined to the units where they are created. TCAB initiatives can be spread to other areas of the organization. Furthermore, the TCAB process can engage teams in reaching solutions in multiple areas, or organizationally when the challenge is shared on a larger scale. When organizations are introduced to TCAB they are encouraged to spread the initiative after successful implementation on a pilot unit. Well-developed TCAB programs engage nursing and operational departments throughout the organization.

The TCAB journey started at St. Joseph's Regional Medical Center in 2009. The New Jersey State Hospital Association (NJHA) initiated a 50-hospital cohort in collaboration with the American Organization of Nurse Executives (AONE). TCAB was piloted on a 33-bed medical-surgical unit.

The pilot unit realized immediate success with TCAB. The team successfully initiated tests of change that were quick wins for the staff that fostered immediate engagement. Early, simple successes included the creation of a maintenance log that eliminated redundancy in following up on unit repairs and became a vehicle for staff to build the physical environment to facilitate work flow. The addition of shelving and a phone in the medication room allowed the staff to communicate with pharmacy and prepare medications simultaneously, eliminating disruptive trips to the desk.

The staff engaged in larger process changes. Through the TCAB process they went on to implement bedside reports, which reduced incidental overtime by 30%. Initiating Team Admissions significantly reduced the time-consuming process of admitting patients to the unit. The average admission time was reduced from an average of 90 minutes to 10 to 15 minutes among three nurses working on an admission together.

The engagement of the staff on the pilot unit was palpable. During the implementation of TCAB overall patient satisfaction scores rose 11 points over two quarters, earning the unit recognition as the most improved by the organization. The staff and nurse manager on the pilot unit embarked on the task of spreading TCAB throughout the organization.

Spreading TCAB throughout the organization provided the opportunity to merge TCAB with the hospital's nurse practice model Relationship-Based Care (RBC).

CLINICAL CORNER—cont'd

As teams engaged in RBC, they were required to establish advisory councils that represented 20% of the staffing mix on the units. The unit-based advisory councils had to meet specific milestones and drive autonomic nursing practice. TCAB training was added as one of the milestones. TCAB became the performance improvement tool for the advisory councils and RBC overall.

The nurse manager and staff of the pilot unit provided TCAB training throughout the organization. Training was organized by specialties, and even provided to the organization's smaller sister hospital. TCAB training included interdisciplinary departments, such as radiology and pharmacy.

The TCAB initiative at St. Joseph's Regional Medical Center has resulted in over 200 staff-led improvements to patient care. Here are some examples:

- Radiology installed slide boards in their procedure rooms, eliminating back injuries
- Pharmacy altered medication delivery times to the automated medication dispensers so as to not interfere with heavy medication pass times.

- Several units reorganized supply locations, reducing hunting and gathering times.
- Medical Surgical Division collaboration on hourly rounding initiative, increasing patient satisfaction.
- Psychiatric unit converted to 12-hour shifts, reducing call outs by 90%.
- Staff developed a rounding and curtain changing schedule with housekeeping, reducing hospital acquired infections.
- Staff developed a medication delivery system, reducing time spent searching for medication by 30 minutes per nurse per shift.
- Several units created equipment parking spots, keeping necessary items clean and ready to use.
- Several units implemented adopt-a-room programs where staff maintain designated areas for survey readiness.

St. Joseph's has become a leader in TCAB on a state and national level.

Eddie A. Perez, RN, MHA, NE-BC
Director of Nursing
Medical Surgical Services
St. Joseph's Regional Medical Center, Paterson, NJ

EVIDENCE BASED PRACTICE

New Health Care Delivery Models Are Redefining the Role of Nurses

www.nursezone.com/nursing-news-events/more-features/new-health-delivery-models-are-redefining-the-role-of-nurses_29442.aspx

Hospitals, health systems, medical clinics, and health plans are attempting to do more with less in today's health care system. Nurses have become key integrators, care coordinators, and efficiency experts. Some of the most innovative nursing-driven models of health care involved elevating the role of nurses from caregivers to "care integrators." New health care delivery models were developed. With more than $700,000 in grant money from the Robert Wood Johnson Foundation, the task was to identify innovative, nursing-driven models of health care delivery. Eight common themes among the care delivery models are:

1. Elevating the role of nurses and transitioning from caregivers to "care integrators."
2. Taking a team approach.
3. Bridging the continuum of care.
4. Defining the home as a setting of care.
5. Targeting high users of health care.
6. Sharpening focus on the patient, including an active engagement of the patient and family in care planning and delivery, and a greater responsiveness to patient wants and needs.
7. Leveraging technology.
8. Improving satisfaction, quality, and cost.

As with anything, changes did not happen overnight, but nurses felt the importance of the care delivery models, and were supported by their management for their endeavors.

NCLEX® EXAMINATION QUESTIONS

1. A model of care in which the nurse assumes full accountability for care of a group of patients is:
   A. Case management
   B. Primary nursing
   C. Functional nursing
   D. Total patient care

2. A schematic description of a theory, phenomenon, or system that depicts how nurses practice, collaborate, communicate, and develop professionally to provide the highest level of care (American Nurses Credentialing Center, 2013) is:
   A. Professional practice model
   B. Care delivery system
   C. Case management model
   D. Functional system

3. Which type of structure is a hierarchy that follows a chain of command concept and is characterized by top-down decision making?
   A. Decentralized
   B. Organizational
   C. Functional
   D. Matrix

4. A decentralized leadership structure would be one that allows decision making:
   A. At senior levels
   B. By the board of trustees
   C. At the point of care
   D. By all involved

5. Which of the following is a disadvantage of primary nursing?
   A. Improved quality and continuity of care
   B. Simplified communication
   C. Increased nurse satisfaction
   D. Increased number of hours of care per day requires greater number of registered nurses

6. Which of the following structures arranges services and departments according to their function?
   A. Organizational
   B. Functional
   C. Primary
   D. Centralized

7. The type of patient care in which the nurse caring for the patient makes most decisions is:
   A. Functional
   B. Team
   C. Case management
   D. Total patient care

8. Which model of nursing mixes both process and delivery?
   A. Modular
   B. Case management
   C. Primary care
   D. Team nursing

9. Which of the following describes an integrated structure?
   A. Providers agree to accept the risk of caring for a particular patient segment or population for a pre-established fee
   B. Combines both function and service line
   C. Arranges services and departments according to function
   D. The nurse is responsible to the nurse manager and vice president of nursing

10. The reorganization of health care systems were developed to:
    A. Provide for care throughout the various transitions of care
    B. Change the levels of nursing authority in the institution
    C. Provide for care in one facility at a time
    D. Prevent partnerships, which would lead to less income

Answers: 1. D   2. A   3. B   4. C   5. D   6. B   7. D
8. B   9. A   10. A

3

Strategic Management and Planning

OBJECTIVES

- Define strategic management and strategic planning.
- Discuss the importance of the strategic planning process.
- Identify the components of the strategic plan.
- Compare and contrast the various types of strategic planning processes.
- Distinguish between short- and long-term plans and objectives.
- Identify the role of the nurse manager in the strategic planning process.

OUTLINE

KEY TERMS

environmental scan analysis of the political, demographic, social, regulatory, and technologic environments of the organization

goals statement of direction of the organization

mission statement statement defining the purpose of the organization

objectives measurable statements related to the goals of the organization

performance measures quantitative tools that allow for measurement of the achievement of goals

stakeholders all groups that may be affected by an organization's services, actions, and outcomes

strategic context competitive environment of the organization

values philosophy or behaviors determined to be vital to the organization

vision future-oriented statement of where the organization sees itself

WHAT IS STRATEGIC PLANNING?

Simply put, strategic planning is the process by which an organization/nursing department or unit decides where it is going over the next year or longer and how it is going to get there. Typically, the process is organization-wide and the outcome of the process, on an organizational level, cascades down to the patient care department and the individual units and employees. The strategic plan is the "map" of where the organization, department, or unit is going over the next year or longer.

Strategic management is the process of setting goals and **objectives** for the organization/department/unit, determining the resources that are necessary to meet the goals, creating an action plan, and evaluating progress towards meeting the goals. It involves defining the long-term objectives of the organization and setting priorities. The timeline is future-oriented and predicts organizational activities over several years (Rundio & Wilson, 2013, p. 37).

Strategic planning used to be the domain of the financial managers of many institutions. This philosophy has changed, and strategic planning now includes all stakeholders of the organization. Nurse managers have an important role in the strategic plan of the organization and in the implementation of action plans at the unit level that assist the organization in meeting its goals.

Leaders of an organization need to focus on a series of key questions as they begin the strategic planning process (Finkler, Kovner, & Jones, 2007, p. 216):

- Why does the organization exist?
- What is the organization currently?
- What would it like to be?
- How can we make the transformation to what we want to be?
- How will we know when the transformation is done?

In answering these questions, the leaders will find that the answers lead to other questions, such as: What are the strengths and challenges faced by the organization? What is its competitive status? Who are the primary stakeholders for the organization? How does the organization measure its performance? How does it learn from its performance? Do we make a difference? What is the value to our stakeholders?

ELEMENTS OF A STRATEGIC PLAN

The elements of a strategic plan include the following (Finkler et al., 2007, p. 217):

- Mission statement.
- Statement of competitive challenges and strategy.
- Statement of short- and long-term goals.
- Statement of organizational policies.
- Statement of needed resources.
- Statement of key assumptions.

Mission and Vision Statements

The first step in strategic management is the development of a mission statement for the organization. The mission statement focuses on the definition of

what the organization does and aspires to do. The mission statement for some organizations is further divided into a vision, which tells the reader where the organization wants to be in the future. Many organizations also create a values statement, which includes the behaviors of importance within the organization. Some organizations include the mission, vision, and values statement in one document. An example is the Mission, Vision and Values of Henry Ford Health System (HFHS) (2011):

Mission: To improve human life through excellence in the science and art of health care and healing.

Vision: Transforming lives and communities through health and wellness; one person at a time.

Values: We serve our patients and our community through our actions that always demonstrate: Each patient first, respect for people, high performance, learning and continuous improvement, and a social conscience

This mission, vision, and values set the direction for HFHS and serves as the basis for their strategic planning and management of operations.

The mission and vision of an organization are consistent with the organizational structure. For example, the mission statement for a small critical access hospital with no primary care services will reflect that reality. Large academic medical centers will have statements that focus on their teaching and research role.

Statement of Competitive Environment and Strategy

As part of the strategic planning process, it is vital for an organization to be aware of its competitive environment. This is accomplished through strategic analysis. Sometimes this is also called an environmental scan. This activity can include conducting a review of the organization's environment (e.g., a review of the political, social, economic, and technical environment). Planners carefully consider various driving forces in the environment, such as increasing competition, changing demographics, and so forth. Planners also look at the various strengths, weaknesses, opportunities, and threats regarding the organization; an acronym for this activity is SWOT. Such information forms the strategic context of the organization. As nurse managers, you will participate in the patient satisfaction initiatives of your institution. Most nurses are aware of the performance of the other units in the hospital in relation to patient satisfaction, and some are aware of the performance of the similar units in the area. An example of changing demographics and their impact on hospital planning would be a population shift to large numbers of families moving into the local area served by the institution. This information from the environmental scan might result in a facility increasing the number of services for a pediatric population. An example of technical and regulatory changes occurring is the introduction of electronic medical records and their meaningful use.

Other information collected for the strategic planning process comes from past performance and information collected from all stakeholders through a variety of means. These involve satisfaction surveys (patient, employees, physicians, community), focus groups with members of the community to determine issues of importance, and other means of listening to the expressed desires of the local community.

The organization then determines its strategic challenges and strategic opportunities. Examples of such challenges and opportunities from (2011) follow:

Strategic Challenges and Advantages

Challenges

SC1: Accelerating pressures requiring cost control, revenue growth, and diversification.

SC2: Growing transparency of results and aligning physicians to drive accountability for improvement.

SC3: Potential increased competition caused by possible mergers and acquisitions.

SC4: Increased publicly available information and the effect on consumer decision making.

SC5: Redesigning care to maximize health and effective outcomes while reducing costs.

SC6: Addressing health care needs of our diverse population including the uninsured and underinsured.

SC7: Retaining, training, and engaging an effective, collaborative workforce and developing leaders.

Advantages

SA1 "Can Do" spirit: a focus on workforce engagement, talent development, and recognition creates unique energy and a "can do" culture to continuously improve the quality and safety of our services.

SA2 Strategic geographic positioning: HFHS's provider and insurance representation in all Southeast Michigan (SEM) regions, growing into other Michigan markets, is fundamental to the integration model and growth.

SA3 Long-term presence in and support of our communities: HFHS has been an active community member in Detroit since 1915 while also creating relationships and facilities in each of our suburbs.

SA4 Commitment to diversity and equity: HFHS is located in a highly diverse community, and this commitment creates a desirable environment in which to work and receive care.

SA5 System integration: a vast continuum of services, unique in health care, provides a means of achieving success across all seven performance pillars.

SA6 Academic mission: our extensive clinical training and research programs attract physicians and allied professionals to HFHS from around the globe.

Many organizations use pillars to organize and measure performance. HFHS uses seven pillars. The seven pillars represent the areas most important to our success: people; service; quality and safety; growth; research and education; community; and finance. The framework aligns system strategic objectives, strategic initiatives, and related performance measures and targets for the system and within business units from the top of the organization to the individual employee. Most organizations use six pillars: people, service, quality, community, finance, and growth (Studer, 2008), but with the academic teaching role of this medical center, a seventh pillar was added reflecting that activity.

The competitive strategy is the organization's plan for achieving its goals. It states what services will be provided to whom. It is decided on as a direct result of the information provided by the strategic analysis and environmental scan. The organization evaluates its mission, vision, and goals in light of the information provided by the environmental scan, the identified strengths and challenges, and the demand for service. Based on this competitive strategy, the organization makes a plan that allows it to take advantage of the identified strengths and needs of the various stakeholders. The product of this process is conclusions about what the organization must do as a result of the major issues and opportunities facing the organization. These conclusions include the overall accomplishments (or *strategic goals*) the organization should achieve.

Statement of Short-Term and Long-Term Goals

According to Carter McNamara (2006), the long- and short-term goals are the overall methods (or strategies) to achieve the strategic goals of the organization. An example of a short-term goal of an organization might be to improve performance on the core measures for cardiac failure, increasing from 80% to 85% compliance by the end of the year. A long-term goal might be to consistently perform at 98% to 100% at the end of 3 years. Goals should be designed and worded as much as possible to be **S**pecific, **M**easurable, **A**cceptable to those working to achieve the goals, **R**ealistic, **T**imely, **E**xtending the capabilities of those working to achieve the goals, and **R**ewarding to them, as well. (A mnemonic for these criteria is "SMARTER.")

Action Planning

Action planning is the process by which the specific goals are matched with each strategic goal. The overall organization-wide strategic goals cascade down to all departments and units and, in some cases, the individual employees. Action planning requires specifying expected outcomes with each strategic goal. These outcomes then form the basis of the performance scorecards used in most organizations. The anticipated outcomes are usually based on the competitive strategy of the organization and are often benchmarked against "best in class performers" or to where the organization wants to be in terms of performance.

Often, each objective is associated with a tactic, which is one of the methods needed to achieve an objective. Therefore, implementing a strategy typically involves implementing a set of tactics along the way; in that sense, a tactic is still a strategy, but on a smaller scale.

Action planning also includes specifying responsibilities and timelines with each objective, or who needs to do what and by when. It should also include methods to monitor and evaluate the plan, which includes knowing how the organization will know who has done what and by when.

It is common to develop an annual plan (sometimes called the operational plan or management plan), which includes the strategic goals, strategies, objectives, responsibilities, and timelines that should be implemented in the coming year. These are the short-term goals of the organization. The difference between short- and long-term plans and objectives relates to the time expected to accomplish them. These times vary from institution

to institution, but short-term plans usually extend up to 1 year. Long-term plans vary from 3 to 5 years.

Usually, budgets are included in the strategic and annual plan, and with individual departmental and unit plans. Budgets specify the funds needed for the resources that are necessary to implement the annual plan. Budgets also show how the funds will be spent. (See Chapter 4 for information on budgets.)

The strategic planning process of HFHS is diagrammed in Figure 3-1 and an example of their broad strategic plan is shown in Figure 3-2. Note that the goals are organized by the seven pillars identified by HFHS. The goals relate to the strategic challenges and opportunities developed by the organization. The performance indicators list the measures that will be used to measure progress toward achievement of the goals. The benchmarks relate the performance of the competitors or "best in class," and the targets are the short- and long-term goals.

As this organizational plan cascades down to the departments and units, it becomes more specific with action plans and timelines for measures of achievement. The action plan in Figure 3-3 is a departmental action plan for another organization. Note that it is also organized according to the pillars, but is is much more department specific than a broader organization-wide strategic plan. Also note the action steps and the outcome results.

UNIT-BASED PLANNING PROCESS

Planning typically includes several major activities or steps in the process. Different organizations often have different names for these major activities and often conduct them in different orders. Strategic planning is very individualized according to the organization. The organizational strategic plan cascades down to the departmental plans, which cascade to the unit plans, and end with the individual employee performance plan.

On a unit-based level, the nurse manager will oversee the unit-based planning process. Things to accomplish include the following:

1. Identify your purpose (mission statement): The mission statement for your unit should carefully mirror that of the overall organization. Remember, it is important that all levels of the organization are "on the same page." If the unit goals are different than those of the organization, there is a potential conflict.

Strategic Challenge / Advant.*	Strategic Objectives by Pillar (Key Stakeholders*)	System Strategic Initiatives (Core Competencies*)	Key Short-Term (ST) and Long-Term (LT) Plans (Bold = most important)	Key Performance Measures (Results Figures) (Bold = most important)	Performance Targets 2011	Performance Targets Stretch 2013	Best Comp 2013
SC7 SA1, 4, 6	**People:** National leader in healthcare employee retention and engagement (KS1,2)	Develop a competent, agile workforce and build a culture of development (C1, C2, C3)	**Develop & implement a flexible staffing model; internal staffing pool (ST)** **Enhance 1st yr. retention programs (LT)**	**Overall Employee Turnover** *(Fig. 7.3-3)*	CONFIDENTIAL		7.3%
		Develop a high-performance work environment with a highly engaged workforce (C1, C3)	**Focus on increasing engagement scores for bottom quartile leaders (ST)** Conduct semi-annual pulse surveys for employees including toolkits and support for all managers (LT)	**Overall & Nursing Engagement Index, 1-5 scale** *(Fig. 7.3-15)*			4.35
SC3,4 SA1, 4, 5	**Service:** Best-in-class service to our customers among U.S. healthcare organizations (KS1,2,3)	Create consistency of The Henry Ford Experience at all HFHS facilities (C1, C2, C3)	**Share lessons and customer feedback to spread best practices (ST);** **Roll-out Culture of Service plan (LT)**	**HCAHPS results at/above national benchmarks** *(Fig.7.2-5)*			100%
				% Top Box, "Likelihood to Recommend" *(Fig. 7.2-3,8,10)*			90%ile
SC2, 5 SA1, 4, 5	**Quality & Safety:** National leader in delivering safe, reliable, high-quality, & highly coordinated care to each individual patient (KS1,2,3)	Fully implement the HFHS No Harm Campaign via System and local collaborative teams (C1,C2,C3)	**Implement best practices for reducing harm in each of the 6 harm categories (LT)**	**Harm events per 1000 acute care patient days** *(Fig.7. 1-1)*			n/a
		Reduce readmissions via discharge and post-acute coordination (C2)	**Implement readmissions avoidance tactics at all sites (ST); System-wide case management system (LT)**	**Readmissions within 30 Days** *(Fig. 7.1-13)*			8.0%
SC1, 2 3, 6 SA1 - 5	**Growth:** Dominant health system in Michigan (KS1,2,3)	Execute growth plans for hospitals to capture market share (C2, C3)	**Implement strategies to attract new business to HFWBH and HFH (LT) and HFMH-WC (ST)** **Expand HFMG ambulatory centers in high growth markets; recruit needed physicians (LT)**	**Tri-County IP Market Share** *(Fig. 7.5-11)*			20.2%
		Execute physician integration and access improvements (C1, C2, C3)		**IP Admissions** *(Fig. 7.5-9)*			116,686
				OP Visit Volume (Fig. 7.5-14)			n/a
		Alter insurance product mix to offset shrinking HMO market (C1, C2, C3)	**Launch new HAP products in preparation for 2012-2013 enrollment periods (LT)**	**Total HAP membership** *(Fig. 7.5-15)*			n/a
SC 2, 5, 7 SA1, 2, 4, 5, 6	**Research & Education:** Leading independent academic medical center and nationally preferred clinical research partner (KS1,2,3)	Strengthen research and education programs through new medical school affiliation(s) and fully integrated allopathic and osteopathic GME programs (C1, C3)	Expand research capabilities and clinical trials to attract new NIH and other external funding (LT)	NIH research grants and contracts *(7.1b(1)✱)*			$33M
			Integrate Medical Education System-wide (LT)	Trainee Satisfaction *(Fig. 7.3-14)*			n/a
				Ready for independent practice *(Fig. 7.3-14)*			n/a
SC5, 6 SA1, 3, 4	**Community:** National leader in community health advocacy and involvement (KS1,2,3)	Improve access to care/services for the Underinsured/Uninsured (C2, C3)	Increase support and utilization of community clinics	Visits to Community Clinics *(Fig. 7.4-8)*			n/a
		Leverage the refreshed CHNA report at all BUs and address identified community needs. (C2,C3)	Implement Community Benefit management and reporting structures for all BUs (ST); link to CHNA (LT)	Community Benefit *(Fig. 7.4-11)*			n/a
SC1, 2, 3, 5, 6 SA1 - 5	**Finance:** Financial strength to fund clinical services, health management, people, research, and education strategies (KS1,2,3)	Achieve operating profit and philanthropic donations sufficient to fund 3-year capital plans (C3)	**Continue revenue and cost management programs at all sites (LT)**	**System Operating Net Income** *(Fig. 7.5-1)*			n/a
				Cost per Unit of Service *(Fig. 7.5-2)*			n/a
			Continue philanthropic campaigns targeting external donors and employee contributors (ST)	% Philanthropic Donor Renewal *(Fig. 7.4-7)*			n/a
				Philanthropy Cash Collected *(Fig. 7.5-8)*			n/a

***Strategic Challenges**: SC1=Cost Control/Revenue Growth, SC2= Phys. Align/Accountable, SC3=Increased Competition, SC4=Increased Consumerism SC5= Care Redesign SC6= Care Needs Diverse Population SC7= Workforce Support **Strategic Advantages**: SA1="Can Do" Spirit, SA2=Strategic Geographic Positioning SA3=Community Support SA4=Commitment to Diversity/Equity SA5=System Integration SA6=Academic Mission **Key Stakeholders:** KS1=Patients (IP, OP, ED, CCS) KS2=Community (Detroit, Regional service areas), KS3=Purchasers (Employers, Health Plan Members) **Core Competencies:** C1=Innovation, C2=Care Coordination, C3=Collaboration/Partnering

FIGURE 3-1 The strategic planning process of Henry Ford Health System (2011). (http://patapsco.nist.gov/Award_Recipients/PDF_Files/2011_Henry_Ford_Health_System_Award_Application_Summary.pdf, figure 2.1-1, p. 6.)

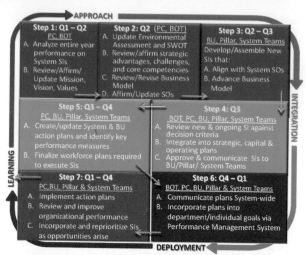

FIGURE 3-2 An example of the HFHS broad strategic plan. http://patapsco.nist.gov/Award_Recipients/PDF_Files/2011_Henry_Ford_Health_System_Award_Application_Summary.pdf, figure 2.1-2, p. 8.

2. Select the goals your organization must reach if it is to accomplish your mission: The unit and personal goals of each employee must relate to accomplishment of the mission of the unit and organization.

3. Identify specific approaches or strategies that must be implemented to reach each goal: Identify realistic activities that you and your staff will do to accomplish the goals.

4. Identify specific action plans to implement each strategy: Identify the things necessary for you and your staff to achieve the goals. This is related to the development of the budget to assist you in the identification of resources necessary to achieve the goals.

5. Monitor and update the plan: As you see in the department plan, there is a 90-day monitoring of results. The careful monitoring of performance allows you and your unit to determine if your action plans are working or if they need reworking. Most strategic plans are fluid documents allowing for changes to be made as necessary.

Sample 90-Day Action Plan • Women's and Children's Service Line (1/06-3/06)			
CSF	**Goal**	**Action steps**	**90-Day result report**
People	Maintain FT turnover rate	• Leader rounding x2 areas each day • Review rounding information at weekly manager meetings. • Implement 90-day AP with direct reports.	• Turnover rate at >1.6% • One 90-day AP per unit
Service	Acheive 90th percentile on inpatient satisfaction	• Nurse rounding • Bi-weekly meeting with Women/Children's patient satisfaction team	• 90th percentile or higher in patient satisfaction
Quality	Reduce practice variation in DRG 372, 373	• Physician champion identified • OM to perform CPA DRG 372-373 • PA to perform documentation analysis	• Decrease DRG 372 LOS • Assure appropriate DRG assignment
	Pediatric asthma	• Physician champion identified • Perform CPA on asthma DRG	• Decrease readmissions for pediatric asthma patients
Financial	Maintain expenses within budget	• Review OB/GYN financials with OBs • Nurse managers analyze and report OT needs to SLL	• BAR at or above 80 • Overtime below 3.0% • Expenses below budget
Growth	Develop a vision for pediatric services	• Set up meeting with LeBonheur Children's Hospital to discuss increase in pediatric subspecialties • Develop cost-benefit analysis with marketing for branding of pediatric services	• Presented draft of vision to March SLOG • Pediatric branding identified and cost-benefit reported to SLOG w/in 30 days
	Implement Women/Children's Community Advisory Board	• Recruit Advisory Board members • Develop agenda for first meeting	• First Advisory Board meeting March, 2006

FIGURE 3-3 Action plan. North Mississippi Medical Center. (2006). Application for the Malcolm Baldrige Performance Excellence Award. http://baldrige.nist.gov/PDF_files/NMMC_Application_Summary.pdf.

As a nurse, you will also deal with action plans that address the Joint Commission Core Measures (see Chapter 5), the National Patient Safety Goals (see Chapter 10), the Centers for Medicare and Medicaid Services (CMS) Hospital Consumer Assessment of Healthcare Providers and Systems (HCAHPS) measures, the National Database of Nursing Quality Indicators (NDNQI) nursing outcome measures, infection control measures, patient satisfaction, and particular issues of concern within your institution. Action plans for specific clinical concerns are usually managed by the performance improvement department of the clinical department, but the nurse manager and staff should be aware of these action plans and their role in the achievement of the overall organizational goal. An example of an action plan for a clinical goal is shown in Figure 3-4.

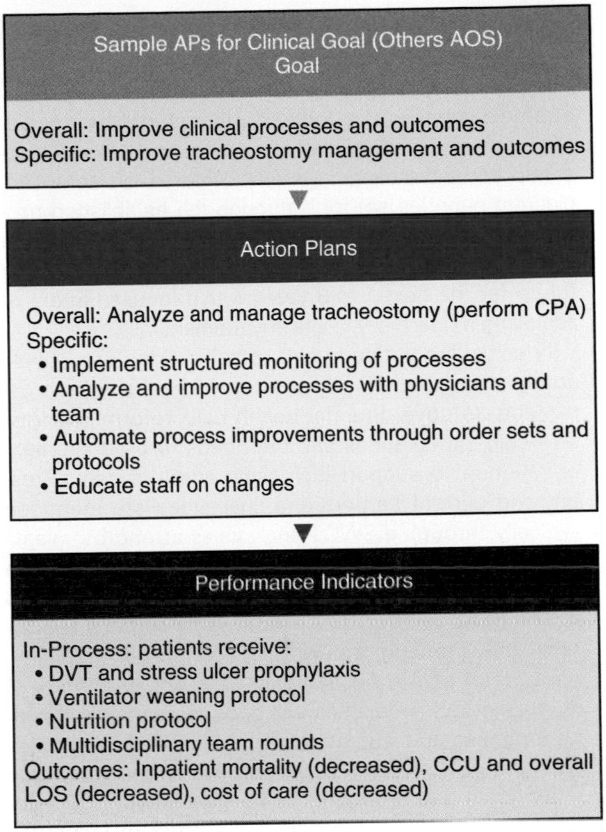

Purposes of Planning

- Increases the chances of success by focusing on results and not on activities.
- Forces analytical thinking, knowledge of current evidence, and evaluation of alternatives.
- Establishes a framework for decision making that is consistent with organizational strategic objectives.
- Orients people to action rather than re-action.
- Includes day-to-day and future-focused managing.
- Helps to avoid crisis management and provides decision-making flexibility.
- Provides a basis for managing organizational and individual performance.
- Is cost effective.

(Adapted from Rousel, 2013)

Sample APs for Clinical Goal (Others AOS)
Goal

Overall: Improve clinical processes and outcomes
Specific: Improve tracheostomy management and outcomes

▼

Action Plans

Overall: Analyze and manage tracheostomy (perform CPA)
Specific:
- Implement structured monitoring of processes
- Analyze and improve processes with physicians and team
- Automate process improvements through order sets and protocols
- Educate staff on changes

▼

Performance Indicators

In-Process: patients receive:
- DVT and stress ulcer prophylaxis
- Ventilator weaning protocol
- Nutrition protocol
- Multidisciplinary team rounds
Outcomes: Inpatient mortality (decreased), CCU and overall LOS (decreased), cost of care (decreased)

FIGURE 3-4 An example of an action plan for a clinical goal. North Mississippi Medical Center. (2006). Application for the Malcolm Baldrige Performance Excellence Award. http://baldrige.nist.gov/PDF_files/NMMC_Application_Summary.pdf.

SUMMARY

Strategic planning is a continually evolving process in most organizations, with constant monitoring of performance to goal, achievement of strategic objectives, and updating of the plan as changes occur within the environment. As a nurse manager, it is your responsibility to always be aware of the plan and your role in the plan and, as a staff nurse, to be aware of your role in assisting the organization and your unit in the achievement of the strategic goals.

CLINICAL CORNER

The Chief Nursing Officer's Role as a Participant in Strategic Planning

Strategic planning is a focused process in which senior management, medical staff leadership, and hospital leadership address changing needs centered on approved, planned priorities set forth through the established mission, vision, and values of an organization. Typically, a plan is a developed path representative of the immediate future for the next 1 to 3 years with a focused intent of achieving a financially viable environment.

By achieving defined goals, organizations proactively address the needs for the successful health of an organization as governmental health care reform changes strategic expectations and the needs to produce higher revenue to support increasing costs of care. Present and current barriers and challenges are identified typically through a SWOT analysis as strengths, weaknesses, opportunities, and threats are identified. The prospect of lighter margins requires strategic plans to now include cost control initiatives to address regulations and spending caps without compromising quality. As a result of the Accountable Care Act, the influx of newly insured Americans will boost demand for hospital inpatient and outpatient services. Medicare policy changes will continue to have an effect on health care settings as briefer lengths of hospital stays, less inpatient hospital occupancy, and the move to increased outpatient care, leave organizations with lower margins that will continue to shift nursing manpower and labor costs to outpatient services.

Continuity of patient care requires well-trained high-quality inpatient and outpatient programs and facilities where clinical practitioners can practice in a financially viable environment. The local and national surplus of physician specialists and the increased need for primary care physicians shows a growing trend of teaching and community-based hospitals that are buying and managing physician practices. To ensure continuity of health care in the community, primary care physicians and their locations are particularly important as a referral base for physician specialists and acute care admissions.

2015 is the first year that hospitals will be penalized more than 3% of their Medicare revenue if they are not achieving Medicare quality and safety incentive programs that are now fully in effect. These include hospital-based readmission rates, hospital acquired conditions, and value-based purchasing rates that are now an integrated measure of quality. Hospitals have the potential of being docked large percentages of their Medicare payments if not compliant. Financial viability is a growing concern.

Strategic planning priorities have changed and developing a patient-centered culture is now on the front burner of all health care organizations. The achievement of governmental standards now weighs heavily on patient centeredness and nursing's interventions to meet patient satisfaction as the core measures and high quality analytical outcomes of the Centers for Medicare & Medicaid Services (CMS) are now transparent in the public domain. Developing a patient-centered culture requires the organization and its physicians and nursing staff to be passionate about transforming the experience of every patient. This requires a commitment of all staff to deliver innovative and creative programming that provides an exemplary experience for patients and their families. Care, now more than ever, needs to be integrated, coordinated, and an exceptional experience across the continuum of care. New care models and payment systems will hold the reimbursement of organizations if the cost of care is not controlled. This includes the managed cost of referrals post-hospitalization to skilled nursing faculties (SNFs), nursing homes, and rehabilitation facilities as CMS pilot payment models hold acute care facilities responsible for managing the cost of those referrals. Other price-sensitive providers will follow to continually drive down health care costs as these pilots prove to be successful.

The strategic planning committee also evaluates the competition of local facilities for inpatient and low-cost ambulatory care services, which include numerous physician-owned ambulatory surgeries, imaging, rehabilitation and pain-management centers, a growing trend in the last 10 years. Improving the performance of the emergency department, including the measurement and daily analysis of wait times, triage times, and treat and release, and admission length of stay is an imperative for addressing a competitive stance and patient's perceptions of care, and is a direct reflection of patient future choice.

Annual reviews of goals, objectives, and strategies to ensure the perceived strengths of the organization evolve from daily and monthly data analysis. Physician and nurse practice feedback, including interviews and surveys as well as actual clinical comparative outcomes of national nursing data, must be transparent and carried out at least annually. These outcomes include benchmark data of best practice in fall rates, falls with injury, pressure ulcer rates, national CMS reportable core measures outcomes of acute

CLINICAL CORNER—cont'd

myocardial infarction (AMI), pneumonia, congestive heart failure (CHF) and ventilated assisted pneumonia (VAP) rates, infection rates, CMS perinatal standards, and psychiatric assessment standards compliance.

Members of the strategic planning committee (made up of key trustees, senior executive and management, and key department heads) must review the hospital's previous mission and strategic direction as an initial process to evaluate what was achieved, the organization's success and still-existing and new initiatives identified to overcome threats, to fulfill its mission to the community.

The process includes the following tasks and activities:

- Review of the existing vision, mission, and values.
- Strategic planning committee appointments.
- Environmental and competitor demographic data collection and analysis.
- Review of payer mix and hospital margins.
- Key physician supply and primary care and specialty projections.
- Interviews with physicians and key leadership regarding the current state and future direction of the organization's clinical programs and services.
- Analysis of preliminary findings and conclusions.
- Development options.

- Strategic goals, objectives, and action strategies.
- Facility planning and prioritizing of needed capital and plant improvements.
- Draft and finalization of a plan and the development of an executive summary for board review and approval.

The chief nursing officer should involve nurse members of practice and governance councils to contribute their professional goals to the organization's strategic plan. Developing new, clear, and measurable expectations regarding pillars of quality, service, people, growth, and costs needs to be understood by all. Communicating these pillars in monthly reports to the board of trustees, employees, and affiliated and employed physicians maintains the focus needed to actually achieve what is important and strives to ensure a financially strong organization, with frontline staff aware that everyone can make a contribution to ensuring the highest quality care while decreasing cost. In a culture that values accountability, once finalized, the strategic plan becomes a living, breathing, transparent document that has focus and involves all of its vested staff in achieving its written goals and quality outcomes.

Bonnie Michaels, RN, MA, NES-BC, FACHE

EVIDENCE-BASED PRACTICE

Drenkard, K. (2012). Strategy as solution developing a nursing strategic plan. *Journal of Nursing Administration,* *42*(5), 242-243.

The Executive Director of the American Nurses Credentialing Center discussed the importance of having a nursing strategic plan, especially when working to create a research agenda. Having a strategy for the implementation of evidence-based practice and the creation of a research agenda in nursing is critical.

Strategic planning includes:

- envisioning a facility's future
- creating a shared vision
- understanding the current state of nursing services provided
- identification of strengths and weaknesses
- development of action plans
- input from nurses
- use of technology in the process
- prioritization

The representatives of the strategic plan should include:

- human resources
- marketing
- strategic planning
- finance

Formal planning of measurement and outcomes for each item in the plan is then done. Strategic planning is critical for the future of nursing. It can encompass nursing research, clinical issues, and concerns. Magnet organizations use the following in the gathering of information: flipcharts, contests, lunch and learn, and technology. Finally, the strategic plan integrates all members of the health care team, aligns resources, drives innovation, and builds excitement.

The planning process of a strategic plan includes a shared vision, understanding the current state of nursing services, and conducting a gap analysis. The next phase is developing action plans. Including key partners, such as human resources, marketing, and finance is essential. For each strategy there must be a measurement. Strategy can drive innovation and build excitement.

NCLEX® EXAMINATION QUESTIONS

1. The mission of an organization:
   A. Sets the competitive tone
   B. States what is done by the organization
   C. Measures the performance of a unit
   D. Defines the philosophy of an institution
2. The vision of an organization is:
   A. A statement defining the purpose of the organization
   B. A future-oriented statement of where the organization sees itself
   C. Philosophy or behaviors determined to be vital to the organization
   D. An analysis of the political, demographic, and social environment of the organization
3. An environmental scan is:
   A. An analysis of the political, demographic, social, regulatory, and technological areas of the organization
   B. The measurable statements related to the goals of the organization
   C. The quantitative tools that allow for measurement of achievement
   D. The competitive environment of the organization
4. A specific action plan should be used for each:
   A. Strategy
   B. Goal
   C. Outcome
   D. Performance improvement
5. Identifying purpose, selecting goals, identifying approaches are all part of:
   A. Unit-based planning
   B. Hospital-wide planning
   C. Organization-wide planning
   D. Decentralized planning
6. An annual plan includes:
   A. People, service, budget, community, finance, and growth

   B. People, service, quality, community, finance, and growth
   C. People, service, quality, objectives, finance, and growth
   D. People, service, quality, community, finance, and perseverance
7. _____is the process by which the specific goals are matched with each strategic goal.
   A. Action planning
   B. Short-term goal planning
   C. Long-term goal planning
   D. Core-measure planning
8. According to Studer, 2003 most organizations use six pillars for organization and performance measures. The six pillars include:
   A. People, satisfaction, quality, community, finance, and growth
   B. People, service, quantity, community, finance, and growth
   C. People, service, quality, community, finance, and growth
   D. People, service, quality, community, diversity, and growth
9. Which of the following is not an element of a strategic plan?
   A. Mission statement
   B. Competitive challenges and strategy
   C. Organizational policies
   D. Unit-specific goals
10. Strategic planning does not include:
    A. A plan to decide where the organization will go in the next year
    B. An organization-wide plan
    C. Effects on patient care and patient units
    D. A community plan

Answers: 1. A   2. B   3. A   4. A   5. A   6. B   7. A
8. C   9. D   10. D

REFERENCES

Finkler, S., Kovner, C., & Jones, C. (2007). *Financial management for nurse managers* (3rd ed.). Philadelphia: W. B. Saunders.

Henry Ford Health System. (2011). *Application for the Malcolm Baldrige Performance Excellence Award.* http://patapsco.nist.gov/Award_Recipients/PDF_Files/2011_Henry_Ford_Health_System_Award_Application_Summary.pdf.

McNamara, C. (Authenticity Consulting, LLC). Copyright © 1997-2006. Adapted from the *Field Guide to Nonprofit Strategic Planning and Facilitation.* www.managementhelp.org/plan_dec/str_plan/models.htm.

North Mississippi Medical Center. (2006). *Application for the Malcolm Baldrige Performance Excellence Award.* http://baldrige.nist.gov/PDF_files/NMMC_Application_Summary.pdf.

Rousel, L. (2013). *Management and leadership for nurse administrators.* Sudbury, MA: Jones & Bartlett.

Rundio, V., & Wilson, A. (2013). *Nurse executive review and resource manual* (3rd ed.). Silver Spring, MD.

Studer, Q. (2003). *Hardwiring excellence: Purpose, worthwhile work, making a difference.* Gulf Breeze, FL: Fire Starter Publishing.

4

Financial Management in Health Care

OBJECTIVES

- Define health care.
- Identify factors influencing today's health care system.
- Discuss the economic realities of U.S. health care.
- Identify the major forms of reimbursement for health care.
- Describe the U.S. health care system.
- Define budgeting.

- Differentiate between types of budgets.
- Discuss the advantages of various budget processes.
- Describe the key elements of budget preparation.
- Identify the responsibilities of the nurse manager in budget preparation.
- Discuss the responsibilities of the nurse manager in budget review.

OUTLINE

KEY TERMS

Accountable Care Organization one billing occurs across the transition of care. Generally the better the quality of care, the better the reimbursement

bottom line income of an organization that is the result of revenue (money earned) minus expenses

budget detailed financial plan for carrying out the activities of an organization or unit

budget variance difference between actual budget and actual spending

capital budget financial plan that deals with purchases of capital assets (equipment, land, etc.)

KEY TERMS—cont'd

cash budget financial plan that tracks cash received and spent

cash on hand amount of cash readily available to the organization

Centers for Medicare & Medicaid Services (CMS) formerly known as the Healthcare Financing Administration, the federal agency that administers Medicare, Medicaid, State Children's Health Insurance Program (SCHIP), and several other health-related programs

continuum of care matching an individual's ongoing needs with the appropriate level and type of medical, psychological, health, or social care or service within an organization or across multiple organizations

for-profit organizations organizations with stated financial structures that include profit goals and tax liabilities

health care system all of the structures, organizations, and services designed to deliver professional health and wellness services to consumers

Health Maintenance Organization (HMO) geographically organized system that provides an agreed-on package of health maintenance and treatment services

indirect costs generalized costs (housekeeping, information technology, etc.) for support of the program and billed to the program; often called support costs

managed care linkage between the financing and delivery of services in such a way as to permit payers to exercise control over the delivery of services

Medicaid joint federal and state assistance program designed to pay for medical long-term care assistance for individuals and families with low income and limited resources

Medicare health insurance program for people age 65 and older or under age 65 with certain disabilities or any age with end-stage renal disease

not-for-profit organizations organizations with financial structures that project financial goals with particular tax and legislative protection or shelters

operating (expense) budget financial plan for the day-to-day activities of the organization

personnel budget part of the operating budget that deals with personnel needed to deliver care; composed of salary and benefit costs

preferred provider organization (PPO) managed care company that contracts with health care providers (both physicians and hospitals) and payers (self-nsured employers, insurance companies, or managed care organizations) to provide health care services to a defined population for predetermined fixed fees

revenues income received for goods or services provided

value-based purchasing reimbursement for health care services based on quality of care

variable costs costs that vary in relation to volume and productivity

HEALTH

With the advent of health care delivery services organized under hospitals and care-giving facilities in the early nineteenth century, there has been movement toward standardizing care and financial practices within these institutions. It was not until the early twentieth century that hospitals began a pay-for-service financial plan. In this arrangement, the patient pays for services received. Insurance companies paid for the services rendered by most institutions. As the cost of health care in the United States rose exponentially, insurers began exploring more cost-effective ways to pay for health care. This has resulted in the health care plans, insurance plans, and federal plans that exist today. This change in reimbursement for health care services has dramatically affected all aspects of health care delivery in the United States driven by changes in Medicare reimbursement. Reimbursement is now based on the quality of care (value-based purchasing) whereby hospitals are fined if they do not meet the benchmark level of performance for identified patient outcomes.

This has also affected the way nursing care is provided. For example, today, patients who are hospitalized have a much higher acuity than they did 20 years ago. Today, the norm is for many patients to be treated at home or in ambulatory care settings; only the critically ill remain in the hospital. Nursing has been expected to meet these challenges both in acute care and in home care. Today there are more ambulatory services, shorter inpatient stays, and an increase in care for chronic illnesses. The greatest challenge facing the U.S. health care system is the high cost of care and services. Technology enables the survival of premature infants weighing 2499 g or less. Some of the infants are kept alive with life support, which may include ventilators and/or feeding tubes. These infants may have a lifetime connection with pediatricians, nurses, specialists, and therapists. Many of them are placed in early intervention programs, whereby the nurses and therapists visit the child and family in the home setting. Once these "preemies" are 3 years old, they are placed in preschool programs for children with special needs. There are also transitions in the continuum of care in which patients with chronic illnesses, such as congestive heart failure, receive care of various levels of acuity during the transitions of the chronic condition. The more recent role of the nurse navigator working with these single populations of patients (such as congestive heart failure) has an expected outcome of increasing the quality of care for that population and decreasing the readmission rates. These are two examples of the trend of health care in the United States. Health care is paramount, but at what expense? At an insurmountable expense. So not only are older adults living longer, the chronically ill are living longer and the preemies are kept alive on life support. Individuals in severe motor vehicle accidents are air lifted to trauma centers and kept alive. What is the cost to the families and to the nation? The costs affect employers, health care providers, the government, and the public sector.

In 2012, the Institute for Healthcare Improvement (IHI) described an approach to optimizing health system performance. It is the IHI's belief that new designs must be developed to simultaneously pursue three dimensions called the "Triple Aim":

- Improving the patient experience of care (including quality and satisfaction).
- Improving the health of populations.
- Reducing the per capita cost of health care.

Health care systems in attempting to meet the "Triple Aim" must focus on the individuals and families that use their services, design and integrate services to meet patient and family needs across the continuum of care, and do all in a cost-effective manner while delivering high-quality care as evidenced by patient and organizational outcomes.

FACTORS THAT INFLUENCE THE FINANCIAL BURDEN OF HEALTH CARE IN THE UNITED STATES

There are numerous factors that influence the continuing financial burden of health care within the United States.

Demographic Influences

The United States is culturally diverse. There is a continuous influx of people from all countries of the world. It is crucial for the U.S. health care system to deliver culturally competent care. The United States spends more on health care per capita than any other industrialized Western nation, but the United States has disproportionately more people without access to appropriate health care (Yoder-Wise, 2011). The numbers of individuals without health care insurance has dropped since the implementation of the Affordable Care Act in 2013, and the health care system is changing to meet the current demands of the health care environment.

Steep population growth and an aging population will increase the need for health care services in the future. The U.S. population age 65 years and over is predicted to reach 82 million in 2050, a 137% increase over 1999. Between 2011 and 2030, the number of older adults could rise from 40.4 million (13% of the population) to 70.3 million (20% of the population) as Baby Boomers begin turning 65 (U.S. Census Bureau, 2000; www.census.gov/).

The U.S. health care system is the most costly in the world, accounting for 17% of the gross domestic product with estimates that this percentage will grow to nearly 20% by 2020 (National Healthcare Expenditure Projections, 2010-2020. Centers for Medicare & Medicaid Services, Office of the Actuary).

As the amount of GDP devoted to health care rises, the amount of monies available for other services declines, and the more vulnerable to outside influences the health care industry becomes (Yoder-Wise, 2011).

Health care costs are a function of the prices of materials, personnel, and services as well as the use of health care services. Economic interests shape the evolution of technology and health care. The types of health care services delivered continue to be limited by multiple factors, most notably cost constraints and reimbursement (Wywialowski, 2004, p. 33). Financial resources have become the focus of much of the clinical decision making within health care and the success or failure of a health care organization depends on the extent that its structures have changed to the extent necessary to deliver high-quality care.

Uninsured Individuals

According to data released by the U.S. Census Bureau, about 48.6 million people were uninsured in 2012 (www.kaiserhealthnews.org/daily-reports/2012/september/13/census-numbers.aspx). One reason is that their place of employment does not provide health care coverage; another reason is that they cannot afford the high cost of health care. The uninsured and underinsured populations affect hospitals as well as the communities in which health care is sought.

This places an added burden on the facilities to provide "charity care." When a patient who is uninsured receives care, the cost of the care trickles down to other payers, to the government, or to private insurance companies. This added cost is then passed down to the customers and to taxpayers. In the end, the uninsured population affects everyone, not just the uninsured. Bankruptcy in the United States has had a direct correlation to medical expenses and depleted savings.

Medical Technology

The expansion of medical technology and specialty medicine also affects the economics of health care. For example, diagnostic and therapeutic techniques such as magnetic resonance imaging, organ transplantation, and electronic medical records enhance the capabilities of health care while increasing costs.

Health Care Payment Sources

There are rising expectations about the value of health care services in the United States. It is the cultural norm in America that we will all receive the highest quality of health care at all times. To this end, the United States spends a great deal of money on health care services. The people of the United States are covered by Medicare, Medicaid, insurance companies, and managed care companies, although 16.1% of the U.S. population is not insured, as of January 2014, down from 17.3% before the American Affordable Care Act's requirement

for Americans to have health insurance took effect on January 1, 2014 (www.gallup.com/poll/166982/uninsured-rate-shows-initial-decline-2014.aspx).

The United States continues to rely on a free-market approach to health care, with the private sector providing insurance coverage (through employers) and the federal sector providing for some individuals who are unable to pay.

Medical insurance began in 1847 with payments made to offset income loss that resulted after an accident. Blue Cross Blue Shield originated the reimbursement of general health costs in the 1930s. The private health care industry has changed dramatically with the advent of managed care. In the private sector, the following five types of organizations fund health care costs:

- Traditional insurance companies, which includes Blue Cross Blue Shield for profit commercial insurance companies.
- Preferred provider organizations (PPOs), which act as brokers between insurers and health care providers.
- Health maintenance organizations (HMOs), which are independent prepayment plans.
- Point of service (POS) plans, which combined features of classic HMOs with client choice characteristics of PPOs.
- Self-funded plans in which the employer takes on the role of insurer.

PRIVATE INSURANCE

The majority of insured Americans received health care insurance through their place of employment. The focus of such coverage has moved from the straight fee-for-services rendered model to managed health care. Managed health care organizations provide for both the delivery and the financing of health care for their members. The principal force behind the movement away from fee-for-service was the belief that health care costs can be controlled by "managing" the way in which health care is delivered and used.

The foundation of the managed care organization is the primary care provider (PCP). The PCP can be a physician or a nurse practitioner. This provider serves as the gatekeeper to coordinate and manage the patient's use of resources and referrals and protects the patient from unnecessary overtreatment.

HMOs deliver comprehensive health maintenance and treatment services for a group of enrolled

BOX 4-1   Types of Health Maintenance Organizations

Staff model	Self-contained organization Majority of physicians are on staff and paid by health maintenance organizations (HMOs)
Group model	Single, large multispecialty group that is the sole or major source of care for enrollees
Network model	Two or more group practices contract to care for the majority of patients enrolled in HMO plan
Independent practice association (IPA)	Contractual agreements with a wide variety of care providers Members have greater choice

individuals. Several models of the HMO structure have evolved. The group model is one in which practitioners employed by the insurer spend all their time caring for patients of that particular HMO. An example of this model is the Kaiser-Permanente health care system. Another model is Independent Practice Associations (IPAs) in which independent practitioners (not employed by the HMO) provide care for HMO members and are reimbursed for that care. Practitioners in an IPA contract may be restricted to caring only for members enrolled in that IPA, but some contracts allow practitioners to provide for nonmembers as well. Many IPAs have ceased existence because they were unable to remain financially viable. In a network model, HMOs contract with individual practitioners and practitioner groups for both primary and specialty services. In a capitation system, each organization is paid a fixed negotiated rate per member per month for each patient regardless of how often services are used. Box 4-1 provides various types of HMOs.

SOCIAL HEALTH MAINTENANCE ORGANIZATION

A social health maintenance organization (SHMO) is a demonstration model conducted under Medicare to determine the value and feasibility of combining health and medical services in one payment. Services provided include those of traditional Medicare and Medicaid as well as adult day care, homemaker services, respite care, hospice care, transportation, and chronic care in a nursing facility without prior hospitalization (Rundio & Wilson, 2013).

POINT OF SERVICE PLANS

POS plans evolved in response to patient concerns about their lack of choice in choosing providers in the previously mentioned plans. These plans allow members to pay additional fees to use providers outside of the individual network.

PPOs agree to deliver services to members for a fee-for-service negotiated price. Members must receive care exclusively from within the PPO or incur additional costs. To control costs, the health care agency must receive pre-authorization from the PPO for a member to be hospitalized, and second opinions are required before all major procedures.

U.S. GOVERNMENT

The federal government oversees plans that assist older adults, the disabled, and some uninsured individuals.

Medicaid

Medicaid is a joint federal and state assistance program designed to pay for medical long-term care assistance for individuals and families with low income and limited resources. Medicaid is available only to certain low-income individuals and families who fit into an eligibility group that is recognized by federal and state law. Medicaid sends payments directly to health care providers. Over time amendments to the Act have been made to include people with developmental disabilities and other low-income groups including the elderly, children, and pregnant women. Medicaid went into effect in 1966 and is known as Title XIX of the Social Security Administration. Each state sets its own guidelines regarding eligibility and services. These may include age, disabilities, income, financial resources (e.g., bank accounts, real property, or other items that can be sold for cash), and citizenship status; whether the individual is a U.S. citizen or a lawfully admitted immigrant. There are special rules for those who live in nursing homes and for children with disabilities living at home. Children may be eligible for coverage if they are U.S. citizens or lawfully admitted immigrants. Eligibility for children is based on the child's status, not the parents'.

State Children's Health Insurance Program (SCHIP)

Of all developed countries, the United States continues to have a high proportion of uninsured individuals. The lack of health insurance is greatest for blacks and Hispanics, younger Americans age 18 to 34, and men more than women. Most of the uninsured have at least one family member who is working full-time, but they do not obtain coverage because the cost of premiums is high. The State Children's Health Insurance Program (SCHIP) is a plan that targets uninsured children who are not eligible for Medicaid. These programs were implemented at the state level to provide insurance for all children.

Medicare

Medicare is the government's largest health care financing program. In 2012, Medicare paid out $77 billion to more than 880,000 medical providers (http://projects.wsj.com/medicarebilling/?mod=medicarein). Medicare is the name given to a health insurance program administered by the U.S. government, covering people who are either age 65 and over or who meet other special criteria. There have been numerous changes to the Medicare system since its introduction. It was expanded in 1972 to include people of any age with end-stage renal disease. Many of these changes have been attempts to deal with the high cost of Medicare expenditures.

Administration of Federal Insurers

The Centers for Medicare & Medicaid Services (CMS), a component of the Department of Health and Human Services (HHS), administers Medicare, Medicaid, and SCHIP. The Social Security Administration is responsible for determining Medicare eligibility and processing premium payments for the Medicare program.

Benefits

The "Original Medicare" program has two parts: Part A (Hospital Insurance) and Part B (Medical Insurance). Only a few special cases exist where prescription drugs are covered by Original Medicare, but as of January 2006, Medicare Part D provides more comprehensive drug coverage. Medicare Advantage plans are another way for beneficiaries to receive their Part A, B, and D benefits.

Part A: Hospital Insurance

Part A covers hospital stays. It also will pay for stays in a skilled nursing facility if certain criteria are met:

1. The hospital admission must be at least 3 days, 3 midnights, not counting the discharge date.
2. The nursing home admission must be for a condition diagnosed during the hospital stay or for the main cause of hospital stay. For instance, a hospital stay for broken hip and then nursing home stay for physical therapy would be covered.
3. If the patient is not receiving rehabilitation, but has some other ailment that requires skilled nursing supervision, then the nursing home condition would be covered.
4. The care being rendered by the nursing home must be skilled. Medicare Part A does not pay for custodial, nonskilled, or long-term care activities, including activities of daily living (ADLs) such as personal hygiene, cooking, cleaning, etc.

The maximum length of stay that Medicare Part A will cover in a skilled nursing facility per diagnosis is 100 days. The first 20 days would be paid for in full by Medicare with the remaining 80 days requiring a co-payment (as of 2014, $152.00 per day). Many insurance companies have a provision for skilled nursing care in the policies they sell.

If a beneficiary uses some portion of their Part A benefit and then goes at least 60 days without receiving skilled services, the 100-day clock is reset and they qualify for a new 100-day benefit period.

Part A is financed by taxes paid by employers and working individuals. Medicare Part A (Hospital Insurance) helps cover inpatient care in hospitals, including critical access hospitals and skilled nursing facilities (not custodial or long-term care). It also helps cover hospice care and some home health care. Beneficiaries must meet certain conditions to get these benefits.

Part B: Medical Insurance

Part B medical insurance helps pay for some services and products not covered by Part A, generally on an outpatient basis. Part B is optional and may be deferred if the beneficiary or their spouse is still actively working. There is a lifetime penalty (10% per year) imposed for not taking Part B if not actively working.

Part B coverage includes physician and nursing services, radiographs, laboratory and diagnostic tests, influenza and pneumonia vaccinations, blood transfusions, renal dialysis, outpatient hospital procedures, limited ambulance transportation, immunosuppressive drugs for organ transplant recipients, chemotherapy, hormonal treatments, such as Lupron, and other outpatient medical treatments administered in a physician's office. Medication administration is covered under Part B only if it is administered by the physician during an office visit.

Part B also helps with durable medical equipment (DME), including canes, walkers, wheelchairs, and mobility scooters for those with mobility impairments. Prosthetic devices, such as artificial limbs and breast prostheses following mastectomy, as well as one pair of eyeglasses following cataract surgery, and oxygen for home use, are also covered. As with all Medicare benefits, Part B coverage is subject to medical necessity. Complex rules are used to manage the benefit, and advisories are periodically issued that describe coverage criteria. On the national level, these advisories are issued by CMS and are known as national coverage determinations (NCDs). Local coverage determinations (LCDs) only apply within the multistate area managed by a specific regional Medicare Part B contractor, and local medical review policies (LMRPs) were superseded by LCDs in 2003.

Part B Medical Insurance is a supplementary voluntary medical insurance financed by general tax revenues and by required premium contributions. Medicare Part B (Medical Insurance) helps cover physicians' services and outpatient care. These may include:

- Outpatient surgery.
- Diagnostic tests.
- Radiology and pathology services.
- Emergency services.
- Outpatient rehabilitation services.
- Renal dialysis.
- Medical equipment and supplies.
- Preventive services (mammography).

Part C: Medicare Advantage Plans

With the passage of the Balanced Budget Act of 1997, Medicare beneficiaries were given the option to receive their Medicare benefits through private health insurance plans, instead of through the Original Medicare plan (Parts A and B). These programs were known as "Medicare+Choice" or "Part C" plans. Pursuant to the Medicare Prescription Drug, Improvement, and Modernization Act of 2003, the compensation and business practices changed for insurers that offer these plans, and

"Medicare+Choice" plans became known as "Medicare Advantage" (MA) plans. In addition to offering comparable coverage to Part A and Part B, Medicare Advantage plans may also offer Part D coverage.

Part D: Prescription Drug Plans

Medicare Part D went into effect on January 1, 2006. Anyone with Part A or B is eligible for Part D. It was made possible by the passage of the Medicare Prescription Drug, Improvement, and Modernization Act in 2003. To receive this benefit, a person with Medicare must enroll in a stand-alone prescription drug plan (PDP) or MA plan with prescription drug coverage (MA-PD). These plans are approved and regulated by the Medicare program, but are actually designed and administered by private health insurance companies. Unlike Original Medicare (Parts A and B), Part D coverage is not standardized. Plans choose which drugs (or even classes of drugs) they wish to cover and at what level (or tier) they wish to cover and are free to choose not to cover some drugs at what level (or tier) they wish to cover and are free to choose not to cover some drugs at all. The exception to this is drugs that Medicare specifically excludes from coverage, including, but not limited to, benzodiazepines, cough suppressants, and barbiturates. Plans that cover excluded drugs are not allowed to pass those costs on to Medicare, and plans are required to repay CMS if they are found to have billed Medicare in these cases.

Prescription Drug Coverage

Most people pay a monthly premium for this coverage. Since 2006, Medicare prescription drug coverage has been available to everyone with Medicare. Medicare prescription drug coverage is insurance.

Private companies provide the coverage. Beneficiaries choose the drug plan and pay a monthly premium. Like other insurance, if a beneficiary decides not to enroll in a drug plan when they are first eligible, they may pay a penalty if they choose to join later.

Hospice

In 1983, Medicare added hospice benefits for the last 6 months of life to cover services for the patient who is terminally ill. An organized program consists of services provided and coordinated by an interdisciplinary team at a frequency appropriate to meet the needs of individuals who are diagnosed with terminal illnesses and have a limited life span. Hospice workers view death as a normal part of the life cycle. Hospice emphasizes living the remaining months of life as fully and as comfortably as possible.

The hospice specializes in palliative management of pain and other physical symptoms, meeting the psychosocial and spiritual needs of the individual and the individual's family or other primary care person(s). The program also includes a continuum of interdisciplinary team services across all settings where hospice care is provided, the availability of 24-hour access to care, utilization of volunteers, and bereavement care to the survivors, as needed, for an appropriate period of time.

CHARITY CARE ASSISTANCE

As an example, the New Jersey Hospital Care Payment Assistance Program (Charity Care Assistance) provides free or reduced-charge care to patients who receive inpatient and outpatient services or care in an acute care hospital throughout New Jersey. Hospital assistance and reduced charge care are available only for necessary hospital care.

Hospital care payment assistance is available to New Jersey residents who:

- Have no health coverage or have coverage that pays only for part of the bill; and
- Are ineligible for any private or government-sponsored coverage; and
- Meet both the listed income and assets eligibility criteria.

The reimbursement for charity care varies from state to state, so be aware of the charity care regulations at your workplace. Income criteria that are related to the percentage of hospital charge to be paid by patients are listed in Box 4-2.

The federal government also operates health care networks, such as the Veterans Health Administration and the Indian Health Service.

VETERANS HEALTH ADMINISTRATION

The goal of the Veterans Health Administration (VHA) is to provide excellence in patient care, veterans' benefits, and customer satisfaction. The VHA strives for high-quality, prompt, and seamless service to U.S. veterans. Of the 25 million veterans currently alive, nearly three of every four served during a war or an official period of hostility. About a quarter of the nation's population (approximately 70 million people) are potentially

BOX 4-2 **Income Criteria for Health and Human Services Poverty Income Guidelines**

Income as a Percentage of HHS Poverty Income Guidelines	Percentage of Charge Paid by Patient
≤200%	0%
>200% but ≤225%	20%
>225% but ≤250%	40%
>250% but ≤275%	60%
>275% but ≤300%	80%
>300%	100%

From *New Jersey Hospital care payment assistance fact sheet.* (January 2014). www.state.nj.us/health/charitycare/documents/charitycare_factsheet_en.pdf.

eligible for VA benefits and services because they are veterans or family members or survivors of veterans.

INDIAN HEALTH SERVICE

The Indian Health Service (IHS), an agency within the Department of Health and Human Services, is responsible for providing federal health services to American Indians and Alaska Natives. The IHS is the principal federal health care provider and health advocate for Indian people, and its goal is to raise their health status to the highest possible level. The IHS provides a comprehensive health service delivery system for American Indians and Alaska Natives who are members of 566 federally recognized tribes across the U.S.

TYPES OF HEALTH CARE SERVICES

With the continuing focus on the cost effectiveness of delivery of care, health care has moved from the acute care hospital to a full continuum of services within the community and the hospital. Twenty years ago, it was not uncommon for a community hospital to attempt to provide all services for a majority of patients. Length of stays (LOS) were long and expensive. As the cost improvement model advanced, health care services have been divided into primary, secondary, and tertiary centers of care.

Health promotion and disease prevention are a focus of many HMOs. Practitioners' offices provide many health maintenance activities, as do community centers for education and health assessment.

BOX 4-3	Types of Health Care Services	
Type of Care	**Description**	**Examples**
Primary	Decreases risk for disease	Immunizations
	Health maintenance	Nutrition counseling
Secondary	Disease prevention through early intervention	Surgery
Tertiary	Long-term care	Durable medical equipment
		Education

There are three types of health care services: primary, secondary, and tertiary care (Box 4-3). Primary care is health maintenance that decreases the risk for disease; secondary care encourages disease prevention through early intervention; and tertiary care is long-term care.

Many diagnostic services, such as colonoscopies, are now being provided in ambulatory care settings and physicians' offices. Many surgical procedures are also now being provided in ambulatory care settings. Secondary and tertiary care is provided in a number of settings across the health care continuum. Health care is provided by the types of agencies and facilities listed in Box 4-4.

It is important for you as a nurse to realize that different levels of care are paid for at differing rates by both private and federal insurers. This differentiation in financial reimbursement for these services results in "type-specific" staffing, standards of care, and services rendered. Each type of service also has to meet differing accreditation requirements (see Chapter 5).

FOR-PROFIT AND NOT-FOR-PROFIT HEALTH CARE AGENCIES

Although the majority of the health care facilities in the United States function as not-for-profit organizations, there is a movement toward hospitals becoming for-profit organizations. An example of a for-profit entity would be a physician opening their own same-day surgery center. There are examples of hospitals that have become for-profit institutions where the profit is funneled back to either the hospital or an overseeing corporation.

With health care costs continuing to escalate, it will be important for you as a nurse to be aware of the economic forces that affect your day-to-day nursing care.

BUDGETING PROCESS

Budget review and management represent one of the most important responsibilities of the nurse manager in this era of escalating health care costs and decreasing reimbursements. The economic stability of an organization depends on the management of the resources that are required to deliver care in a cost-effective and safe manner. The earlier content of this chapter provided a review of the essentials of health care reimbursement.

Health care institutions are businesses, and one of the largest costs is the actual delivery of patient care. The resources required to deliver that patient care are costly and most often managed at the point of service (the unit). Nurses need to understand how to manage the cost of patient care as it relates to their clinical practice as well as to the workings of their particular unit. Also, accrediting agencies require collaborative input from staff in the development of annual budgets (The Joint Commission, 2014).

In most institutions, there is a well-defined process for the development, implementation, and evaluation of the budget. The budgeting process is a part of the overall strategic planning process (see Chapter 3). The organizational budget cascades down to individual departments and units. Budgets are usually developed annually for a 12-month period. The budget cycle is based on the organization's definition of the fiscal year (calendar [January 1–December 31] or fiscal [July 1–June 30]).

There are two major types of budgeting processes: zero-based budgeting and incremental budgeting. Zero-based budgeting requires the entire budget to be re-created annually starting from zero. This type of budgeting allows for the consideration of alternatives in the delivery of the service. All portions of the zero-based budget need to be justified annually. This type of budgeting also demands the proactive evaluation of the need for the services. Incremental budgeting is the more traditional approach, building on the previous year's budget. If a 10% increase in funds is available, the budget may be increased by 10%. This is an easier process, but at times it allows budgets to become bloated with minimal justification of the service or at times it does not reflect the actual changes that may be anticipated for the unit.

BOX 4-4   Agencies and Facilities That Provide Health Care

Health Care Facility	Examples	Health Care Facility	Examples
Acute care	Hospitalization for episode of illness *Example: patient suffering an acute myocardial infarction*	Rehabilitation	Post-injury focus on restoration of function *Example: patient with spinal cord injury re-learning activities of daily living*
Subacute care	Continued hospitalization after initial acute stage has passed *Example: patient requiring long-term ventilatory assistance*	Home health care	Post-hospitalization support within the home *Example: post congestive heart failure patient requiring medication and dietary follow-up*
Long-term care	Continued hospitalization after stabilization of chronic long-term condition *Example: patient in end-stage Alzheimer disease*	Hospice services • Inpatient • Outpatient	Care of the dying patient and family *Example: in-home care for dying patient* *Example: in-home care for dying patient*
Residential care	Living facilities for patients in need of basic support *Example: group home for individual with mental retardation*	Health care centers	Full range of preventative health care services *Example: federally qualified health care center*
Assisted living	Living facilities with an option of basic support *Example: 85-year-old independent patient with occasional falls*	Local health departments	Preventative health services in support of *Healthy People 2010* *Examples: blood pressure screenings, immunizations*
Ambulatory care	Diagnostic testing screenings Low-acuity surgery *Example: same-day operations*	Urgent care centers	Treatment of non-urgent injuries *Examples: physical examinations and first aid*

The budgeting process can be divided into phases (Finkler, Kovner, & Jones, 2007):

- Information gathering and planning.
- Development of organizational and unit budgets.
- Development of cash budgets, negotiation, and revision.
- Evaluation.

Information Gathering and Planning

In the information gathering and planning phase, the nurse manager is provided with data necessary to the development of the budget. An environmental assessment is done. This assessment provides the organization and the nurse manager with information about the changing needs of the community, changing professional requirements, economic changes that will affect the unit's function, community demographics, stakeholder needs and requirements, regulatory changes, and other items. This assessment provides the context of the needs that the unit budgets for during the next fiscal year. This environmental assessment provides the materials for the reassessment of the organization's mission, goals, and priorities. As organizational priorities are set, financial objectives are created, allocating resources to all units.

Development of Organizational and Unit Budgets

Organizational and unit budgets are then created to match the financial objectives of the organization. It is important that both the financial and overall objectives of the particular unit are in concert with the organization-wide objectives and goals. The basic assumptions of the organization need to be part of the development of both organizational and unit objectives. Such assumptions may be the negotiated union contract raise for all employees, the cost of a new electronic record system, or similar items. Such assumptions are an important part of the development of the unit budget.

Development of Cash Budgets, Negotiation, and Revision

The cash budget is developed after the operating and capital budgets of the unit or department are developed. It is at this stage that the unit manager's negotiating and revising skills come into play. This cash budget is usually prepared by the chief financial officer. It is the plan for the actual anticipated cash receipts and disbursements of the organization; the cash flow. An organization must have sufficient cash to meet its monthly obligations. This reflects the *cash on hand*. Ideally, the nurse manager needs to be able to predict when budgeted items will be needed. Unexpected expenditures do occur and may put a strain on a cash-poor system.

Evaluation

Evaluation of the budget occurs at both the organizational and unit levels. Many organizations have created dashboards that allow for monitoring of progress in meeting department goals. These dashboards provide a quick visual display of the unit's performance. An example of an organization-wide financial dashboard is shown in Figure 4-1. Evaluation of the budget performance is usually obtained through a process known as variance analysis. A variance is the difference between planned and actual costs. A positive variance (favorable) may be seen when the budgeted amount was greater than that which was actually spent. A negative variance may be seen if the budgeted amount was less than the actual spending. Variance analysis is a complex process in which the unit environment is fully investigated. Variances may be characterized in four ways. A volume variance in a hospital setting may occur in response to fluctuating in-patient days. An efficiency variance may be expressed in changes from the anticipated hours per patient day (HPPD). Rate variances reflect the difference between the budgeted hourly rate of pay and the actual rate paid. A non-salary expenditure variance may be caused by changes in patient mix, supply quantities and costs, and price paid. A negative variance may be seen in the number of staff required during a 2-week period. However, on further investigation, it may be determined that the patient acuity was higher than anticipated, and expenses were increased in response to this increased acuity. It is the role of the nurse manager to be aware of the variances related to the unit and the reasons for the alteration in expected performance. These variance data are often used in the preparation of the next year's budget. Examples of such variable costs seen in unit budgets are:

- Increased overtime related to greater-than-anticipated use of sick time.
- Increased use of part-time personnel related to an unanticipated increase in patient acuity.
- Increased expense for minor equipment because of an electrical malfunction that destroyed equipment.
- Increased expenses caused by resignation of staff and orientation of replacement staff.

Many health care organizations have flexible budgets that automatically adjust to environmental changes. A goal of most organizations is to proactively anticipate challenges through the collection of the information in an environmental assessment. An example of a proactive budget process would be the budgeting of increased staff during the influenza season.

Most organizations provide the nurse manager with fiscal reports on a routine basis (weekly, monthly, or quarterly depending on the organization). This allows each cost center manager to carefully monitor the financial activity of the unit. The budget process is a continually evolving work requiring evaluation and continual improvement.

TYPES OF BUDGETS

The overall budget is composed of a number of smaller budgets that represent specific areas of concern in the financial objective setting of an organization. The operating (expense) budget includes (1) the personnel budget, (2) costs other than for personnel, and (3) the revenue budget. Not all units prepare a revenue budget; that may be done by the finance department.

The personnel budget requires that the nurse manager forecast the anticipated workload for the year. This is done based on information gathered from the environmental assessment, review of the previous workload, and identification of the services to be provided. The calculation of staff needs is a complex procedure. First, the average daily census and occupancy rate are calculated. The total required patient-care hours are calculated (Figure 4-2). Then, the number of full-time equivalents (FTEs) required to provide care is calculated based on the expected number of hours. An FTE is calculated as 2080 hours of work per year. Then, the number of full-time employees, part-time employees, and shifts needs to be calculated. Adjustments need to be made for employee

HELPING HANDS HOSPITAL DASHBOARD RESULTS

	Q1	Q2	Q3	Annual Goal	Top 10%
QUALITY					
1. Overall patient satisfaction	88%	90%	93%	92%	95%
CORE MEASURES					
2. Acute Myocardial Infarction					
A. AMI Beta Blocker on discharge	90%	95%	98%	100%	100%
B. Smoking Cessation Advice/Counseling	98%	98%	100%	100%	100%
C. Heart Attack patients given aspirin on arrival	99%	98%	97%	100%	100%
D. Heart Attack patients given aspirin on discharge	100%	100%	100%	100%	100%
E. Heart Attack patients given thrombolytic medication within 30 min of arrival	100%	99%	100%	99%	100%
3. Surgical Care Improvement Project (SCIP)					
A. Surgery patients who received preventative antibiotic 1 hour before incision	94%	92%	91%	96%	98%
B. Surgery patients whose preventative antibiotic are appropriately selected	98%	92%	94%	96%	96%
FINANCIAL					
Days Cash on Hand	150	175	170	180	184
Inpatient net receivables (000s)	69,500	65,000	68,000	69,000 (per Qtr)	73,000 (per Qtr)
Average L.O.S.	4.1	3.9	4.3	3.9	3.85
Inpatient gross charges (000s)	70,000	68,000	69,500	70,050 (per Qtr)	75,000 (per Qtr)
Market Share	42%	48%	47%	49%	56%
PEOPLE					
Nursing Full-Time Equivalents	400	385	396	400	400
Employee satisfaction (overall)	79%	82%	81%	88%	91%
Injury/Illness Last Time per 100 employees	5%	6%	4%	4%	2%

Interpretation   **Red** – below goal   **Orange** – within 2% of goal   **Green** – at goal   **Blue** – top 10% at goal

FIGURE 4-1 An example of an organization-wide financial dashboard. Indiana Rural Health Association. (2008). *Inpatient scorecards*. www.indianaruralhealth.org/Sample%20Dashboard%20_(3_).pdf.

benefits and nonproductive time (vacation, orientation, education, sick time, etc.) (Figure 4-3).

The next step is to prepare a daily staffing plan. This plan includes the staff mix of individuals required to provide the patient care (registered nurses, licensed practical nurses, unit clerks, patient care associates, etc.). Remember that the skill mix of staff and the staffing requirements are regulated. It is important that the nurse manager maintain compliance with all regulatory boards while determining the budget. Once the nurse manager has decided on the positions required to deliver care, the other labor costs can be included in the personnel budget. These other labor costs include benefits, shift differential, overtime, raises, premium pay, and so forth. Benefits are often calculated at close to an additional 40% to 50% of an individual's pay.

For costs other than personnel costs, the nurse manager will have to calculate supply and expense costs, such as supplies, education, travel to conferences, telephone, electricity, and minor equipment. Some health care

WORKLOAD CALCULATION (TOTAL REQUIRED PATIENT-CARE HOURS)				
Patient Acuity Level*	Hours of Care Per Patient Day (HPPD)†	× Patient Days‡	=	Workload§
1	3.0	900		2,700
2	5.2	3,100		16,120
3	8.8	4,000		35,200
4	13.0	1,600		20,800
5	19.0	400		7,600
Total		10,000		82,420

*1, Low; 5, high.
†HPPD is the number of hours of care on average for a given acuity level.
‡1 patient per 1 day = 1 patient day.
§Total number of hours of care needed based on acuity levels and numbers of patient days.

FIGURE 4-2 Calculation of patient-care hours.

Productive Hours Calculation

Method 1:   Add all nonproductive hours/FTE and subtract from paid hours/FTE
  Example: Vacation   15 days
         Holiday   7 days
         Average sick time 4 days
         TOTAL   26 days

   26 × 8* hours = 208 nonproductive hours/FTE
   2080 – 208 = 1872 productive hours/FTE

Method 2:   Multiply paid hours/FTE by percentage of productive hours/FTE
  Example: Productive hours = 90%/FTE
         (1872 productive hours of total 2080 = 90%)
         2080 × 0.90 = 1872 productive hours/FTE

Total FTE Calculation

Required Patient-Care Hours ÷ Productive Hours Per FTE = Total FTEs Needed

82,420   ÷ 1872   = 44 FTEs

*Based on an 8-hour shift pattern.

FIGURE 4-3 Productivity calculation.

institutions also require support services (indirect costs) to be included in the budget; an example would be information technology services provided by an in-house department to a unit. These are all examples of indirect costs.

The nurse manager is dealing with only minor equipment purchases in this budget. For major items there is a capital expenditure budget. A capital expenditure must have a life span of at least 1 year, and there is usually a dollar limit for determining if an equipment request is capital or minor. A capital expenditure usually costs more than $500 or $1000 (depending on the institution) and includes equipment and renovation expenses needed to meet long-term goals. Organizations often perform long-term planning with capital expenditures. In this manner, the organization determines priorities for such expenditures.

Each nursing unit is usually called a cost center. The cost center is the organizational unit for which costs can be identified and managed. Although in most large health care organizations the revenue budget is prepared by the chief financial officer, the nurse manager must be aware of the revenue anticipated by the unit. Nurses working in smaller outpatient centers may be responsible for the development of the revenue budget. The calculation of the revenue budget requires knowledge of the anticipated reimbursement expected for patient care and the time of the expected reimbursement.

The majority of health care institutions orient the nurse manager to the financial aspects of the position. This also includes an orientation to the budget process of the institution and the role of the nurse manager in this process. Some health care agencies have changed the organizational structure of the unit management to include a clinical nurse manager and a business manager. The business manager may not be a nurse, but they work with the unit director to maintain financial efficiency in operations.

STAFF NURSE ROLE IN BUDGET PROCESS

Although the nurse manager or director oversees the budget, the staff nurse also has a role in the financial management of the unit. The clinical nurse, through the organization's shared governance process, participates in the budget process. In Magnet institutions, the

TABLE 4-1   Strategies for Cost-Conscious Nursing Practice
1. Understanding what is required to remain financially sound
2. Knowing costs and reimbursement practices
3. Capturing all possible charges in a timely manner
4. Using time efficiently and effectively
5. Discussing the costs of care with the patient
6. Meeting patient rather than provider needs
7. Evaluating cost effectiveness of new technologies and equipment
8. Predicting and using nursing resources efficiently
9. Using research to evaluate standard nursing practice
10. Consistently evaluating practice based on evidence

Adapted from Yoder-Wise (2011, p. 239).

clinical nurse is expected to advocate for resources that result in actual allocation of such resources to support a nursing unit goal (American Nurses Credentialing Center, Magnet, 2013). The staff nurse needs to be aware of the financial costs and reimbursement of the care delivered on the unit. Table 4-1 delineates strategies for cost-conscious nursing practice.

SUMMARY

Health care has undergone many changes in the past 10 years. The rapid pace of change shows no signs of abating, and it is important for nurses to be aware of the rules and regulations of payment, reimbursement, and the various types of health care systems and care available to patients and their families. The nurse usually is the advocate for the care that the patient receives and works with the case manager to determine the level of services necessary for the patient. Sadly, the reimbursement method often dictates much of the care available to the patient, so it is

imperative for nurses to be aware of all of the ramifications of the payers, so that appropriate care can be planned and implemented for the duration of the patient's need.

The financial management of a clinical unit, as well as the entire health care institution, is the responsibility of the nurse leaders as well as clinical nurses. The careful balance of delivery of quality health care and financial stewardship is a delicate balance that nurse leaders juggle daily. This is a goal of the "Triple Aim." It is a learning system that all nurses work with on a daily basis.

CLINICAL CORNER

Changing Reimbursements for Accountable Care Organization—Nursing Perspective

The structure of the Accountable Care Act (ACA) is changing reimbursements for **Accountable Care Organizations** (ACOs) through a system of quality and financial incentives to encourage improvement of care while lowering cost to consumers and payers. These reimbursement modifications significantly increase demands on the role of nursing as we are in the forefront to improve overall care for health care consumers in the hospital and the community. Nursing's potential to improve and eliminate complications along with lowering length of stay (LOS) directly influences the ACO's ability to receive enhanced reimbursement. By demonstrating our value to improve patient outcomes, nursing is in an excellent position to become leaders in the ACO's ability to provide services to patients and enable it to remain a viable organization while thriving in today's ever changing health care environment.

The most significant changes that effect reductions in reimbursement are based on preventing hospital acquired infections, other quality outcomes and **HCAHPS (Hospital Consumer Assessment of Healthcare Providers and Systems)**. Preventing hospital-acquired infections gives the role of the nurse greater importance. Hospital quality performance is coupled to its financial reimbursement; therefore nursing's role must be to improve the overall care that we give to our patients by using best practices and research to demonstrate our ability to make comprehensive contributions to the financial **bottom line** of the ACO.

Advanced nursing research has brought more scientific models of nursing care to our arsenal of health care delivery and practice. With each intellectual investigation, evaluation, and improvement, we expand our body of knowledge while building new foundations of our professional nursing practice. In these pursuits, not only are we improving the vocation of nursing, but we are fulfilling nursing's responsibility to humanity within the art and science of nursing: caring, compassion, and knowledge.

Infections acquired by patients while in the hospital, such as catheter-associated urinary tract infections (CAUTIs) and central line-associated bloodstream infections (CLABSIs), take a significant toll on the health of a patient who is already dealing with a comprising illness. These infections place the ACO at substantial risk of lost revenue in the form of extra costs to care for the patient, for which hospitals do not receive reimbursement. A report from the Centers for Disease Control and Prevention stated that an estimated cost for each CLABSI is around $17,000 per case.[1]

Reducing clinical variation by all clinicians through use of established interventions and best practices enhances the overall quality outcome for the patient and brings other cost savings. Nurses can help lead their reluctant colleagues into improvement in practices by means of protocols, pathways, and care plans, which nursing has used for many years now. Standardization in practices to eliminate variability of the care that each patient receives will represent a cost saving for the patient and the ACO.

Along with educating nursing staff and care givers in best practices to improve the nursing process and skill level, we have an obligation to improve accurate documentation for the electronic health record (EHR). The EHR has become an even more important tool for the documentation of care provided to the patient. Health care medical records continue to evolve; nevertheless, the massive amount of money to build EHR systems and the inconsistency of different IT systems throughout the country demonstrate the vulnerability of documentation. There is no prefect EHR technology system, at least not yet.

Certainly, one can argue the EHR gives the interdisciplinary team, the nurse and other care partners, the ability to communicate better and have more timely information that can lead to more appropriate changes in the care for each patient. But at what cost? Many clinicians feel they cannot spend as much time interacting with their patient because of the need to spend so much time at the computer. Point of care documentation is here to stay; therefore, there needs to be more standardization of EHRs to optimize the documentation process.

It is no longer acceptable to not perform a thorough head-to-toe assessment of the patient at admission to look for and document any existing conditions, such as decubitus ulcers and urinary tract infections and to evaluate the patient's fall rate score. Any preventable condition discovered after entry into the hospital that was not documented at the time of admission will lead the organization to be charged with a hospital-acquired adverse event. The inevitable outcome of the failure to complete documentation is loss of reimbursement.

The same EHR documentation requirement applies to the education of the patient and their family and/or partner, which should start at time of admission. Discharge instructions, which have been viewed in the past by nurses as an onerous chore to be rushed through as quickly as possible to get the patient out the door, become an even more important method to prevent readmission. We cannot think only of what happens inside the walls of our organization, we must now think "outside the walls." (This is a term I created several years ago. My intent was

Continued

CLINICAL CORNER—cont'd

to demonstrate to clinicians the necessity of realizing patient outcomes and readmissions have a severe reimbursement impact on the ACO. Clinicians must partner with all levels of care providers for continuity of care.)

ACOs are penalized with lost reimbursement for readmissions within 30 days after hospital discharge. If nurses are thinking outside the walls of the hospital, then patients and their care givers should receive comprehensive aftercare education to prevent hospital readmission and to assist the patient to return to optimal health. Several methods can be used to follow up with the patient after discharge, for instance by the use of discharge phone calls, home visits from a nurse, and on-line communication (chat) with a nurse. Furthermore, effective communication after discharge should include the next level of care where the patient will be living; this must include nursing homes and assisted living situations. All strata of patient care have a responsibility for linkage of care.

Link together all the documentation nurses need to do along with all the quality nursing indicators now required, and it is a wonder nurses have any time to provide actual nursing care for a patient. Currently, with the loss of reimbursement, ACOs are in the unenviable positions of having to reduce their most valuable assets: employees. Nurses are not immune to having their positions eliminated, and they are currently being required to work harder with reduced amounts of resources. With all the requirements for added value, HCAHPS, patient safety, quality, and prevention measures, one can safely justify that more and better-educated nurses are needed at the bedside—not fewer. ACOs should invest in continuous education for nurses and other hands-on care givers.

Nursing leaders have an obligation to team up with their colleagues, nurse managers, and nursing staff to combine our talents and other resources to articulate the importance of additional nurses at the bedside, which adds value to the ACO. If the ACO will fully acknowledge that nurses have the ability to contribute by developing and implementing plans, and reinventing how care is delivered to the patient on multiple levels, then nurses will significantly demonstrate that increasing nursing staff will help the ACO reach expected quality and financial performance goals.

Shirley Bennett Thompson, RN, BSN,
BSBA, MSHA, FACHE
Bennett Thompson LLC, February 01, 2015

[1]Centers for Disease Control and Prevention (CDC), Morbidity and Mortality Weekly Report (MMWR), Vital Signs: Central Line-Associated Blood Stream Infections — United States, 2001, 2008, and 2009. March 2011. www.cdc.gov/mmwr/pdf/wk/mm60e0301.pdf.

EVIDENCE BASED PRACTICE

Douglas, K. (2010). Taking action to close the nursing-finance gap: Learning from success. Staffing unleashed. *Nursing Economics*, 28(4):270–272.

Executive Summary
- Nurse leaders control the largest part of a hospital labor budget, in some cases the largest part of the overall budget.
- The effectiveness of overseeing this responsibility can mean the difference between an organization's financial stability and financial turmoil.
- The nursing department at Northwestern Memorial Hospital took ownership of its financial performance.
- Over the past 2 years their financial performance saved $4.9 million in productivity while reducing nurse turnover costs by $7.6 million.
- Valuable lessons from their experience are offered for improving health care's financial and operational outlook.
  Thoughts on Reasons for the Gap Between Nursing and Finance
- The role of the nurse leader has evolved to require greater business and financial skills.

- Nursing's ownership, or lack thereof, of financial performance.
- How well, or not, our education systems prepare nurses to become part of leadership in business; the business of health care.
- How we orient and educate nurses as they are promoted into positions with greater business responsibilities.
- The conflict some nurses feel between being a care giver and patient advocate with embracing the business and financial side of care delivery.
- Nurses not understanding the language of finance.
- Finance not understanding the role and realities of nursing.
- Retrospective reporting of business analytics, decreasing value, and relevance.
- Surely there are more . . .

The author states that hospitals should invest more in financial education for nurses as they are promoted into positions requiring financial oversight. There also should be a better relationship between nursing and finance.

NCLEX® EXAMINATION QUESTIONS

1. An example of an indirect cost is:
   A. Cost center
   B. Information technology
   C. Nursing staff
   D. Delivery of care

2. The difference between actual budget and actual spending is referred to as:
   A. Budget variance
   B. Fixed cost
   C. Cash on hand
   D. Revenues

3. _____deliver comprehensive health maintenance and treatment services for a group of enrolled individuals.
   A. Health maintenance organizations (HMOs)
   B. Preferred provider organizations (PPOs)
   C. Independent Practice Associations (IPAs)
   D. Primary Care Providers (PCPs)

4. An example of an indirect cost would be:
   1. Housekeeping staff
   2. Ink for a printer on the unit
   3. Uniform allowance for licensed practical nurses
   4. Registered nurse salary

5. An example of a direct cost is:
   A. Telephone costs for the entire facility
   B. Copy paper for a specific unit
   C. Room use for a hospital event
   D. Housekeeping staff

6. The operating expense budget does not include:
   A. The personnel budget
   B. The costs other than personnel
   C. The revenue budget
   D. Off-site registered nurse continuing education seminars

7. _____originated the reimbursement of general health costs in the 1930s.
   A. Blue Cross Blue Shield
   B. United Health Care
   C. Medicare
   D. Medicaid

8. According to the United States Census Bureau, there were _____people uninsured in 2012.
   A. 30.2 million
   B. 48.6 million
   C. 50.2 million
   D. 52.2 million

9. Which country spends more on health care per capita than any other industrialized Western nation?
   A. United States
   B. United Kingdom
   C. China
   D. Canada

10. In 2012, the Institute for Healthcare Improvement described an approach to optimizing health system performance. It is their belief that new designs must be developed to simultaneously pursue three dimensions called the "Triple Aim." This includes:
    A. Improving the patient experience of care, improving the economy, and reducing the per capita cost of health care
    B. Improving the patient experience of care, improving the health of populations, and reducing the per capita cost of health care
    C. Improving the patient experience of care, improving the health of populations, and reducing the per diem cost of health care
    D. Improving the patient experience of care, improving the health of certain groups, and reducing the per capita cost of health care

Answers: 1. A   2. A   3. A   4. A   5. B   6. D   7. A   8. B   9. A   10. B

REFERENCES

American Nurses Credentialing Center. (2013). *2014 Magnet application manual.* Silver Spring, MD: Author.

Grohar-Murray, M. E., & DiCroce, H. R. (2011). *Leadership and management in nursing* (3rd ed.). Upper Saddle River, NJ: Prentice Hall.

Institute for Healthcare Improvement. (2014). Triple aim initiatives, www.ihi.org/engage/initiatives/TripleAim/Pages/default.aspx.

Kelly-Heidenthal, P. (2003). *Nursing leadership and management.* Clifton Park, NY: Delmar Thompson Learning.

National Healthcare Expenditure Projections, 2010-2020. Centers for Medicare & Medicaid Services, Office of the Actuary.

New Jersey Hospital Care Payment Assistance Program (Charity Care Assistance). (2013). www.nj.gov/health/cc/documents/ccfactsh.pdf.

Rundio, A., & Wilson, V. (2013). *Nurse executive: Review and resource manual.* Silver Spring, MD: ANCC.

Stiefel, M., & Nolan, K. (2012). *A guide to measuring the triple aim: Population health, experience of care, and per capita cost.* IHI Innovation Series white paper. Cambridge, MA: Institute for Healthcare Improvement. www.IHI.org.

The Joint Commission. (2014). *Comprehensive accreditation manual — Hospitals.* Oak Book, IL: Author.

U.S. Census Bureau (2000). U.S. Census Data. www.census.gov.

U.S. Census Bureau. (2010). U.S. Census Data. www.census.gov.

Veterans Health Administration. (2008). www.va.gov/about_va.

Veterans Health Administration. (2008). *Healthcare.* www1.va.gov/health/AboutVHA.asp.

Wall Street Journal. (2014). *Medicare billing.* http://projects.wsj.com/medicarebilling/?mod=medicarein. http://www.medicare.gov/coverage/skilled-nursing-facility-care.html. http://www.ihs.gov/aboutihs/overview/.

Wywialowski, E. F. (2004). *Managing client care* (3rd ed.). St. Louis: Mosby.

Yoder-Wise, P. S. (2006). *Beyond leading and managing nursing administration for the future.* St. Louis: Mosby.

Yoder-Wise, P. S. (2011). *Leading and managing in nursing* (4th ed.). St. Louis: Mosby.

5

Health Care Regulatory and Certifying Agencies

OBJECTIVES

- Identify health care regulatory and certifying agencies.
- Explain the nurse's role in relation to hospital surveys.
- Differentiate among The Joint Commission, Det Norske Veritas, and Healthcare Facilities Accreditation.
- Define accreditation.

- Discuss strategies for implementation of proper procedures for an upcoming hospital survey.
- Discuss strategies for implementation of proper procedures using appropriate regulatory and certifying agency guidelines.
- Differentiate between accreditation and awards for performance.
- Discuss the nurse's role in accreditation and awards for excellence.

OUTLINE

KEY TERMS

accreditation a self-assessment and external peer assessment process used by health care organizations to accurately assess their level of performance in relation to established standards and to implement ways to continually improve

American Osteopathic Association (AOA) Healthcare Facilities Accreditation Program osteopathic accreditation program that ensures health care facilities meet standards of care while also meeting the Medicare conditions of participation

Centers for Disease Control and Prevention (CDC) agency charged with the promotion of health and quality of life by preventing and controlling disease, injury, and disability; has created multiple infection control standards that are now part of standard Joint Commission accreditation

compliance to act in accordance with stated requirements, such as standards. Levels of compliance include noncompliance, partial compliance, and substantial compliance

Det Norske Veritas a healthcare accreditation agency that integrates the International Organization for Standardization's ISO 9001 quality management system with the Medicare conditions of participation

The Joint Commission (TJC) accreditation organization that strives to continuously improve the safety and quality of care provided to the public through the provision of health care accreditation and related services that support performance improvement in health care organizations

National Institute for Occupational Safety and Health (NIOSH) federal agency responsible for conducting research and making recommendations for the prevention of work-related injury and illness. NIOSH is part of the CDC within the U.S. Department of Health and Human Services

Occupational Safety and Health Administration (OSHA) U.S. Department of Labor agency that ensures the safety and health of America's workers by setting and enforcing standards; providing training, outreach, and education; establishing partnerships; and encouraging continual improvement in workplace safety and health

State departments of health departments that foster accessible and high-quality health and senior services to help all people to achieve optimal health, dignity, and independence in an attempt to prevent disease, promote and protect well-being at all life stages, and encourage informed choices that enrich the quality of life for individuals and communities

U.S. Department of Health and Human Services (USDHHS) U.S. government's principal agency for protecting the health of all Americans and providing essential human services, especially for those who are least able to help themselves

REGULATORY AGENCIES

Health care organizations work with myriad accrediting and regulatory agencies so that optimum standards of care and delivery of care can be met. Regulatory agencies are charged by federal and state governments to.

- Set standards for the operation of health care organizations;
- Ensure compliance with federal and state regulations developed by government administrative agencies; and
- Investigate and make judgments regarding complaints brought by consumers of the services and the public.

Licensing of health care agencies to maintain practice occurs through state departments of health. State departments of health usually oversee outcomes of care within health care facilities, investigate consumer complaints, and deal with issues of importance to the public health. These agencies monitor basic compliance with the specific health care regulations of that state. Compliance with regulatory standards on both national and state levels is mandatory, and fines can be leveled against organizations for noncompliance.

Accreditation agencies evaluate health care organizations against a set of standards that have been validated against best practice. Accreditation is voluntary, but mandatory for continued Centers for Medicare & Medicaid Services (CMS) reimbursement. The Medicare conditions of participation require that hospitals be accredited by an organization with "deeming authority." "Deeming authority" is authority granted by CMS to accrediting organizations to determine, on CMS's behalf, whether an organization evaluated by the accreditor is in compliance with corresponding Medicare regulations.

ACCREDITATION

Accreditation agencies were initially founded to set a minimum of standard of care. As they have matured, their mission has expanded to "continuously improve health care for the public, in collaboration with other stakeholders, by evaluating health care organizations and inspiring them to excel in providing safe and effective care of the highest quality and value" (The Joint Commission, 2014). They have moved from compliance agencies to agencies that hope to drive improvement and quality of care.

Accrediting agencies move beyond basic compliance and look to the continual improvement of operational systems critical to patient care and safety. Although accreditation is listed as a voluntary process, federal reimbursement of health care is dependent on accreditation. The three major health care organization accrediting agencies are The Joint Commission, Det Norske Veritas, and the American Osteopathic Association Healthcare Facilities Accreditation Program.

THE JOINT COMMISSION

The mission of The Joint Commission (previously known as the Joint Commission on Accreditation of Healthcare Organizations) is to continuously improve the safety and quality of care provided to the public through the provision of health care accreditation and related services that support performance improvement in health care organizations. The Joint Commission evaluates and accredits more than 25,000 health care organizations and programs in the United States. An independent, not-for-profit organization, The Joint Commission is the country's predominant standards-setting and accrediting body in health care. Since 1951, The Joint Commission has maintained state-of-the-art standards that focus on improving the quality and safety of care provided by health care organizations. The Joint Commission's comprehensive accreditation process evaluates an organization's compliance with these standards and other accreditation requirements.

The Joint Commission's evaluation and accreditation services are provided for the following types of organizations:

- General, psychiatric, children's, and rehabilitation hospitals.
- Critical access hospitals.
- Health care networks, including managed care plans, preferred provider organizations, integrated delivery networks, and managed behavioral health care organizations.
- Home care organizations, including those that provide home health services, personal care and support services, home infusion and other pharmacy services, durable medical equipment services, and hospice services.
- Nursing homes and other long-term care facilities, including subacute care programs, dementia special care programs, and long-term care pharmacies.
- Assisted living facilities that provide or coordinate personal services, 24-hour supervision and assistance (scheduled and unscheduled), activities, and health-related services.

- Behavioral health care organizations, including those that provide mental health and addiction services, and services to persons with developmental disabilities of various ages, in various organized service settings.
- Ambulatory care providers, such as outpatient surgery facilities, rehabilitation centers, infusion centers, group practices, and office-based surgery.
- Clinical laboratories, including independent or freestanding laboratories, blood transfusion and donor centers, and public health laboratories.

Accreditation by The Joint Commission is recognized nationwide as a symbol of quality that reflects an organization's commitment to meeting certain performance standards. To earn and maintain The Joint Commission's Gold Seal of Approval, an organization must undergo an on-site survey conducted by The Joint Commission at least every 3 years. Laboratories must be surveyed every 2 years.

Benefits of Accreditation

There are many benefits to accreditation, but those specific to health care accreditation include:

- Leads to improved patient care.
- Demonstrates the organization's commitment to safety and quality.
- Offers an educational on-site survey experience.
- Supports and enhances safety and quality improvement efforts.
- Strengthens and supports recruitment and retention efforts.
- May substitute for federal certification surveys for Medicare and Medicaid.
- Helps secure managed care contracts.
- Facilitates the organization's business strategies.
- Provides a competitive advantage.
- Enhances the organization's image to the public, purchasers, and payers.
- Fulfills licensure requirements in many states.
- Is recognized by insurers and other third parties.
- Strengthens community confidence.

Standards and Performance Measurement

The Joint Commission standards address an organization's level of performance in key functional areas, such as patient rights, patient treatment, and infection control. The standards focus not simply on an organization's ability to provide safe, high-quality care, but also on its actual performance. Standards set forth performance expectations for activities that affect the safety and quality of patient care. If an organization does the right things and does them well, there is a strong likelihood that its patients will experience good outcomes. The Joint Commission develops its standards in consultation with health care experts, providers, measurement experts, purchasers, and consumers. See Box 5-1 for an overview of The Joint Commission Hospital Accreditation Standards.

There are also disease-specific certifications, such as The Joint Commission's certificate of distinction for primary stroke centers. This certification program was developed in collaboration with the American Stroke Association. The disease-specific certifications evaluate programs that provide clinical care directly to participants. Examples include, but are not limited to, services provided in hospitals, long-term care health care settings, home care organizations, health plans, integrated delivery systems, rehabilitation centers, physician groups, and disease management service companies. They also evaluate programs that provide comprehensive clinical support and that interact directly with participants on site, by telephone, or through online services or other electronic resources. Examples include, but are not limited to, disease management companies and health care plans with disease management services. There are 143 disease-specific certifications available from The Joint Commission.

Disease-specific care certifications focus on:
- Creating an organized comprehensive approach to disease-specific performance improvement;
- Using comparative data to evaluate disease-specific program processes and patient outcomes;
- Evaluating the patients' perception of care quality; and
- Maintaining data quality and integrity.

The Joint Commission survey is considered a "rite of passage" for any new nurse manager. Before 2008, the survey would occur every 3 years and was announced. In 2008, The Joint Commission started making unannounced visits. This change requires that all health care institutions be in a state of "constant readiness." As a consequence, nurses are required to be aware of accreditation standards, best practice, and current evidence and to deliver nursing care that meets and exceeds standards at all times (Box 5-2).

The importance of the nurse's role in ensuring patient safety and delivering quality care is emphasized through key nursing activities such as:
- Influencing improved design of care processes.
- Creating a nonpunitive environment to enhance error reporting.
- Participating in error reporting and analysis.
- Maintaining knowledge of current levels of performance and relationship to goals and benchmarks.
- Practicing based on most current evidence.

The importance of the nurse's position is further elaborated by their leadership role in complying with the necessary standards for medication management, infection control, pain management, and the environment of care.

BOX 5-1 The Joint Commission Hospital Accreditation Standards Overview

Accreditation Standards fall into the following categories:
- Accreditation Participation Requirements (APR)
- Care, Treatment, and Services (CTS)
- Document and Process Control (DC)
- Environment of Care (EC)
- Emergency Management (EM)
- Equipment Management (EQ)
- Human Resources (HR)
- Infection Prevention and Control (IC)
- Information Management (IM)
- Leadership (LD)
- Life Safety (LS)
- Medication Management (MM)
- Medical Staff (MS)
- National Patient Safety Goals (NPSG)
- Nursing (NR)
- Provision of Care, Treatment, and Services (PC)
- Performance Improvement (PI)
- Quality System Assessment for Nonwaived Testing (QSA)
- Record of Care, Treatment, and Services (RC)
- Rights and Responsibilities of the Individual (RI)
- Transplant Safety (TS)
- Waived Testing (WT)

Joint Commission (2013) Comparison Between Joint Commission Standards, Malcolm Baldrige National Quality Award Criteria, and Magnet Recognition Program Components. www.jointcommission.org/assets/1/6/Comparison_Document2013.pdf

Daily adherence to current standards is of the utmost importance. During a site visit from the accrediting agencies, nurses will be asked to participate in interviews or team meetings with representatives from the accrediting bodies. These site evaluators will also talk with patients to evaluate the patient-centeredness of the care delivered.

One of the most common standards of The Joint Commission that affects nursing care deals with the management of pain. The standard includes the following:

- Documentation of assessment of pain.
- Documentation of the relief of pain.
- Use of therapeutics to manage pain.
- Assessment of the use of therapeutics.

Documentation of this standard will be reviewed for compliance with the standard. Under this standard, organizations will be required to (The Joint Commission, February 2001):

- Recognize patients' rights to the assessment and management of pain.
- Assess the nature and intensity of pain in all patients.
- Establish safe medication prescription and ordering procedures.
- Ensure staff competency and orient new staff in pain assessment and management.
- Monitor patients post-procedurally and reassess patient problems appropriately.
- Educate patients on the role of pain management in treatment.
- Address patients' needs for symptom management in the discharge planning process.
- Collect data to monitor performance.

Accreditation surveyors measure an institution's compliance through the following:

- Interviews with patients, families, and clinical staff.
- Review of policies, procedures, protocols, and practices for effective pain management.
- Review of clinical records.
- Educational materials for patients, family, and staff.
- Statement of patient rights or other statements reflecting the organization's commitment to effective pain management.

As a nurse, it is important for you to remember that you may be interviewed and your patient charts may be reviewed and evaluated by the team.

DET NORSKE VERITAS

Hospitals across the United States are choosing Det Norske Veritas (DNV) Healthcare for a new approach to accreditation, one that focuses on quality, innovation, and continual improvement. Although the standards are similar to those of TJC, there is an integration of ISO 9001 standards moving the institution toward continual improvement. There are also disease-specific certifications, such as primary stroke center, comprehensive stroke center, and management of infection risk. There are 364 health care institutions that participate in DNV accreditations.

DNV accreditation requires an annual survey and the organization's continual compliance with the DNV accreditation process.

THE AMERICAN OSTEOPATHIC ASSOCIATION

The American Osteopathic Association (AOA) Healthcare Facilities Accreditation is a recognized alternative to accreditation by The Joint Commission or DNV. This accrediting agency deals primarily with osteopathic hospitals with approximately 174 accredited institutions across the United States participating. It also certifies institutions as "stroke ready" and as primary stroke centers and comprehensive stroke centers.

OTHER ACCREDITING AGENCIES

There are also specialty certifications for specialty care units, and nurses will be asked to participate in these evaluations.

- American College of Surgeons Commission on Cancer: Accrediting agency that evaluates cancer treatment in hospitals and outpatient and freestanding facilities. In addition to participating in a TJC and state licensing survey, nurses may also be asked to participate in a specialty survey such as this, depending on their area of practice or expertise.
- Commission on Accreditation of Rehabilitation Facilities (CARF): Accrediting agency that evaluates hospital-based or freestanding medical rehabilitation, employment, and community services.
- Community Health Accreditation Program (CHAP): Evaluates home care and community health organizations.
- Accreditation Association for Ambulatory Health Care (AAAHC): Evaluates ambulatory surgery centers, medical and dental group practices, diagnostic imaging centers, and student health centers.
- American Association for Accreditation of Ambulatory Surgery Facilities (AAAASF): Accreditation of ambulatory surgery settings.
- Commission on Accreditation of Ambulance Services (CAAS): Accreditation of medical transportation services.

- National Commission for Correctional Health Care (NCCHC): Accreditation of U.S. prisons, jails, and juvenile detention facilities.
- National Committee for Quality Assurance (NCQA): Accreditation and evaluation of quality management systems and managed care organizations.

EDUCATIONAL ACCREDITATION

If your hospital participates in the education of health care personnel, nurses, and physicians, nurses will also be exposed to visits by the accrediting agencies used by the schools working with your hospital. The schools are usually responsible for the compliance with standards in these situations. Your role will be to respond to the role of the students in the provision of care on your unit. Examples of such agencies include the Accreditation Commission of Education in Nursing (ACEN), the Commission on Collegiate Nursing Education (CCNE), the Liaison Committee on Medical Education (medical schools), the American Osteopathic Association (osteopathic schools), and the Commission on Accreditation in Physical Therapy.

REGULATORY AGENCIES

In addition to these accrediting agencies, there are multiple regulatory and advisory agencies that have an impact on standards of health care. As discussed in Chapter 17, agencies, such as the Occupational Safety and Health Administration (OSHA), regulate the manner in which a hospital implements workplace safety standards. These standards then become part of the accreditor's management of the environment of care standard. The Centers for Disease Control and Prevention (CDC), an agency charged with the promotion of health and quality of life through the prevention and control of disease, injury, and disability, has created multiple infection control standards that are now part of standard accreditation as well as the practice standards of most hospitals. The U.S. Food and Drug Administration (FDA) is a federal agency that regulates drugs, medical devices, and radiation-emitting products. These regulations also form the basis of the medication management standard of the accreditors.

LICENSING BODIES

Health care organizations are licensed to perform services by the state department of health. Most state departments of health undertake the following:

- Regulate a wide range of health care settings for quality of care, such as hospitals, nursing homes, assisted living residences, ambulatory care centers, home health care, medical day care, and others.
- Investigate complaints received from patients, other consumers, and other state and federal agencies.
- Provide consumer information in the form of report cards and other performance information.

Nurses are often called to assist hospital administrators regarding complaints lodged with the state department of health.

GOVERNMENT AGENCIES

There are a number of government agencies that will provide oversight for some of the functions within health care. Examples of these agencies follow.

Occupational Safety and Health Administration

OSHA's mission is to ensure the safety and health of America's workers by setting and enforcing standards; providing training, outreach, and education; establishing partnerships; and encouraging continual improvement in workplace safety and health.

OSHA staff establish protective standards, enforce those standards, and reach out to employers and employees through technical assistance and consultation programs. An example of an OSHA guideline of importance to nursing was the September 12, 2005, guideline for the recommendation to minimize patient lifting to prevent health care musculoskeletal injuries. OSHA recommended that manual lifting of patients be minimized in all cases and eliminated where feasible (OSHA, 2015). This standard has also been implemented in the work safety standards and has resulted in a decline in nursing back injuries.

The U.S. Department of Health and Human Services

The U.S. Department of Health and Human Services (USDHHS) provides 115 programs across 11 divisions covering a wide spectrum of activities including the following (U.S. Department of Health and Human Services [USDHHS], 2014):

- Health and social science research.
- Preventing disease, including immunization services.
- Ensuring food and drug safety.
- Medicare (health insurance for older adults and disabled Americans) and Medicaid (health insurance for low-income people).
- Health information technology.
- Financial assistance and services for low-income families.
- Improving maternal and infant health.
- Head Start (preschool education and services).
- Faith-based and community initiatives.
- Prevention of child abuse and domestic violence.
- Substance abuse treatment and prevention.
- Services for older Americans, including home-delivered meals.
- Comprehensive health services for Native Americans.
- Medical preparedness for emergencies, including potential terrorism.

CENTERS FOR DISEASE CONTROL AND PREVENTION

The CDC, an agency within the USDHHS, is charged with the promotion of health and quality of life by preventing and controlling disease, injury, and disability. The CDC seeks to accomplish its mission by working with partners throughout the country and the world to:

- Monitor health;
- Detect and investigate health problems;
- Conduct research to enhance prevention;
- Develop and advocate sound public health policies;
- Implement prevention strategies;
- Promote healthy behaviors;
- Foster safe and healthful environments; and
- Provide leadership and training.

Nurses come in contact with the CDC in the development of policies and in the possible investigation of disease outbreaks. One notable example was the 2014/2015 Ebola outbreak in West Africa. Nurses in the United States were called upon to treat nurses and health care workers who had contracted the disease. The CDC developed specific policies for the care of such patients.

Other agencies with health care oversight are known by the acronyms shown in Table 5-1.

TABLE 5-1   Glossary of Acronyms

Acronym	Full Name
AAAASF	American Association for Accreditation of Ambulatory Surgery Facilities
AAAHC	Accreditation Association for Ambulatory Health Care
AAHCC	American Accreditation Health Care Commission
ACHC	Accreditation Commission for Health Care, Inc.
ACR	American College of Radiology
ACS-CoC	American College of Surgeons Commission on Cancer
ALS	American Lithotripsy Society
AOA	The American Osteopathic Association
CAAS	Commission on Accreditation of Ambulance Services
CAP	College of American Pathologists Commission on Inspections and Accreditation
CARF	Commission on Accreditation of Rehabilitation Facilities
CCAC	Continuing Care Accreditation Commission
CDC	Centers for Disease Control and Prevention
CHAP	Community Health Accreditation Program, Inc.
CMS	Centers for Medicare & Medicaid Services
COA	Council on Accreditation
COLA	Commission on Office Laboratory Accreditation for Blood Banks and Transfusion Services
DHHS	U.S. Department of Health and Human Services
DNV	Det Norske Veritas
FDA	United States Food and Drug Administration
FEMA	Federal Emergency Management Agency
HAP	Hospital Accreditation Program
NCCHC	National Commission for Correctional Health Care
NIOSH	The National Institute for Occupational Safety and Health
OSHA	Occupational Safety and Health Administration
TJC	The Joint Commission
URAC	Utilization Review Accreditation Commission

Modified from George Mason University. (2007). *Accreditation agencies in United States.* http://gunston.gmu.edu/healthscience/547/MajorAccreditationAgencies.asp.

OTHER GROUPS RECOGNIZING HEALTH CARE PERFORMANCE AND EXCELLENCE

In this time of heated hospital competition, many institutions are attempting to differentiate their performance from the norm through recognition in other areas of performance. Such levels of recognition demonstrate excellence beyond accreditation, regulatory, and licensing areas.

- The most significant group, in terms of nursing performance, is the American Nurses Credentialing Center (ANCC), which oversees the Magnet Award; the highest level of recognition that the ANCC can award to organized nursing services in the national and international arena. Through this award, the ANCC recognizes nursing-sensitive outcomes as a predictor of quality of patient care and values the retention and recruitment of highly competent nurses (American Nurses Credentialing Center [ANCC], 2008).
- The Malcolm Baldrige Award for Performance Excellence recognizes health care institutions that demonstrate performance excellence across all areas of the organization. The requirements for excellence must exist in seven categories: Leadership, Strategic Planning, Customer and Market Knowledge, Information Management, Workforce Focus, Process Management, and Results (Baldrige National Quality Program, 2014).
- *U.S. News and World Report* annually ranks the "best hospitals in the U.S." This ranking rates hospitals across the nation in terms of breadth of expertise and quality. In 2007, 5462 hospitals were screened. Just 173 made it to the rankings, and 18 made it to the honor role (U.S. News and World Report, 2007). Of the hospitals listed in the 2007 rankings, 7 of the top 10 were also Magnet hospitals.
- J. D. Power and Associates recognizes hospitals for service excellence. The firm's Distinguished Hospital Program expands the traditional evaluation of quality by recognizing hospitals that achieve a notable level of satisfaction with services that are provided. This program helps consumers identify hospitals that provide outstanding service excellence and may serve as a competitive advantage when consumers are looking for service excellence (J. D. Power and Associates, 2008).

The Joint Commission accreditation standards, the Malcolm Baldrige National Quality Award, and the ANCC's Magnet Award contain many parallels. All three share the following characteristics:

- Developed using a consensus-building approach.
- Built upon a core set of values and principles.
- Use a framework of important functions (patient care) that cross internal structures (departments) of an organization.

- Recognize the "systemness" of organizations.
- Focus on continuous improvement and organizational performance.
- Are not prescriptive.
- Promote the use of organizational self-assessment. (The Joint Commission [2014]. Comparison Between Joint Commission Standards, Malcolm Baldrige National Quality Award Criteria, and Magnet Recognition Program Components. p. 1.)

SUMMARY

It is important to realize that the integration of regulation, accrediting standards, and licensing requirements forms a major part of the health care accreditation in the United States. As with all regulatory and accrediting bodies, there are multiple standards for each regulation or level of accreditation. As a nurse, it is your responsibility to understand your role in the accreditation process, your role in the adherence to regulatory standards, and your role in meeting accreditation standards. Although many of the accreditations are "voluntary," hospitals cannot receive reimbursement unless they are accredited. The accreditation process validates the effectiveness and safety of the care being rendered. Also, in this era of highly competitive hospitals, the levels and amounts of accreditation may be a way of marketing the excellence of one particular hospital compared with another.

CLINICAL CORNER

Benefits of Det Norske Veritas Germanischer Lloyd National Integrated Accreditation for Healthcare Organizations Accreditation

Benefits of DNV (Det Norske Veritas) GL (Germanischer Lloyd) NIAHO® (National Integrated Accreditation for Healthcare Organizations) accreditation can be summarized as follows:

- Integration of International Organization for Standardization (ISO) 9001 Quality Management Certification recognizes organizational excellence beyond the minimum requirements of the Centers for Medicare & Medicaid Services (CMS) Conditions of Participation (CoPs).
- Annual Survey drives continuous improvement.
- Annual Survey encourages a collaborative approach to accreditation.
- NIAHO® accreditation process fosters a culture that focuses on process improvement and addressing nonconformance, rather than criticizing individual performance.
- Process improvement encourages the organization to ensure that all employees understand the "why" behind the change, thus fostering engagement.

Hospitals seek accreditation to demonstrate compliance with the CMS CoPs. Accreditation allows the hospital to receive federal reimbursement for services provided. Most third-party payers require compliance with the CMS CoPs as a prerequisite for reimbursement. Accreditation validates a level of competence appreciated by patients as well as health care professionals employed by the organization.

Nonetheless, compliance with the CMS CoPs is a minimum performance expectation in today's accountable health care environment.

DNV GL-Healthcare was granted deeming authority by CMS in 2008. DNV GL's NIAHO® hospital accreditation program is the only accreditation choice that aligns the Quality Management System requirements of ISO 9001 with the CMS CoPs.

The ISO 9001 standards, a series of five international criteria, published in 1987 by the ISO of Geneva, Switzerland, outline the components of a Quality Management System that incorporate W. Edwards Deming's Plan Do Study Act (PDSA) (see Chapter 18) cycle of continuous improvement. ISO 9001 outlines a systematic approach to managing quality.[1] NIAHO®-accredited hospitals use the ISO 9001 standards to define for the organization what requirements are needed, in concert with the CoPs, to maintain an efficient quality conformance system. For example, the ISO standards describe the need for an effective quality system, ensuring that measuring and testing equipment are calibrated regularly, and for maintaining an adequate record-keeping system.[2]

ISO 9001 requires that all members of the workforce understand the "why" behind their actions to drive systematic improvement. Nursing, typically the largest segment

Continued

Benefits of Det Norske Veritas Germanischer Lloyd National Integrated Accreditation for Healthcare Organizations Accreditation

of the hospital workforce, is central to successful implementation of an integrated Quality Management System. Nurses must participate in the measurement, monitoring, analysis, and improvement of key processes throughout the organization: at the bedside, in Quality Management Oversight (an ISO requirement) activities, and as patient (customer) advocates. Nurse leaders are key to encouraging a culture that focuses on process improvement and addressing nonconformance rather than criticizing individual performance.

ISO 9001 registration validates that an organization identifies and complies with its own quality system requirements. Thus, choosing NIAHO® accreditation supports a hospital's efforts to create and manage an efficient quality compliance process with a quality management system focused on continuous performance improvement and organizational excellence. Adoption of the NIAHO® accreditation process can stand alone in a hospital's effort to create and manage an efficient quality conformance system or function as the impetus for developing a holistic system for organizational performance and sustainability, such as that reflected in the Baldrige Criteria for Performance Excellence.[3]

The ISO alignment mandates that DNV GL survey (audit) organizations to the NIAHO® requirements on an annual basis. The annual survey and resulting nonconformance reports enable the actualization of continuous readiness within the organization; there is no "ramp down" because surveyors return to check on progress every year. As a result, there is an urgency for the organization to develop meaningful corrective action plans that drive improvement. Accreditation becomes a management asset for quality and patient safety improvement. Because the focus is on systematic quality management, all employees are empowered to participate in ongoing improvement activities. DNV GL's approach to accreditation has been described as collaborative rather than prescriptive. DNV GL offers training programs relating to the NIAHO® accreditation process

but does not provide consultation services. Customer satisfaction surveys for 2014 indicated that more than 90% of clients ranked the NIAHO® accreditation program better than their previous accreditation programs.[4]

Compliance with the CMS CoPs is a minimum performance expectation in today's accountable health care environment. Visionary health care leadership knows that a sustainable presence in the hospital management environment relies on an integrated management system that aligns organizational design, strategy, systems, and human capital to create long-term effectiveness in an institutionalized high-performance culture.[5]

Five choices are available to hospital organizations seeking to validate compliance with the CMS CoPs. As the health care industry continues to systematically focus on achieving and sustaining quality outcomes, more choices are likely to emerge. For those organizations actively seeking to align accreditation activities with the desire to integrate a sustainable systematic quality management organizational focus with the CoPs, the NIAHO® accreditation program is the logical accreditation choice.

References

1. Reid, R.D. From Deming to ISO 9000:2000. Qual Prog, June, 2001. http://asq.org/quality-progress/2001/06/standards-outlook/from-deming-to-iso-9000-2000.html.
2. Schulingkamp, R. C. (2013). *Study of Malcolm Baldrige Health Care Criteria Effectiveness and Organizational Performance*. New Orleans, Louisiana. Tulane University Theses and Dissertations Archive p. 72.
3. www.asahq.org/resources/publications/newsletter-articles/2014/may-2014/quality-and-regulatory-affairs.
4. issuu.com/dnvbaus/docs/dnvgl_hc_brochure_americas.
5. www.asahq.org/resources/publications/newsletter-articles/2014/may-2014/quality-and-regulatory-affairs.

Maureen Washburn, RN, ND, CPHQ, FACHE
Chief Clinical Officer
DNV GL Business Assurance, Healthcare Accreditation Services

EVIDENCE-BASED PRACTICE

Drenkard, K. (2013). Magnet perspectives: The value of Magnet. *Journal of Nursing Administration*, *43*(10), S2–S3

The American Nurses Credentialing Center (ANCC) is the recognized leader in global credentialing services, committed to driving nursing excellence, quality care, and improved outcomes.

This article discusses outcomes-focused research. The research offers evidence of better outcomes in Magnet organizations. Best practices are driving innovative nursing study and scholarly advancements. The article discusses findings from McHugh et al. (2013) at the University of Pennsylvania. The research demonstrated that Magnet hospitals have significantly better work environments and higher proportions of nurses with bachelor's degrees and specialty certifications. There are lower mortality rates. The Magnet culture stimulates quality and positive organizational behavior and this improves outcomes.

McHugh and Ma (2013) studied the relationship between a hospital's nursing work environment, staffing, and education levels and its 30-day readmission rate for patients with heart failure, acute myocardial infarction, and pneumonia. The conclusion was that improving nurses' work environments, staffing levels, and educational levels can be effective in preventing readmissions.

Abraham et al. (2011) identify the characteristics that distinguish Magnet-recognized hospitals within the framework of diffusion theory; the spread of innovation, ideas, and technology through a culture. The authors identify Magnet designation as an organizational innovation and recommend its diffusion as a strategic imperative for hospitals to continue to create a competitive advantage for nurse recruitment.

In a national survey of hospital nursing research, McLaughlin et al. (2013) and Kelly et al. (2013) describe scholarly outcomes for registered nurses (RNs) and find that nursing output is greater in Magnet organizations than in non-Magnet organizations. They identified the presence of a mentor to guide nurses through research projects as most influential factor in improving scholarly output.

Wilson et al. (2013) shared four creative approaches to research and evidence-based practice implementation in Magnet and Magnet-aspiring organizations. These articles look at the importance of integrating nursing research into clinical practice.

Research by Zrelak et al. (2012) reviews the critical effects that nurses have on the prevention and early recognition of potential complications and adverse events. The article shows that nursing's influence on outcomes can be used to improve patient care.

References

Abraham, J., Jerome-D'Emilia, B., & Begun, J. W. (2011). The diffusion of Magnet hospital recognition. *Health Care Management Review*, *36*(4), 306–314.

Kelly, K. P., Turner, A., Gabel Speroni, K., McLaughlin, M. K., & Guzzetta, C. E. (2013). National survey of hospital nursing research, part 2: Facilitators and hindrances. *Journal of Nursing Administration*, *43*(1), 18–23.

McHugh, M. D., Kelly, L. A., Smith, H. L., Wu, E. S., Vanak, J. M., & Aiken, L. H. (2013). Lower mortality in Magnet hospitals. *Medical Care*, *51*(5), 382–388.

McHugh, M. D., & Ma, C. (2013). Hospital nursing and 30-day readmissions among Medicare patients with heart failure, acute myocardial infarction, and pneumonia. *Medical Care*, *51*(1), 52–59.

McLaughlin, M. K., Gabel Speroni, K., Kelly, K. P., Guzzetta, C. E., & Desale, S. (2013). National survey of hospital nursing research, part 1: Research requirements and outcomes. *Journal of Nursing Administration*, *43*(1), 10–17.

Wilson, B., Kelly, L., Reifsnider, E., Pipe, T., & Brumfeld, V. (2013). Creative approaches to increasing hospital-based nursing research. *Journal of Nursing Administration*, *43*(2), 80–88.

Zrelak, P. A., Utter, G. H., Sadeghi, B., Cuny, J., Baron, R., & Romano, P. S. (2012). Using the Agency for Healthcare Research and Quality patient safety indicators for targeting nursing quality improvement. *Journal of Nursing Care Quality*, *27*(2), 99–108.

NCLEX® EXAMINATION QUESTIONS

1. What agency provides national and world leadership to prevent work-related illnesses and injuries and conducts a range of efforts in the areas of research, guidance, information, and service?
   A. The Centers for Disease Control and Prevention (CDC)
   B. National Institute for Occupational Safety and Health (NIOSH)
   C. The Joint Commission (TJC)
   D. Centers for Medicare & Medicaid services (CMS)

2. _____is a health care accreditation agency that integrates the International Organization for Standardization's ISO 9001 quality management system with the Medicare conditions of participation.
   A. Det Norske Veritas (DNV)
   B. The Joint Commission (TJC)
   C. American Osteopathic Association (AOA)
   D. National Institute for Occupational Safety and Health (NIOSH)

3. The Joint Commission standards address an organization's level of performance in key functional areas, such as:
   A. Patient rights, patient treatment, high-quality care
   B. Patient rights, patient assessment, pain control
   C. Infection control, pain control, falls
   D. Infection control, safe care, injection safety

4. The Occupational Safety and Health Administration (OSHA) has provided guidelines for minimizing patient lifting to prevent health care musculoskeletal injuries. Within these guidelines, OSHA recommends that:
   A. Patients be allowed to decide whether safe lifting equipment should be used when transferring out of bed
   B. Manual lifting of residents be minimized and eliminated when feasible
   C. Only specific types of lifting equipment be used, such as a ceiling-mounted patient lift with a sling
   D. Institutions should be allowed to decide based on patient population whether safe lifting equipment should be used

5. One benefit of accreditation by The Joint Commission is that it:
   A. Leads to improved patient care and demonstrates the organization's commitment to safety and quality
   B. Allows for increased financial gain through Medicare and Medicaid reimbursement and offers employee assistance programs
   C. Influences the improved design of care processes, creating a nonpunitive environment to enhance error reporting and allow participation in error reporting and analysis
   D. Offers an educational off-site survey experience

6. The Joint Commission's evaluation and accreditation services are provided for the following types of organizations:
   A. State department of health and town senior housing services
   B. Physicians' offices and freestanding laboratory service agencies
   C. Home hemodialysis and peritoneal dialysis
   D. Critical access hospitals, home care organizations, and nursing homes

7. The U.S. Department of Health and Human Services (USDHHS) is the most important federal actor in health care. What are some of the other federal agencies with major health services roles?
   A. Department of Veterans Affairs
   B. Department of Treasury and Taxation
   C. Department of Corrections and Law
   D. Department of Agriculture and Taxation

8. The mission of the U.S. Department of Health and Human Services (USDHHS) is:
   A. To protect and promote the health and social economic well-being of legal immigrants by helping them and their families develop and maintain productive and independent lives
   B. To support legal immigrants both financially and legally
   C. To protect and promote the health and social and economic well-being of Americans by helping them and their families develop and maintain productive and independent lives
   D. To deport all illegal immigrants to their countries in an effort to maintain alliances with those countries

9. An example of what the Centers for Disease Control and Prevention (CDC) would evaluate is:
   A. A toxic spill on a state highway
   B. An outbreak of rubella at a school
   C. A flu shot clinic at a pharmaceutical company
   D. An outbreak of respiratory syncytial virus in a neonatal intensive care unit
10. The National Institute for Occupational Safety and Health (NIOSH) is:
   A. The agency that works closely with The Joint Commission and hospital accreditation
   B. A local agency that coordinates patient care and patient services
   C. A state agency that is part of the Centers for Disease Control and Prevention (CDC) in the U.S. Department of Health and Human Services
   D. The federal agency responsible for conducting research and making recommendations for the prevention of work-related injury and illness.

Answers: 1. A   2. A   3. A   4. B   5. A   6. C   7. A   8. C   9. B   10. D

REFERENCES

American Nurses Credentialing Center [ANCC]. (2008). www.nursecredentialing.org/Magnet/ProgramOverview.aspx.

Baldrige National Quality Program. (2014). *Health care criteria for performance excellence*. Gaithersburg, MD: Baldrige National Quality Program.

J.D. Power and Associates. (2008). *Turning information into action*. www.jdpower.com/corporate/healthcare/hospital.aspx.

Joint Commission. (2001). Pain assessment and management. *Perspectives, 8*, 10 Oct 2001, 4, 11.

Joint Commission. (2014). *The Joint Commission mission-related commitments*, January 1, 2009. www.jointcommission.org/about_us/about_the_joint_commission_main.aspx.

Occupational Safety and Health Administration (OSHA) guideline. (2003). www.osha.gov/ergonomics/guidelines/nursinghome/final_nh_guidelines.html.

U.S. Department of Health and Human Services (HHS). (2015). What we do. www.hhs.gov/about/whatwedo.html/.

U.S. News and World Report. (2007). http://health.usnews.com/sections/health/besthospitals.

Yoder-Wise, P. S. (2006). *Beyond leading and managing nursing administration for the future*. St. Louis: Mosby.

WEBSITES

www.state.nj.us/health/

www.osha.gov/oshinfo/mission.html

www.cdc.gov/niosh/

www.osha.gov/oshinfo/mission.html

http://gunston.gmu.edu/healthscience/547/MajorAccreditationAgencies.asp

www.hhs.gov/about/whatwedo.html

www.osha.gov/ergonomics/guidelines/nursinghome/final_nh_guidelines.html

Health and Human Services Program Inventory. (2014). http://www.hhs.gov/budget/2013-program-inventory/federal-program-inventory.html.

Joint Commission. (2013). *Comparison Between Joint Commission Standards, Malcolm Baldrige National Quality Award Criteria, and Magnet Recognition Program Components.* www.jointcommission.org/assets/1/6/Comparison_Document2013.pdf

Structural Empowerment

SECTION OUTLINE

Nurses within Magnet organizations are actively involved in shared governance and decision making to establish standards of care and opportunities for improvement. The flow of information and decision making among professional nurses with Magnet institutions is multidirectional among nurses at the bedside, nursing leadership, interdisciplinary teams, and senior leadership. Nurses throughout such organizations are "empowered" to continually advocate for superior patient and nursing outcomes through structures and processes that are designed to encourage the voice of the nurse in decision making.

This section will deal with shared governance structures, professional decision-making structures, flow of information and policy, and professional development structures that support nursing autonomy.

6

Organizational Decision Making and Shared Governance

OBJECTIVES

- Differentiate among the various structures of shared governance.
- Identify the types of decisions made at the various levels of the organization.
- Recognize the role of senior nursing leadership in the clinical decision making.
- Identify the various functions represented in the shared governance structures.

- Define the four primary principles of shared governance: partnership, equity, accountability, and ownership.
- Discuss the responsibility of the staff nurse in shared governance.

OUTLINE

KEY TERMS

accountability willingness to invest in decision making and express ownership in those decisions

board of trustees responsible for overseeing the activities of a nonprofit organization, ranging from huge foundations to small local charities. A board of trustees usually has between 5 and 20 members. Many members of a Board of Trustees hold other external positions, but the Board of Trustees may also include senior management of the nonprofit.

equity maintains a focus on services, patients, and staff; is the foundation and measure of value; and says that no one role is more important than any other.

ownership recognition and acceptance of the importance of everyone's work, and of the fact that an organization's success is bound to how well individual staff members perform their jobs.

partnership health care providers and patients along all points in the system; a collaborative relationship among all stakeholders and nursing required for professional empowerment.

senior leadership senior management group or team. In many organizations this consists of the head of the organization and his or her direct reports (also called C-suite leaders).

shared governance is shared decision making based on the principles of partnership, equity, accountability, and ownership at the point of service. This management process model empowers all members of the health care workforce to have a voice in decision making, thus encouraging diverse and creative input that will help advance the business and health care missions of the organization.

Decision making occurs throughout all levels of any organization. Strategic planning initiatives usually occur at the senior leadership level with input from all stakeholders. Organizations are usually designed to facilitate such communication and decision making. Organizational design is a formal, guided process for integrating the people, information, and technology of an organization, and serves as a key structural element that allows corporations to maximize value by matching their corporate design to overall strategy (Burton, 2004).

Health care organizations are a complex mix of stakeholders: patients/families, communities, physicians, nurses, other health care disciplines, and so on. The major goal of all organizations is the delivery of effective, efficient care, while enhancing the patient experience.

Though many hospitals may differ in framework, particularly between large and small organizations, or those with for-profit or nonprofit missions, most follow accepted models of hierarchy well established in the business realm.

A board of directors (Board of Trustees) is invariably at the top of most organizational structures in health care. This board may be formed by a vote of trustees in a founding organization or by stakeholders in the hospital franchise. Typically it contains more tenured hospital professionals like doctors, nurse members, community members, and researchers, but many are also populated with local lawyers, entrepreneurs, politicians, and even celebrities who might help to lend the hospital a competitive edge.

A hospital's president or chief executive officer (CEO) is usually responsible for answering to the board and carrying out its funding, regulatory oversight, and research initiatives. This chief often serves as an ex officio member as does the Chief Nurse. Many nonprofit facilities will populate the board in alignment with its particular mission. For instance, the board of a Catholic hospital will often have faith and medical leaders serving, each focused on a different element of the mission.

The senior leadership team is usually the first link in the chain connecting organizational alignment to the strategic goals. The Chief Nurse is the link for the planning, alignment, and implementation of the nursing strategic plan, as discussed in Chapter 3. The Chief Nurse is strategically positioned within the organization to effectively influence and communicate with other executive stakeholders, including the board of trustees. Senior level nursing leaders serve at the highest levels of the organization, with the Chief Nurse typically reporting to the CEO.

Communication between senior leaders and the other stakeholders of the organization is of vital importance to its success. The central roles of the senior leadership are (Porter-O'Grady & Malloch, 2015, p. 146) the following:

- Link between Board and staff.
- Inform the Board and translate strategy to the system.
- Provide good linkage between the various loci of control.
- Create a positive context for worker relationships.
- Build the infrastructure of decisions and action.

The senior leadership is interested in the effectiveness of the system in decision-making actions and outcomes. The actual decisions and actions are usually made at the level of the point of care. A shared governance model forms the basis of decision making throughout most institutions. Shared governance is the vehicle through which nurses at all levels of the organizations make and share decisions.

SHARED GOVERNANCE

Governance is about power, control, authority, and influence. It answers the question in an organization, "Who rules?" Nursing shared governance extends that rule to nurses (Hess, 2004). Nursing shared governance models have always focused on nurses controlling their professional practice. It's a theme that flows consistently through shared governance research and literature. Structure is of vital importance to the success of shared governance. The American Nurses Credentialing Center (ANCC) (2013) states that shared leadership/participative decision making is a model in which nurses are formally organized to make decisions about clinical practice standards, quality improvement, staff and professional development, and research (p. 74). As one of the early Magnet Hospitals noted, "unlike participatory management environments, [shared governance structures] ensure that the practicing nurse has not only the right but the power to make practice decisions" (Hess, 2004; George et al., 2002).

This power to make practice decisions characterizes the autonomy of nurses to control nursing practice. Shared governance activities may include participatory scheduling, joint staffing decisions, and/or shared unit responsibilities (e.g., every registered nurse [RN] is trained to be "in charge" of their unit or area, and shares that role with other professional team members, perhaps on a rotating schedule) to achieve the best patient care outcomes. The same control over practice, at the unit level, requires a transition from the historically hierarchical design of heath care decision making to a more decentralized decision-making process. To make that happen, employee partnership, equity, accountability, and ownership must occur at the point of service (e.g., on the patient care units).

Partnership

Partnership links health care providers and patients along all points in the system, and is a collaborative relationship among all stakeholders and nursing required for professional empowerment (Batson, 2004). Partnership is essential to building relationships, involves all staff members in decisions and processes, implies that each member has a key role in fulfilling the mission and purpose of the organization, and is critical to the health care system's effectiveness (Porter-O'Grady & Hinshaw, 2005).

Equity

Equity is the best method for integrating staff roles and relationships into structures and processes to achieve positive patient outcomes. Equity maintains a focus on services, patients, and staff; is the foundation and measure of value; and says that no single role is more important than any other. Although equity does not equal equality in terms of scope of practice, knowledge, authority, or responsibility, it does mean that each team member is essential to providing safe and effective care (Porter-O'Grady & Hinshaw, 2005).

Accountability

Accountability is a willingness to invest in decision-making and express ownership in those decisions. Accountability is the core of shared governance. It is often used interchangeably with responsibility, and allows for evaluation of role performance It supports partnerships and is secured as staff produce positive outcomes (Porter-O'Grady & Hinshaw, 2005).

Ownership

Ownership is recognition and acceptance of the importance of everyone's work and of the fact that an organization's success is bound to how well individual staff members perform their jobs. To enable all team members to participate, ownership designates where work is done, and by whom. It requires all staff members to commit to contributing something, to own what they contribute, and to participate in devising purposes for the work (Porter-O'Grady & Hinshaw, 2005; Koloroutis, 2004).

At least 90% of the decisions need to be made at the point of service. Indeed, in matters of practice, quality, and competence, the locus of control in the professional practice environment must shift to practitioners. Only 10% of the unit-level decisions should belong to management (Porter-O'Grady & Hinshaw, 2005). A recent comparative analysis by Kramer and Schmalenburg, (2003), who interviewed 279 nurses at 14 Magnet hospitals, found the highest staff nurse ownership of practice issues and outcomes occurred where there were visible, viable, and recognized structures devoted to nursing control over practice.

Box 6-1 shows the differences between the decentralized shared governance interactions and those of the more centralized decision making structures.

In fact, Florence Nightingale (1992) represented a shared governance model in 1859 with the following quote:

The key provider at point of service, the staff nurse, moves from the bottom to the center of the organization. Nurses are the primary employees who do the work and connect the organization to the recipient of its service. An entirely different sense and set of variables now affect the design of the organization; the only one who matters in a service-based organization is the one who provides its service. All other roles become servant to that role. In this way, the paradigm shifts to a relationship-based,

---

BOX 6-1   Self Governance vs. Shared Governance

Centralized Interactions *(Self Governance)*	Decentralized Interactions *(Shared Governance)*
1. Position based	1. Knowledge based
2. Distant from point of care/service	2. Occurs at point of care/service
3. Hierarchical communication	3. Direct communication
4. Limited staff input	4. High staff input
5. Separates responsibility/managers are accountable	5. Integrates equity, accountability, and authority for staff and managers
6. We-they work environment	6. Synergistic work environment
7. Divided goals/purpose	7. Cohesive goals/purpose, ownership
8. Independent activities/tasks	8. Collegiality, collaboration, partnership

Adapted from Porter-O'Grady, T., & Hinshaw, A.S. (2005). Introduction: The concept behind shared governance. In: Swihart, D. (Ed). *Shared Governance: A Practical Approach to Transform Professional Nursing Practice* (pp. 1–12). Danvers, MA: HCPro.

---

staff-centered, patient-focused professional nursing practice model of care in which nurse managers or supervisors assume the role of servant leaders managing resources and outcomes.

Many structures have evolved over the years to ensure the effectiveness of this nursing decision making.

The most common model is the Councilor Model. In this model, unit-based councils form the decision-making and action bodies at the unit or point of service level. Other councils are formed around major initiatives and strategic priorities. Figure 6-1 shows a schematic of the shared governance councils of The Lahey Clinic with a description of each council's function.

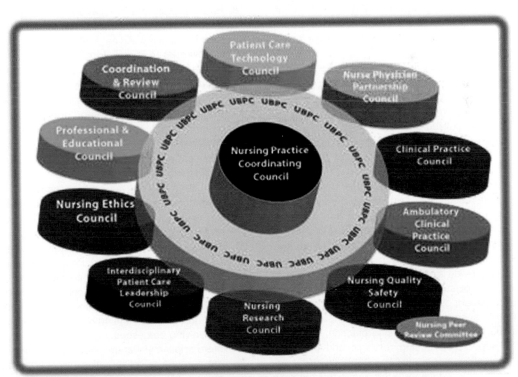

FIGURE 6-1 The Lahey Clinic Nursing Shared Governance Model.

Nursing Governance Councils

Unit-Based Councils

The shared governance structure has evolved to include the Unit-Based Practice Councils (UBPCs) that includes the Nurse Practitioner Committee and Certified Registered Nurse Anesthetists. They meet regularly and identify opportunities for improvement in nursing practice in their respective units that enhance excellence in patient care. The Unit-Based Practice Council structure is the essential process for staff nurse decision making in operational and professional practice issues at the unit level.

Central Councils: The following is a description of the 11 Shared Governance Central Councils and their functions. These councils include nursing staff from all areas in nursing and focus on processes for relationship building and mutual collaboration, and the development and promotion of policies, guidelines, and standards of practice that enhance professional nursing practice, and promote quality in patient care (Glickman et al., 2007).

1. Nursing Practice Coordination Council: The purpose of this council is to provide a forum for shared decision making in nursing practice and best practice initiatives across the organization by representatives from the UBCs and central shared governance councils. All councils will share best practices and solve nursing practice problems, creating linkage across ambulatory and tertiary care.

2. Clinical Practice Council: The purpose is to review all policies and nursing practice guidelines and ensure that they conform to current standards of care, are evidence based, incorporate research, and reflect interdisciplinary collaboration as appropriate.

3. Ambulatory Clinical Practice Council: The purpose of this council is to review all ambulatory policies and practice guidelines and ensure that they conform with current standards of care, are evidence based, incorporate research, and reflect interdisciplinary collaboration as appropriate.

4. Nurse Physician Partnership Council: The purpose of this council is to create a partnership between nurses and physicians to jointly manager and problem solve, to provide a forum of shared ideas, discuss issues, and disseminate new information that will enhance patient outcomes.

5. Nursing Research Council: This council provides the scientific foundation for nursing practice, dedicated to the support of nursing research and evidence-based practice at Lahey Clinic. The council's objectives include educating staff about the research process and evidence-based practice, providing resources and research consultation that facilitate the conduct of nursing research; disseminating research findings from organization, local, and national meetings; and facilitating the use of research findings to improve patient care.

6. Nursing Quality Safety Council: The purpose of this council is to review data related to quality and safety initiatives including National Patient Safety Goals, Core Measures, and Failure Modes and Effects Analysis results. This council makes recommendations that promote and maintain a nursing environment where the best practices in safety and quality are able to be provided for patient care.

7. Patient Care Technology Council: This is a multidisciplinary council that facilitates the implementation of departmental and organization objectives related to technology to enhance patient care. This council develops guidelines and protocols for technology initiatives, ensures that clinical applications reflect standards of care and nursing practice, and solicits input and feedback from end users.

8. Professional and Educational Council: The purpose of this council is to facilitate a culture where learning is viewed as a life-long process, which is essential to the growth and development of all nurses at LC. This council develops and reviews all staff education materials, the nursing practice guidelines, oversees the process of incorporating evidence-based practice and nursing research into patient care practices, and supports professional development through Pathways to Expertise and Certification.

9. Coordination and Review Council: The purpose of this council is to review, revise, and standardize job descriptions; streamline documentation; and approve and revise clinical administrative policies as necessary for accurate nursing functions and process.

10. Nursing Ethics Council: As voted by the Nursing Practice Coordinating and Review Council in February 2008. This council is designated as a central council where staff nurses participate in identifying strategies and educational initiatives to improve the staff nurse knowledge on ethical principles and problem-solving processes.

11. Interdisciplinary Patient Care Leadership Council: The purpose is collaborative discussion and shared decision making on operational patient care issues

Nursing Governance Councils—cont'd

and updates on current patient care initiatives, including Joint Commission Readiness and a review of the status of initiatives related to the organization's strategic plan. This council is incorporated in the shared governance structure and allows collaboration with other disciplines who are invited to discuss organizational initiatives and strategies and seek broad nursing input for the most comprehensive approach to address patient care and operational concerns. (Lahey Clinic Shared Governance Structure www.lahey.org/For_Health care_Professionals/Nursing/Nursing_Governance_Structure.)

Another example of shared governance principles and structures follows:

Shared Governance Structure Mount Sinai/Beth Israel Hospital

Unit-Based Practice Councils

Unit-Based Councils represent their own culture while using the organization's shared governance framework and bylaws. They deal with patient care practices and issues rather than business decisions. Issues identified at the point of patient care are initially addressed within the unit by the Unit Practice Council.

These councils are authorized to make decisions that affect their unit. Decisions are made by consensus and supported by evidence-based practice.

Effective communication is an essential strategy at all the following levels:

Between unit council and staff

Between unit council members

Between unit council and management council

Between unit council and organization-wide councils

Nurse Executive Council

The role of this council is the management of resources as defined in the strategic plan and nursing conceptual framework.

This council examines the delivery of patient care as it is affected by the availability of human, fiscal, material support, and system linkage resources.

Nursing Quality and Patient Safety Council

Provides a forum to develop and review nursing quality indicators. Defines and measures key processes of patient care, performs product evaluation and reviews for safety, monitors performance through data collection, and designs processes to improve efficiency and effectiveness of patient care.

A representative from this council may be assigned to attend any hospital or system-wide Quality and Patient Safety Committee meetings to represent the discipline of nursing, and to coordinate and enhance communication.

Nursing Professional Standards and Practice Council

Defines standards, policies, and procedures for clinical practice, and care delivery. Identifies the need for development of new policies, or revisions to current policies related to research findings, new technology, and/or practice changes. A representative from this council may be assigned to attend any hospital or system-wide committee meeting, which addresses nursing standards and/or practice issues, to represent the discipline of nursing, and to coordinate and enhance communication.

Nursing Staff Development, Education and Research Council

Advances the practice of nursing, and fosters the nursing role in patient education through staff development and evidence-based research initiatives.

A representative from this council may be assigned to attend any hospital or system-wide committee meeting, which addresses nursing professional development and nursing research, to represent the discipline of nursing, and to coordinate and enhance communication.

Nursing Informatics and Communication Council

In collaboration with members from Information Technology and Nursing Informatics, this council will provide guidance and expertise into the development and implementation of the electronic documentation systems, and nursing information systems. A representative from this council may be assigned to attend any hospital or system-wide committee meeting, which addresses nursing informatics and/or impacts nursing communication, to represent the discipline of nursing, and to coordinate and enhance communication.

Advanced Practice Nurse Council

This council provides the opportunity for APNs, with support from the CNO and the director of Ambulatory Services, to identify areas of improvement and to share best practices within this diverse group of clinicians.

A representative from this council may be assigned to attend any unit-based hospital or system-wide committee or council meeting as a clinical resource.

Continued

Shared Governance Structure Mount Sinai/Beth Israel Hospital—cont'd

Nursing Strategy & Vision Coordinating Council	**Entity-Based Council**
This council coordinates the work of all the councils and delivers results from the strategic plan. This council also mediates any conflict that arises for the councils. This council stays appraised of regulatory changes, and any new work that emerges outside the strategic plan, to ensure that the work is assigned to the appropriate councils for action and implementation.	This council serves as a communication link for geographically remote sites within a multi-campus system that uses the same shared governance model. Representatives from the site specific, entity-based council share information discussed in the house-wide councils to ensure that appropriate changes can be applied properly, or adopted at a particular campus or remote setting.

Shared governance structure of Beth Israel. www.bethisraelnynursing.com/patient-care/shared-governance-structure.

Shared governance is much more than a set of committees. The number, titles, and arrangements of committees are not as important as the people who make up the membership. Rather, their expertise and knowledge that guide their actions, what they have power to do, and their commitment to both their profession and the mission of their organization are more likely predictors of success. The meaning of success in terms of shared governance and patient care is the control of practice leading to better patient outcomes (Hess, 2004).

Although definitions, models, structures, and principles of shared governance (or collaborative governance, participatory governance, shared or participatory leadership, staff empowerment, or clinical governance) vary, the outcomes are consistent. The evidence suggests that shared governance processes result in the following:

- Increased nurse satisfaction with shared decision making, related to increased responsibility that is combined with appropriate authority and accountability.
- Increased professional autonomy, as higher staff and nurse manager retention.

- Greater patient and staff satisfaction.
- Improved patient care outcomes.
- Better financial states because of cost savings/cost reductions.

(Anthony, 2004; Hess, 2004; Wilson et al., 2008.)

The first step in participation in shared governance is membership in a unit-based council. This council allows the new nurse to become aware of the major operational and practice issues affecting the unit. It will also allow for the opportunity to contribute to the decisions made impacting the unit. Membership is usually composed of all members of the nursing staff of a particular unit. It is important for nurses to take membership in such councils seriously, and to view them as an opportunity to be empowered to make decisions about their practice, and the practice of the entire institution. They must assume accountability, a willingness to invest in decision making, and express ownership in those decisions. Accountability is the core of shared governance and empowerment as a nurse. As the nurse grows professionally, advancement through the decision-making structure is expected.

CLINICAL CORNER

Shared decision making is an essential part of nursing professional practice as it creates a culture of empowerment for everyone, from clinical staff to executive nursing leadership. Shared governance is a vehicle for professional nurse engagement, fostering new ideas, nursing research, and evidence-based practices. Professional nurse engagement is rewarded through clinical ladder programs, recognition through nursing excellence awards, publications, and conference presentations. The structure we have implement- ed includes a specific council for each level: Directors, Advanced Practice Nurses (APNs), Educators, Nurse Managers, and Clinical Registered Nurses (RNs) to assess practice, implement necessary changes, and evaluate, through data analyses, professional and patient outcomes. Each council meets monthly then moves the policies, projects, and research studies they are working on through all the councils for consideration and input. Nursing Leadership is our highest decision-making council, chaired by the Chief

Nursing Officer (CNO), where all the council chairs, directors, and managers meet to vote.

We value the role of the clinical RN as the health care provider, who is positioned closest to the patient and family to make patient care delivery decisions. The Nurse Practice Council (NPC) is at the heart of shared governance. Each unit sends an RN representative to the monthly meeting as a prescheduled 8-hour business day. The morning session is divided into four core committees: Informatics, Professional Practice, Recruitment & Retention, and Evidence-based Practice & Research, with each council member participating in two of the four meetings. In the afternoon the entire council comes together for Performance Improvement committee and the CNO's State-of-Affairs presentation. Each chair of the four committees then presents the work they are doing to the entire council, eliciting feedback and discussion to make decisions on moving projects forward.

Nurse autonomy and empowerment lead to increased nurse job satisfaction and improved patient outcomes. Shared governance councils also develop skills such as team building, networking, public speaking, and writing proficiency.

A team-building activity used by our NPC was to have each unit create a mosaic using any bits of material found on the unit: medication cups, pieces of disposable gloves, needle caps, and so on. The unit staff needed to think of a message or vision that they feel displays the essence of caring. Each person on the unit contributed material and time to put the mosaic together in their break room. Once completed, all the units displayed their creations in an art exhibit in our main lobby before hanging the mosaics in their units.

With each service line unit so busy in their day-to-day work they are often amazed to hear about the practices, projects, and successes on the other units. The intensive care unit (ICU) was inspired to replicate the Geriatric Unit's bereavement process of placing a wreath on the door of a patient who died, to alert the unit that quiet reflection was needed at this time. This networking encourages nurses to get to know each other as professionals and co-workers, offering opportunity to develop sharing and caring relationships with each other.

Great work needs to be shared. Publications and presentations are excellent venues to use, but public speaking and writing abstracts, or designing creative posters are often a deterrent for many nurses. Our council members have mentored and coached each other to accomplish these skills. By starting small such as presenting to each other, then to the organization, then at state and national levels, our members have experienced professional growth and self-confidence. The above mentioned mosaics were displayed at the National Magnet Conference's Art Exhibit. Our bereavement programs have been published in nursing journals and original research studies conducted by the staff through the shared governance model.

To truly be successful it takes the commitment of each participating member. Choosing membership is a crucial element and should be done at the unit level by the team. The chosen member should be seen as a representative of that unit, bringing needs and ideas from the unit for practice improvements, and bringing back to the unit the information discussed at council. It is a very rewarding opportunity for nurses to be involved in decision making. An old adage says that if you are not part of the solution you must be part of the problem. Complaining about barriers and problems will not improve the situation. It will take a professional and thoughtful approach within shared governance to identify the opportunities and problem solve using evidence-based practices.

Mary Ann Hozak, MSN, RN, NEA-BC,
Magnet Program Director, Director of Nursing Quality and Innovation
St. Joseph's Regional Medical Center, Paterson, NJ

EVIDENCE-BASED PRACTICE

Barden, A., Quinn Griffin, M., Donahue, M., Fitzpatrick, J., (2011). Shared Governance and Empowerment in Registered Nurses Working in a Hospital Setting. *Nurs Admin Q, 35(3), 212-218.*

Abstract
Empowerment of registered nurses through professional practice models inclusive of shared governance has been proposed as essential to improve quality patient care, contain costs, and retain nursing staff. The purpose of this study was to determine the relationship between perceptions of governance and empowerment among nurses working in acute care hospital units in which a shared governance model had been in place for 6 to 12 months. The 158 nurses who participated perceived themselves to be moderately empowered, and in an early implementation stage of shared governance. There was a statistically significant positive relationship between

Continued

EVIDENCE-BASED PRACTICE—cont'd

perceptions of shared governance and empowerment. Recommendations for professional practice and future research are included.

The article discusses empowerment of Registered Nurses (RNs) through professional practice models inclusive of shared governance. The authors feel that shared governance is essential to improve quality patient care, contain costs, and retain nursing staff. In today's world of cutting costs in health care, it is challenging to develop professional practice models in nursing. There are heavy workloads for nurses as a result of many factors such as nurses retiring and hospitals downsizing. This brings about serious concerns with patient safety.

Shared governance brought about in the 1980s led to nurse satisfaction and improved patient outcomes. Magnet-designated organizations from the American

Nurses Credentialing Center (ANCC), is the gold standard of knowledge and expertise. The ANCC model has five components: transformational leadership, structural empowerment, exemplary professional nursing practice, new knowledge, and innovations and improvements, and empirical quality outcomes. Nurses are attracted to hospitals with Magnet status. Hospitals with Magnet status have positive patient outcomes. When nurses are empowered to make decisions, the outcome is nursing excellence. Shared governance has been in existence for more than 20 years. Further research is needed.

Nursing administration needs to identify new strategies to empower nurses in order that nurses will continue to be integral in the health care delivery system of the present and future.

■ NCLEX® EXAMINATION QUESTIONS

1. Shared governance is:
   A. Decision making based on the principles of partnership, equality, accountability, and ownership at the point of service
   B. Decision making based on the principles of partnership, equity, accountability, and ownership at the point of service
   C. Decision making based on the principles of partnership, equity, accessibility, and ownership at the point of service
   D. Decision making based on the principles of patient care, equity, accountability, and ownership at the point of service

2. Which council is concerned with the management of resources as defined in the strategic plan and nursing conceptual framework?
   A. Nurse Executive Council
   B. Unit-Based Council
   C. Nursing quality and patient safety council
   D. Advanced practice nurse council

3. Which council provides the opportunity for APNs, with support from the Chief Nursing Officer (CNO) and the Director of Ambulatory Services, to identify areas of improvement and to share best practices within this diverse group of clinicians?
   A. Advanced Practice Nurse Council
   B. Nurse Executive Council

   C. Unit-Based Council
   D. Nursing Informatics and Communication Council

4. Which council serves as a communication link for geographically remote sites within a multicampus system that uses the same shared governance model?
   A. Nurse executive council
   B. Entity-based council
   C. Unit-based council
   D. Advanced practice nurse council

5. Which council advances the practice of nursing and fosters the nursing role in patient education through staff and development and evidence-based research initiatives?
   A. Nursing Staff Development, Education and Research Council
   B. Nurse executive council
   C. Advanced practice nurse council
   D. Nursing informatics and communication council

6. Who is responsible for answering to the board of trustees in an institution?
   A. Chief executive officer (CEO)
   B. Chief nursing officer (CNO)
   C. Chief financial officer (CFO)
   D. Safety officer

7. Self-governance:
   A. Occurs at the point of care
   B. Is position based
   C. Has high staff input
   D. Integrates equity and accountability
8. Shared governance is:
   A. Knowledge based and occurs at the point of care
   B. Position based and occurs at the point of care
   C. Knowledge based and there is limited staff input
   D. Position based with hierarchical communication
9. _____(2013) states that shared leadership/participative decision making is a model in which nurses are formally organized to make decisions about clinical practice standards, quality improvement, staff and professional development, and research.

A. American Nurses Association
B. American Nurses Credentialing Center
C. National League for Nursing
D. State boards of nursing

10. According to Burton (2004) _____is a formal, guided process for integrating the people, information, and technology of an organization, and serves as a key structural element that allows corporations to maximize value by matching their corporate design to overall strategy.
   A. Organizational design
   B. Decision making
   C. Shared governance
   D. Accountability

Answers: 1. B   2. A   3. A   4. B   5. A   6. A   7. B
8. A   9. B   10. A

REFERENCES

Anthony, M. (2004). Shared Governance Models: The Theory, Practice, and Evidence. *The Online Journal of Issues in Nursing, 9*(1). Manuscript 4. www.nursingworld.org/MainMenuCategories/ANAMarketplace/ANAPeriodicals/OJIN/TableofContents/Volume92004/No1Jan04/SharedGovernanceModels.

Batson, V. (2004). Shared Governance in an Integrated Health Care System. *AORN Online, 80*(3), 493–514. www.aornjournal.org/article/S0001-2092(06)60540-1/abstract.

Burton, R. M., DeSanctis, G., & Obel, B. (2004). *Organizational design: A step-by-step approach.* Cambridge, UK: Cambridge University Press.

George, V., Burke, L. J., Rodgers, B., Duthie, N., Hoffmann, M., Koceja, V., et al. (2002). Developing Staff Nurse Shared Leadership Behavior in Professional Practice. *Nursing Administration Quarterly, 26*(3), 44–59.

Glickman, S., Baggett, K., Krubert, C., Peterson, E., & Schulman, K. (2007). Promoting quality: The health care organization from a management perspective. *International Journal of Quality Health Care, 19*(6), 341–348.

Hess, R. (2004). From bedside to boardroom–nursing shared governance. *Online Journal of Issues in Nursing, 9*(1). www.nursingworld.org/MainMenuCategories/ANAMarketplace/ANAPeriodicals/OJIN/TableofContents/Volume92004/No1Jan04/FromBedsidetoBoardroom.aspx.

Koloroutis, M. (Ed.). (2004). *Relationship based care: A model for transforming practice.* Minneapolis, MN: Creative Health Care Management.

Kramer, M., & Schmalenburg, C. E. (2003). Magnet hospital nurses describe control over nursing practice. Western Journal of Nursing Research, 25(4), 424–452.

Nightingale, F. (1992). *Notes on nursing: What it is, and what it is not.* (Commemorative Edition). Philadelphia: J.B. Lippincott.

Porter-O'Grady, T., & Malloch, K. (2015). *Quantum leadership.* Burlington, MA: Jones & Bartlett Learning.

Porter-O'Grady, T., & Hinshaw, A.S. (2003). Introduction. The concept behind shared governance. In: Swihart, D. (Ed). *Shared Governance: A Practical Approach to Transform Professional Nursing Practice* (pp. 1–12). Danvers, MA: HCPro.

Wilson, B., Squires, M., Widger, K., Cranely, L., & Tourangeau, A. (2008). Job satisfaction among a multigenerational nursing workforce. *Journal of Nursing Management, 16*(6), 716–723.

Professional Decision Making and Advocacy

KEY TERMS

advocacy a political process by an individual or group that aims to influence public-policy and resource allocation decisions within political, economic, and social systems and institutions

policy encompasses the choices that a society, segment of society, or organization makes regarding its priorities, and the ways that it allocates resources to attain those goals

In Chapter 6, the role of the nurse in organizational decision making and accountability was discussed. The Institute of Medicine report The Future of Nursing called for the preparation of nurses to advance health across the nation. Public, private, and governmental health care decision makers at every level should include representation from nursing on boards, on executive management teams, and in other key leadership positions. (American Nurses Credentialing Center [ANCC], 2013, p. 6). American Nurses Credentialing Center (ANCC) states that Magnet nurses "support organizational goals, advance the nursing profession, and enhance professional development by extending their influence to professional and community groups" (ANCC, 2013, p. 35).

Contrary to what many nurses believe, patient and health care is a highly political activity. Nurses are engaged in a continuous competition for scarce resources on behalf of patients. Policy and politics are the ways that nurses can influence the quality, safety, and accessibility of health care in the United States. As the largest single group of health professionals (3.1 million), registered nurses have the ability to be an incredible force by sheer numbers; in addition, policymakers also rely upon nurses' expertise.

Policy has been simply defined as "authoritative decision making" (Stimpson & Hanley, 1991, p. 12). There are many types of policy:

- Public Policy: Policy formed by governmental bodies such as legislation passed by a state legislature, for example, the regulations about mandatory staffing ratios in California.
- Social Policy: Pertains to the policy decisions that promote the welfare of the public. For example, local ordinances that require children to wear helmets while bicycling.
- Health Policy: This includes actions to promote the health of individual citizens, such as health promotion reimbursements to vaccinate all children.
- Institutional Policy: These policies govern workplaces. They include the administrative and nursing polices within a healthcare organization. Such policies govern how you would practice within that institution.
- Organizational policies: This includes the positions taken by professional organizations such as the American Nurses Association (ANA), and specialty organizations. An example would be the position paper calling for the Bachelor of Science in Nursing (BSN) as the entry level for nursing licensure.

There are four major arenas of political action in nursing: the workplace, the government, professional organizations, and the community. The four spheres are shown in Figure 7-1.

Obviously your workplace will be a major arena for your work with policy development. The Magnet model requires that nurses are involved in decision-making groups throughout the organization, and in the community. In Chapter 6 shared governance structures were discussed. One of the common shared governance committees present in most hospitals is the Nursing Practice and Standards Committee. The charge of such a committee usually focuses on the definition of standards, policies, and procedures for clinical practice and care delivery across the institution. The majority of these policies deal with patient care, but there is also policy development on issues of workplace safety, professional development of nurses, staffing, and other issues that impact the delivery of care. Recent examples of issues that have resulted in policy development at the workplace level include:

- Safe patient handling.
- Creation of a just culture (discussed in Chapter 9).
- Prevention of workplace bullying (discussed in Chapter 9).
- Staffing ratios.
- Delegation of nonnursing tasks (discussed in Chapter 13).
- Roles of Advanced Practice Registered Nurses (APRNs).

Policy evaluation usually occurs on 3 year cycles within organizations. One third of existing policies are reviewed each year. New policies are developed as needed and come from new practice issues, new professional guidelines, performance outcomes, research, and other areas. They are rated according to current evidence. They can be brought forward by anyone in the institution.

Table 7-1 demonstrates an algorithm for policy review and decision making.

As a member of the Professional Practice Committee at your institution, a nurse will be asked to review a policy and to make suggestions for changes. This review will include the current practice and a literature review to determine current best evidence. The nurse is responsible for ensuring that the policies that guide your practice are current and based on sound evidence. Nurses will need to keep current through membership in professional organizations, continued professional development, and journal reading.

Another arena for political action will be through a professional organization. As a nurse, it is very important to continue professional development and to belong to a professional organization. Professional organizations play a major role in the continual shaping of nursing practice across the world. They also play a role in the continued upgrading of nursing and health care. Magnet organizations are expected to document that their nurses belong to professional organizations, and improve nursing practice because of such participation.

The American Nurses Association (ANA) represents the interests of nurses regarding many issues. Each year

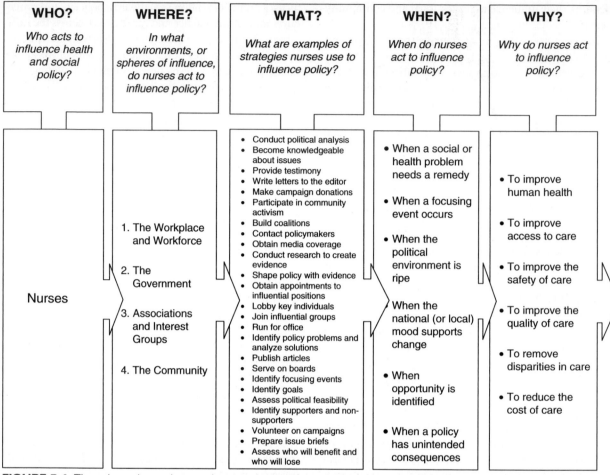

FIGURE 7-1 The who, what, where, when, and why of nursing's policy influence. From Mason, D.J., Leavett, J.K., Chaffee, M. (2016). *Policy and Politics in Nursing and Health Care*, 7th ed. St. Louis: Elsevier.

TABLE 7-1	**Policy and Procedure Algorithm Steps**
Review Steps	**Suggested Actions**
1. Select the policy for revision	Routine review or changes in practice; this process is also applicable for new policies
2. Search for evidence	Suggested approaches and sites
	Research-based evidence:
	• CINAHL and Medline databases
	• Cochrane Library
	• American College of Physicians Pier
	• National Guideline Clearinghouse (www.guideline.gov)
	• Turning Research Into Practice (www.tripdatabase.com)
	Professional Association Guidelines/Standards of Care
	University Health Consortium for other academic hospital policies/procedures
	Local standards or policies
	Expert opinion/clinical expertise
	• Clinical articles
	• Web search
	• Clinical experts

TABLE 7-1 Policy and Procedure Algorithm Steps—cont'd

Review Steps	Suggested Actions
3. Systematic evaluation of the evidence	Critically appraise research evidence • Assign level of evidence: a method of evaluating the strength of the evidence using the Stetler model • Consider a mechanism for organization of evidence, e.g., an evidence table may be constructed
4. Compare evidence to current policy and make a decision	Decision point • Make no changes • Make language more precise or update references • Revise policy to incorporate new evidence • Develop new policy or procedure based on evidence if indicated • Retire or delete policy if no longer effective for quality patient care
5. Policy review by stakeholders/experts	Send revised policy to stakeholders who have reviewed prior versions of the policy or determine who is appropriate to review a new policy
6. Make revisions based on stakeholder/experts' comments	
7. Obtain approval signatures	E-mail signature is accepted at UCH
8. Submit policy to Patient Care Policy and Procedure Subcommittee	**Final recommendations and approval by the committee**
9. Staff education as needed	Present to Nurse Educator Council if needed
10. Web submission	Hospital-wide policies are located on the hospital's intranet

CINAHL, Cumulative Index to Nursing and Allied Health Literature; *UCH,* University of Colorado Hospital. From Oman, K., Duran, C., & Fink, R. (2008). Evidence-based policy and procedures. *Journal of Nursing Administration,* 38(1), 49.

they track over 1000 nursing and health care–related bills across all states, examining priority issues, and trends. They also release position statements on many issues of importance to nursing and health care in the United States. In 2012, the following issues were brought forward to the ANA House of Delegates for policy development.

• Rights of registered nurses handling drugs.
• Reproductive rights of registered nurses handling hazardous drugs.
• Workplace violence.
• Revision of the House of Delegates Policy on Representation of certified medical assistants (CMAs) in the ANA House of Delegates.
• A process for optimal nurse staffing in acute care settings.
• Nurses' roles in recognizing educating and advocating for healthy energy choices.

Full descriptions are available at http://ananet.nursingworld.org/Main-Menu/Governance/HOD-Delegates/Reference-Process-2012/Resolution-Index_1.aspx.

For a listing of the position statements of the ANA go to www.nursingworld.org/positionstatements.

The ANA also supports worthy candidates for federal office who have demonstrated their belief in the legislative and regulatory agenda of the ANA through their Political Action Committee (ANA-PAC).

Although nurses represent one of the largest workforces in the nation at 3.1 million, it is estimated that only 5% belong to the ANA. Many nurses belong to a specialty nursing organization, but the estimate is that they only represent 30% of the total nursing workforce. If you, as a nurse, are to have an impact on policy development that affects your workplace and the health of your community, it is imperative you belong to a professional organization.

The third arena of political activity for nurses is the government. Nurses are increasingly entering government at local, state, and federal levels. There are presently six nurses serving in the U.S. Congress. Government plays an enormously important role in nursing and health care. Nursing practice acts are determined through state legislation. Reimbursements for health care are determined at the federal level.

Issues of importance during the 2013 federal legislative calendar included the following:

SCOPE OF PRACTICE

Advanced Practice Registered Nurses

- Barriers to the Practice of Advanced Practice Registered Nurses.
- Home Health: Plan of Care Designation.
- Medicaid Coverage of Advanced Practice Nursing.

HEALTH CARE INNOVATION

Advanced Practice Registered Nurses

- Provides neutral language.
- Care coordination.

SAFE STAFFING

Appropriate Staffing

- Acute care staffing.

WORK ENVIRONMENT AND HEALTHY NURSE

Workplace Health and Safety

- Safe Patient Handling and Mobility.

QUALITY

Health Care Quality Measures

- Press Ganey Patient Satisfaction Survey

OTHER ISSUES

Gun Violence

- Assault Weapons Ban of 2013 Senate.
- Assault Weapons Ban of 2013 House.
- Safe Communities Safe Schools Act Senate.

Medical Malpractice Liability/Tort Reform
Mental Health Care

- S. 689 the Mental Health Awareness and Improvement Act of 2013.

Patient Safety/Advocacy

- The Affordable Care Act.
- Appropriations.

- Rules and regulations.
- State exchange implementation.

Protection of Medicare/Medicaid

Social Security

NURSING SHORTAGE

- Title VIII: Funding for nursing workforce development programs.
- Immigration and nursing workforce.
  (www.nursingworld.org/MainMenuCategories/Policy-Advocacy/Federal/113th-Congress-Federal-Legislative-Agenda)

One final point is that the nurse can have a tremendous impact on the health of the community. Nursing contributions to improved community health have a historical perspective, and are currently recognized and expected in Magnet organizations. Historically, nurses such as Florence Nightingale improved sanitation services in England, thereby reducing cholera in London. Lillian Wald greatly improved the health care access to services in early 1900s New York through the development of the Henry Street Settlement. Although you may not see yourself as in the same league as these iconic nurses, you have the responsibility of working to improve the health of the community. You may be called upon to support the agenda of communities that are trying to develop a better place for their citizens to live. Nurses are often asked to serve on local boards of health, and boards of education. You may also be asked to serve on local advisory boards/committees such as community planning boards and senior services advisory boards.

The Institute of Medicine (IOM) report challenges nurses and society to ensure that nurses are represented in leadership positions in health care, including governing boards. The sparse data that exist indicate that physicians comprise more than 20% of the governing board members of hospitals, and less than 5% are nurses. In this era of greater accountability for clinical performance, the role of the nurse in improving processes and accountability of care is paramount. A recent study in New York City documented a slight increase in nurse membership on organizational decision making, with 93% of hospitals reporting physicians on their governing boards, compared with 26% with nurses, 7% with dentists, and 4% with social workers, or psychologists. The overrepresentation of physicians declined with the other health care organizations (HCOs). Only 38% of home care agencies had physicians on their governing boards, 29% had nurses, and 24% had social workers. What better representative of the community that an organization serves than the professionally educated nurse? Nurses possess a level of insight into health care issues and policymaking unlike any other health care professional.

What can you as a nurse do to influence policy?

1. Keep abreast of developments. Know what is happening both in your community and in the country generally. Keep up-to-date with public issues by attending public meetings and reading newspapers and journals
2. Write and publish. Well-placed articles can help influence opinion. Keep an eye on newsworthy issues that would benefit from a nursing perspective.
3. Join professional organizations that match your interests and share your positions. Your contribution might be more effective if channeled through a larger group with an established reputation and credibility.
4. Know who key players are such as politicians and officials in local, regional, and national government.
5. Know the key nursing positions and networks that you (or your organization) might work with to have input into policy.
6. Identify nurses in influential positions outside nursing. They may be in policy or senior management positions in departments of health or other health organizations. These groups can be useful resources to help you achieve your health policy goals.
7. Communicate your position through:
   - Ongoing representation on policymaking.
   - Committees or boards.
   - Lobbying.
   - Making submissions.
   - Meeting with people in positions of influence.

CLINICAL CORNER

The Importance of a Nurse on a Board of Trustees

I have been privileged enough to serve as a member of various boards of trustees, overseeing the operations of health care facilities. As a nurse, I feel that I bring a unique perspective to the governing board of a health care organization. It seems natural that a nurse should be a member of such governing boards, yet it is often not the case.

The Institute of Nursing Report (2011) on the Future of Nursing talks of the importance of nursing leadership on governing boards. The report states that "private, public, and governmental healthcare decision makers at every level should include representation from nursing on boards, on executive management teams, and on other key leadership positions" (IOM, 2011). Nurses do indeed serve in leadership positions, serving on executive management teams as chief nursing officers, yet only 6% of board positions were held by nurses; 20% are physicians. (AHA, 2011).

It is interesting that nurses are seldom viewed as leaders in the development of health care systems and delivery (Khoury et al., 2011). But...nurses are consistently rated as the most ethical profession (Gallup, 2012) and survey reports say that nurses should have more input and impact in policy development (Khoury et al., 2011). Respondents from this same survey said that nurses should have more influence in reducing medical errors, increasing the quality of care, and influencing health care efficiency and reducing costs (as cited in Hassmiller & Combes, 2012). Who better than a nurse, then, for a leadership position on a board of trustees?

As a board member, I feel that I bring a unique perspective to the operations of the health care facility. The majority of employees in the system are nurses, so I bring a unique understanding of their perspective to the decision making of the board. I also have a knowledge of the current evidence and best practice in nursing and health care that form important decision points in the strategic plan of the organization.

A nurse also brings a unique broad-based skill and knowledge set to the table. We have experienced the various patient care processes that either facilitate or impede patient care. Such knowledge can assist the health care institution in the development of patient care processes that are efficient and patient friendly. A nurse also understands the complicated world of health care reimbursement and its relationship to patient satisfaction and high-quality care. As a nurse, I have an awareness of the job design of care delivery, the actual work systems, the community orientation, and the accountability of patient care outcomes as well as a documented ability to lead.

I am often asked "What is the nursing perspective" and it is interesting that a this perspective at times is different from that of the larger group. One such difference came with the advent of the electronic medical record (EMR) within a health care facility. The initial timeline of implementation for the EMR project dealt with the physician order being set as the first outcome. These order sets were in the very early stages of implementation and would

Continued

CLINICAL CORNER—cont'd

The Importance of a Nurse on a Board of Trustees

have prolonged the EMR implementation for 18 months. A stronger knowledge of physician ordering patterns was required to fully implement the order sets. The nursing documentation and medication administration system implementation would be able to be implemented within 1 year, and would be able to provide a wealth of information regarding physician ordering. Along with the nursing executive team, I was able to alter the EMR implementation timeline to allow the organization to learn from the rich data being made available from the new EMR. As the physician order sets were evaluated, a wealth of information evaluated against current evidence allowed the organization to more fully integrate best practice with order sets.

Nurse leaders understand the requirements of day-to-day patient care and they understand the constraints on health care quality and outcomes. They have the ability and skills necessary to drive improvement, deal with conflict management, and facilitate decision making, as well as the compassion and capacity to positively impact patient care across all communities. Who better to be a board member, but a NURSE!

References

American Hospital Association. (2011). *AHA hospital statistics*. Chicago AHA.

Gallup Survey. (2011). *Nurses Top Honesty and Ethics List for 11th Year*. Retrieved from www.gallup.com/poll/145043/Nurses-Top-Honesty-Ethics-List-11-Year.aspx. April, 12, 2015.

Hassmiller, S., & Combes, J. (2012). Nurse leaders in the boardroom: A fitting choice. *Journal of HealthCare Management, 57*(1).

Institute of Medicine. (2011). *The future of nursing: Leading change advancing health*. Washington, DC: The National Academies Press.

Khoury, C., Blizzard, R., Moore, L., & Hassmiller, S. (2011). Nursing leadership from bedside to boardroom: A Gallup national survey of opinion leaders. *Journal of Nursing Administration, 41*(7/8), 299–305.

Kathleen M. Burke, PhD, RN

EVIDENCE-BASED PRACTICE

Mason, D., Keepnews, D., Homberg, J., Murray, E. (2013).The Representation of Health Professionals on Governing Boards of Health Care Organizations in New York City, *J Urban Health* 90(5), 888-901.

Mason, D., Leavitt, J., & Chafee, M. (2007, 2014). *Policy and Politics in Nursing and Health Care*. St Louis: Elsevier.

Mason, D., Keepnews, D., Homberg, J., Murray, E. (2013). The Representation of Health Professionals on Governing Boards of Health Care Organizations in New York City. *J Urban Health* (90)5, 888-901.

Abstract

The Representation of Health Professionals on Governing Boards of Health Care Organizations in New York City.

The heightened importance of processes and outcomes of care, including their impact on health care organizations' (HCOs) financial health, translate into greater accountability for clinical performance on the part of HCO leaders, including their boards, during an era of health care reform. Quality and safety of care are now fiduciary responsibilities of HCO board members. The participation of health professionals on HCO governing bodies may be an asset to HCO governing boards because of their deep knowledge of clinical problems, best practices, quality indicators, and other issues related to the safety and quality of care. And yet, the sparse data that exist indicate that physicians comprise more than 20% of the governing board members of hospitals, whereas less than 5% are nurses, and no data exist on other health professionals. The purpose of this two-phased study is to examine health professionals' representations on HCOs—specifically hospitals, home care agencies, nursing homes, and federally qualified health centers—in New York City. Through a survey of these organizations, phase 1 of the study found that 93% of hospitals had physicians on their governing boards, compared with 26% with nurses, 7% with dentists, and 4% with social workers or psychologists. The overrepresentation of physicians declined with the other HCOs. Only 38% of home care agencies had physicians on their governing boards, 29% had nurses, and 24% had social workers. Phase 2 focused on the barriers to the appointment of health professionals to governing boards of HCOs, and the strategies to address these barriers. Sixteen health care leaders in the region were interviewed in this qualitative study. Barriers included invisibility of health professionals other than physicians; concerns about "special interests"; lack of financial resources for donations to the organization; and lack of knowledge and skills with regard to board governance, especially financial matters. Strategies included developing an infrastructure for preparing and getting appointed various health professionals, mentoring, and developing a personal plan of action for appointments.

NCLEX® EXAMINATION QUESTIONS

1. A political process by an individual or group that aims to influence public policy and resource allocation decisions within political, economic, and social systems and institutions is:
   A. Policy change
   B. Advocacy
   C. Institutional policy
   D. Public policy

2. Nurses represent one of the largest workforces in the nation at 3.1 million. It is estimated that only _____% belong to the American Nurses Association.
   A. 5
   B. 10
   C. 15
   D. 20

3. Which of the following would be an example of a policy dealing with workplace safety?
   A. Safe patient handling
   B. Prevention of workplace bullying
   C. Staffing ratios
   D. All of the above are correct

4. There are four major areas of political action in nursing. They are:
   A. The workplace, the government, professional organizations, and the community
   B. The workplace, the educational institutions, professional organizations, and the community
   C. The government, professional organizations, and the state regulators
   D. The government, the community, and nursing boards

5. Which of the following is a policy that pertains to the positions taken by professional organizations such as ANA?
   A. Health
   B. Organizational
   C. Institutional
   D. Health

6. Which of the following is a policy that pertains to the governing of workplaces?
   A. Social
   B. Health
   C. Organizational
   D. Institutional

7. Which of the following is a policy that pertains to the decisions that promote the welfare of the public?
   A. Social
   B. Health
   C. Organizational
   D. Public

8. Which of the following is a policy formed by governmental bodies such as legislation passed by a state legislature?
   A. Social
   B. Health
   C. Organizational
   D. Public

9. Public, private, and governmental health care decision makers at every level should include representation from nursing on:
   A. Nursing boards
   B. Executive management teams
   C. Key leadership positions
   D. All of the above are correct

10. The American Nurses Credentialing Center (ANCC) (2013, p. 35) states that Magnet nurses "support organizational goals, advance the nursing profession, and enhance professional development by:
    A. Extending their influence to professional and community groups
    B. Increasing the number of nurses obtaining ANCC certification
    C. Increasing the number of BSN nurses in their facilities
    D. Speaking at professional conferences

Answers: 1. B   2. A   3. D   4. A   5. B   6. D   7. A   8. D   9. D   10. A

REFERENCES

American Nurses Association [ANA]. (2014). Policy and Advocacy. Retrieved from http://nursingworld.org/MainMenuCategories/Policy-Advocacy. July 19.

American Nurses Credentialing Center [ANCC]. (2013, 2014). *Magnet application manual.* Silver Spring, MD: ANCC.

International Council of Nurses (ICN). (2005). Guidelines for Shaping Effective Health Policy. www.nursecredentialing.org/MagnetApplicationManual www.icn.ch/images/stories/documents/publications/guidelines/guideline_shaping.pdf.

Lyttle, B. (2011). Politics: A natural step for nurses. *American Journal of Nursing, 111*(5), 19–20.

Mason, D., Leavitt, J., & Chafee, M. (2012). *Policy and politics in nursing and health care.* St Louis: Elsevier.

Mason, D., Keepnews, D., Homberg, J., & Murray, E. (2013). The representation of health professionals on governing boards of health care organizations in New York City. *Journal of Urban Health, 90*(5), 888–901.

Oman, K., Duran, C., & Fink, R. (2008). Evidence based policy and procedures. *Journal of Nursing Administration, 38*(1), 47–51.

Stimpson, M., & Hanley, B. (1991). Nurse policy analysis. *Nursing and Health Care, 12*(1), 10–15.

8

Communication in the Work Environment

OBJECTIVES

- Identify the principles of good communication.
- Discuss the importance of good communication in the management of care.
- Identify various means of communication used in health care.
- Review the components of a change-of-shift report.
- Discuss SBAR (situation, background, assessment, recommendation) communication and its use in health care.

- Discuss Team STEPPS (Team Strategies and Tools to Enhance Performance and Patient Safety) and its importance in the safe delivery of care.
- Identify principles of communication when dealing with patients/families and staff members.
- Review communication principles when dealing with conflict resolution.

OUTLINE

KEY TERMS

change-of-shift report process by which patient information is shared by nurses who have taken care of the patient for the previous shift, and are reporting to the incoming care givers.

communication process by which information is shared between and among individuals.

computerized physician order entry process by which clinician orders are entered through electronic information systems.

handoff the transfer of information (along with authority and responsibility) during transitions in care across the continuum; to include an opportunity to ask questions, clarify, and confirm.

huddle ad hoc planning to reestablish situation awareness; reinforcing plans already in place; and assessing the need to adjust the plan.

SBAR template for communication among professionals that includes communication about situation, background, assessment, and recommendation.

Team STEPPS an evidence-based framework to optimize team performance across the health care delivery system.

COMMUNICATION

Communication forms the basic principle when managing and coordinating care. Much of what nurses do needs to be communicated to the patient, family, and fellow staff members. Professional communication sets the tone of our management style, and often the tone of the unit in which we work. Communication and the lack of a consistent process for communication of a patient's condition have been cited as variables in the number of medical errors that occur in hospitals. A recommendation of the Institute of Medicine calls for hospitals to "develop a working culture in which communication flows freely" (1999, p. 180).

Sullivan and Decker (2009) note five principles of effective communication:

- Giving information is not the same as communication, which requires interaction, understanding, and response. For example, if a nurse asks a staff member to do something, but the staff member does not understand, information has been given, but communication has not occurred.
- The sender of the communication is responsible for clarity. Nurses and nurse managers must make sure that their communication is clear; it is not the job of the receiver of the message "to translate." If the receiver of the message has to translate the message, the possibility of error increases. For example, if you expect the unlicensed nursing personnel to report back to you immediately if a patient's temperature increases, you need to specifically say just that.
- Use simple, exact language. The sender of the message needs to use words that are easily understood by the receiver of the communication. The words need to be precise and unambiguous. A word about e-mail communication; "I" message language is inappropriate; professional e-mail needs to avoid the use of all slang and shortcuts.
- Communication encourages feedback. Although feedback is not always positive, it is essential for making sure that the receiver understands the message. It is not enough to ask, "Did you understand?" The answer may be an automatic "yes" because the receiver expects that is what you want to hear. Feedback can be verbal ("I do not understand what you said"), or nonverbal (rolling of eyes when asked to do a task).
- Sender must have credibility. A credible sender is perceived as trustworthy and reliable. Receivers who think the sender is not reliable may ignore the message.
- Use direct communication channels when possible. Direct communication (person to person, face to face, or in writing) is best because there is less chance of the message being distorted as it passes through senders. Face-to-face communication is preferred as it allows the sender to get immediate feedback about the message.

E-mail

In the new technological age, much of interdepartmental and staff-to-staff communication involves electronic mail, or e-mail. Communication using such technology should follow the principles just stated, but also needs to follow the basic principles of e-mail netiquette. Tschabitscher (2005) offers 10 rules for e-mail netiquette, which have been adapted as follow:

1. Use e-mail the way you want everybody to use it: Do not use it to send nonprofessional concerns.
2. Take another look before you send the message: Proofread your comments for appropriateness and confidentiality.
3. Quote original messages properly in replies: Make your e-mail replies easy to read by quoting in a useful manner.
4. Avoid irony, sarcasm, and emotional tones in e-mail: Keep the message objective.
5. Clean up e-mails before forwarding them: Forwarding e-mails is a great way of keeping track of a concern but make sure that the original idea is not lost.
6. Send plain text e-mails: Avoid fancy formatting of e-mails. Cutesy pictures are for personal, not professional, communication.
7. Writing in all capital letters is shouting: Capital letters are also difficult to read.
8. Ask before you send large attachments: Large attachments may clog e-mail systems.
9. The use of "smileys" raises an alarm: Avoid the use of emoticons, instant messaging (IM) language, texting shortcuts, and Internet slang.
10. Avoid "me too" messages: Content needs to be specific and complete.
11. Do not "reply to all": unless that is the intent of the message.

(Adapted from *Top 26 Most Important Rules of Email Etiquette.* Copyright 2009 by Heinz Tschabitscher. http://email.about.com/od/emailnetiquette/tp/core_netiquette.htm. Used with permission.)

COMMUNICATION WITH PATIENTS AND STAFF

Nurses and nurse leaders also communicate with families and staff. Difficult situations often involve patients and staff, and disagreements, or complaints about the delivery of, or assignments of care. According to Sullivan and Decker (2009), nurse leaders need to keep the following in mind when dealing with patient or staff issues:

- Patients and their families are customers and should be communicated to with honesty and respect. Even if the communication involves dealing with a complaint, the customer needs to receive prompt and tactful assistance. The same philosophy is appropriate for an employee; he or she is a stakeholder in the work environment, and also requires honesty and respect in communication.

- Nurses need to find a balance between avoiding medical jargon that is too complex, and using terms that are too simple and condescending. Paying attention to both verbal and nonverbal feedback will help nurse managers negotiate this challenge.

- Provide angry, or upset customers, or staff members a private, neutral place for communicating their concerns.

- When possible, if customers or stakeholders are not native speakers, and/or are not fluent in English, try to provide interpreter service. For patients, professional interpreters and language lines (including those for American Sign Language) should be used. Unless it is an emergency, do not use family members, as the practice is a potential violation of patient privacy. Family members also may have an agenda that will bias their communication with the patient. Each hospital has specific regulations about patient translation and privacy regulations. When communicating to fellow employees with limited language skills, make sure that the message is clear and understood.

- Learn about cultural issues to be able to recognize communication issues with both patients and staff members that are culturally based. Culturally competent responses to patients and fellow staff greatly enhance communication.

There are many modes of communication in the health care organization. One mode is used to communicate with the patient and family. Much of the nursing curricula have been spent on the theories and principles of professional and therapeutic communication. The Joint Commission (2014) also has some very specific regulations dealing with patient/family communication, and the necessity of open and honest communication. It is crucial that patients and families understand the communication that is directed toward them. Cultural competence in communication is a vital skill of every nurse.

Another mode of communication deals with communication about the patient. Hospitals are institutions that are operational on a 24-hour-a-day/7-day-a-week basis and therefore require communication processes that are sound and reliable and can communicate vital patient information. The communication processes also need to follow Health Insurance Portability and Accountability Act (HIPAA) guidelines (see Chapter 17). Processes that are used in the communication of patient care include transcription of orders, change-of-shift report, **SBAR (situation, background, assessment, recommendation) reporting,** and **Team STEPPS (Team Strategies and Tools to Enhance Performance and Patient Safety)** communication methods.

Communication among health care professionals remains one of the most challenging concerns reported by the professionals. There are many reasons for inadequate communication, but there are approaches that have been found to improve patient safety, and to make interprofessional communication more consistent. Table 8-1 reviews

TABLE 8-1 **Barriers to Communication with Suggested Strategies**		
Barriers	**Tools & Strategies**	**Outcomes**
Inconsistency in team membership	Brief Huddle	Shared mental
Lack of time	Debrief	model
Lack of information sharing	STEPP Cross	Adaptability Team
Hierarchy	monitoring	orientation
Defensiveness	Feedback	Mutual trust
Conventional thinking	Advocacy and	Team per-
Complacency	assertion	formance
Varying communication styles	Two-challenge rule	*Patient Safety!!*
Conflict	CUS	
Lack of coordination and follow-up with co-workers	DESC script Collaboration SBAR	
Distractions	Call-out	
Fatigue	Check-back	
Workload	Handoff	
Misinterpretation of cues		
Lack of role clarity		

CUS, Concerned, uncomfortable, safety of the resident is at risk; *DESC,* describe, express, specify, consequences; *SBAR,* situation, background, assessment, recommendation; *STEPP,* Strategies and Tools to Enhance Performance and Patient Safety. Agency for Health care Research and Quality (AHRQ) (2014). Team STEPPS www.ahrq.gov/professionals/education/curriculum-tools/teamstepps/instructor/essentials/pocketguide.html.

TABLE 8-2   Key Principles

Team Structure
Delineates fundamentals such as team size, membership, leadership, composition, identification, and distribution.

Leadership
Ability to coordinate the activities of team members by ensuring team actions are understood, changes in information are shared, and that team members have the necessary resources.

Situation Monitoring
Process of actively scanning and assessing situational elements to gain information and understanding or maintain awareness to support functioning of the team.

Mutual Support
Ability to anticipate and support other team members' needs through accurate knowledge about their responsibilities and workload.

Communication
Process by which information is clearly and accurately exchanged among team members.

AHRQ (2014). www.ahrq.gov/professionals/education/curriculum-tools/teamstepps/instructor/essentials/pocketguide.html.

some of the barriers reported by health care team members and potential strategies to improve communication.

Team STEPPS is an important communication method when working in team situations. The majority of care is delivered in an interdisciplinary manner, and communication among all team members needs to be open, honest, and reliable. The principles of Team STEPPS culture are listed in Table 8-2. The team, whose responsibility it will be to care for the patient over the next 8 to 12 hours, forms during the change of shift. The communication that will occur among this team is a vital process for ensuring patient safety.

An Effective Team Leader Will:

- Organize the team.
- Articulate clear goals.
- Make decisions through collective input of members.
- Empower members to speak up and challenge when appropriate.
- Actively promote and facilitate good teamwork.
- Be skillful at conflict resolution.

Team Events that will Occur During the Shift Include:
Planning

- *Brief*: Short session before start of shift to discuss team formation; assign essential roles; establish expectations and climate; and anticipate outcomes and likely contingencies.

Problem Solving

- *Huddle:* Ad hoc planning to reestablish situation awareness; reinforce plans already in place; and assess the need to adjust the plan. Huddles also occur after unexpected events such as patient falls, and for evaluation of the safety of the situation.

Process Improvement

- *Debrief*: Informal information exchange session designed to improve team performance and effectiveness; after action review. This is important in the culture of continual improvement; a team always needs to consider how to improve their performance.

Brief Checklist
During the brief, the team should address the following questions:
___ Who is on the team?
___ Do all members understand and agree upon goals?
___ Are roles and responsibilities are understood?
___ What is our plan of care?
___ What is staff and provider availability throughout the shift?
___ What is the workload among team members?
___ What is the availability of resources?

Debrief Checklist
The team should address the following questions during a debrief:
___ Communication clear?
___ Roles and responsibilities understood?
___ Situation awareness maintained?
___ Workload distribution equitable?
___ Task assistance requested or offered?
___ Were errors made or avoided? Availability of resources?
___ What went well, what should change, what should improve?

AHRQ. (2014).Team STEPPS. www.ahrq.gov/professionals/education/curriculum-tools/teamstepps/instructor/essentials/pocketguide.html.

The feedback loop is very important in the improvement of care (AHRQ, 2014). Feedback should be a routine component of daily patient care. Feedback is information provided for the purpose of improving team performance.

Feedback, which should be:

Timely: Given soon after the target behavior has occurred.

Respectful: Focus on behaviors, not personal attributes.

Specific: Be specific about what behaviors need correcting.

Directed toward improvement: Provide directions for future improvement.

Considerate: Consider a team member's feelings and deliver negative information with fairness and respect.

Communication About the Patients: Transcription of Orders

The creation of physicians' and nursing orders in patient care forms the basis of the therapeutic regimen for the patient. This was often divided into two processes: the transcription of the physician's orders, and the creation of the nursing care plan. Both of these documents need to be communicated effectively to all members of the health care team. Historically, the nurse has been responsible and accountable for the transcription process. This accountability was, and remains documented by the nurse "signing off" the order as it is transcribed. With the increasing use of computerized physician order entry (CPOE), the role of the nurse in the transcription process is changing (Box 8-1). The order is transmitted directly by the physician or practitioner to the specific patient department, and is automatically placed on the order sheets. A new order alert is highlighted on the computer system when a new order is entered. These orders are then integrated with the existing therapeutic regimen that is part of the computerized record. The electronic medical record (EMR) is further discussed in Chapter 16.

In agencies where there is no CPOE, it will be important to follow the policy for transcription of orders. Each institution has specific guidelines dealing with the transcription of orders, and one must be familiar with the institution's guidelines. A sample policy for the transcription of orders is shown in Figure 8-1.

Examples of communication about orders are also seen in the verbalization of orders with actions, such as in the following examples.

BOX 8-1 Impact of Computerized Physician Order Entry

Handwritten orders have become a thing of the past for patients and their care givers in the John Dempsey Hospital (UConn Health Center, Farmington, CT) intensive care and cardiac step-down units, where an electronic system for entering physicians' orders was recently adopted. The system, introduced on a pilot basis on one of the surgical floors last spring, is designed to improve patient safety and reduce medical errors.

"The electronic physician order entry system not only eliminates handwriting and transcription errors, it provides many online alerts and warnings for clinical caregivers, and distributes orders as they are written directly and immediately to ancillary units," says Roberta Luby, assistant vice president for information technology strategic projects, who supervised the rollout." The process is much safer and more streamlined."

When a physician orders a medication for a patient with the new electronic system, the order goes to the pharmacy with no manual intervention.

Goodnough, K. (2007). Electronic system for physician orders improves patient safety. *UConn Advance, 25*(29).

Call-Out

Strategy used to communicate important or critical information.

- Informs all team members simultaneously during emergent situations.
- Helps team members anticipate next steps.
- Directs responsibility to a specific individual responsible for carrying out the task.
  Example during an incoming trauma:

Leader: "Airway status?"
Resident: "Airway clear"
Leader: "Breath sounds?"
Resident: "Breath sounds decreased on right"
Leader: "Blood pressure?"
Nurse: "BP is 96/62"

Check-Back

Process of using closed-loop communication to ensure that information conveyed by the sender is understood by the receiver as intended.

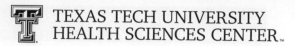

TEXAS TECH UNIVERSITY
HEALTH SCIENCES CENTER.

Ambulatory Clinic Policy and Procedure

Title:	Orders, Receiving and Noting	Policy Number:	3.04
		Version Number	4
Regulation Reference:	Joint Commission, Current Nursing Skills Test	Effective Date:	6/2011
		Original Approval:	4/2002

POLICY STATEMENT:

It is the policy of TTUHSC Ambulatory Clinics to accurately transcribe orders and to implement the orders correctly and efficiently. Orders transcription may be done by an RN or LVN.

SCOPE:

This policy applies to all TTUHSC ambulatory clinic operations conducted through its Schools of Medicine and School of Nursing.

PROCEDURE:

1. **Who May Give or Write Orders** – Only licensed providers (attending physician, consultant, fellow, resident, physician assistant or nurse practitioner) may give or write orders. Orders written by students, authorized as part of their education program, will not be honored by the nursing staff or ancillary personnel unless validated/countersigned by a licensed physician.

2. **Verbal and Telephone Orders** – Verbal orders, except telephone orders, will be accepted in emergencies or when it is not practical for the physician to write the order. Orders must be given to an RN or LVN.

    a. The RN or LVN should record the order directly onto a clinic progress note, labeled "T.O" or "V.O."

    b. The RN or LVN should read back what has been written to the ordering physician, validating the accuracy of the order.

    c. The verbal order and documentation should include:

        1) Date and time received

        2) Patient name, age, weight (when appropriate)

        3) Drug name

        4) Dosage form

        5) Exact strength or concentration

        6) Dose frequency and route

        7) Purpose indication (as appropriate)

3. **Registered Nurse or Licensed Vocational Nurse**

    a. Reviews orders and identifies those needing immediate attention

    b. Documents final validation or orders by signing first initial, last name, title, date, and time (as appropriate to clinic documentation).

    c. The order should be signed by the physician or practitioner as soon as possible.

CERTIFICATION:

This policy was approved by the Deans for the Schools of Medicine and Nursing June 2011.

FIGURE 8-1 Sample policy for transcription of orders. (Texas Tech University Health Sciences Center. [2007]. Orders, receiving and noting. Policy No. 3.04. http://www.ttuhsc.edu/provost/clinic/policies/ACPolicy3.04.pdf.)

The steps include the following:
    Sender initiates the message
    Receiver accepts the message and provides feedback
    Sender double-checks to ensure that the message
        was received

Example:
Doctor: "Give 25 mg Benadryl IV push"
Nurse: "25 mg Benadryl IV push"
Doctor: "That's correct"

AHRQ. (2014).Team STEPPS. www.ahrq.gov/professionals/education/curriculum-tools/teamstepps/instructor/essentials/pocketguide.html.

The communication of these orders to all care givers is the responsibility of the nurse. The order needs to be communicated directly to others as it was entered. The manner in which these orders are communicated varies, but many institutions use a nursing care plan, medication/therapeutic orders, and nursing flow sheet to communicate the plan of care. These plans are also communicated via the change-of-shift report.

Communication About the Patients: Changes in Condition

Nurses are also expected to communicate changes in patient conditions to the team caring for the patient. This communication may be made to the physician to receive a new set of medical orders, to members of the health care team to update them on a patient's condition, or to a rapid response team. SBAR is a communication mechanism useful for framing any conversation, especially those requiring a rapid response from a clinician (Institute for Healthcare Improvement, 2007). Figure 8-2 shows a template for an SBAR report to a physician, which can be used in a number of situations requiring communication about a patient's condition.

The following guidelines need to be followed:
1. Before calling the physician, follow these steps:
   - Have I seen and assessed the patient myself before calling?
   - Has the situation been discussed with the nursing coordinator?
   - Review the chart for the appropriate physician to call.
   - Know the admitting diagnosis and date of admission.
   - Have I read the most recent physician's progress notes, and notes from the nurse who worked the shift before me?
   - Have available the following when speaking with the physician:
     - Patient's chart.
     - List of current medications, allergies, intravenous fluids, and labs.
     - Most recent vital signs.
     - Reporting lab results: provide the date and time test was done and results of previous tests for comparison.
     - Code status.
2. When calling the physician, follow the SBAR process:
   (S) **Situation:** What is the situation you are calling about?
   - Identify self, unit, patient, and room number.
   - Briefly state the problem, what it is, when it happened or started, and the severity.
   (B) **Background:** Pertinent background information related to the situation could include the following:
   - Admitting diagnosis and date of admission
   - List of current medications, allergies, intravenous fluids, and labs
   - Most recent vital signs
   - Lab results: provide the date and time test was done and results of previous tests for comparison
   - Other clinical information
   - Code status
   (A) **Assessment:** What is the nurse's assessment of the situation?
   (R) **Recommendation:** What is the nurse's recommendation, or what does he or she want?
   Examples:
   - Notification that patient has been admitted
   - Patient needs to be seen now
   - Order change
3. Document the change in the patient's condition and physician notification.

Communication About the Patients: Change of Shift

Change-of-shift reports vary across institutions. The purposes of the report are to exchange information that is necessary for future patient care, and to discuss the present status of the patient. These reports occur during the overlapping time between shifts. They occur in a variety of ways, with the most common being (1) change-of-shift

S	**Situation**
	I am calling about <u><patient name and location></u>
	The patient's code status is <u><code status></u>
	The problem I am calling about is_____
	    I am afraid the patient is going to arrest
	
	I have just assessed the patient personally:
	
	Vital signs are: Blood pressure_____ /_____ Pulse_____ Respiration_____ Temperature_____
	
	I am concerned about the:
	    Blood pressure because it is over 200 or less than 100 or 30 mmHg below usual
	    Pulse because it is over 140 or less than 50
	    Respiration because it is less than 5 or over 40
	    Temperature because it is less than 96 or over 104

B	**Background**
	The patient's mental status is:
	    Alert and oriented to person, place, and time
	    Confused and cooperative or noncooperative
	    Agitated or combative
	    Lethargic but conversant and able to swallow
	    Comatose, eyes closed, not responding to stimulation
	The skin is:
	    Warm and dry
	    Pale
	    Mottled
	    Diaphoretic
	    Extremities are cold
	    Extremities are warm
	The patient is not or is on oxygen
	    The patient has been on _____ (l/min) or (percent) oxygen for _____ minutes (hours)

A	**Assessment** This is what I think the problem is: <u><say what you think is the problem></u> The problem seems to be Cardiac infection neurologic respiratory I am not sure what the problem is, but the patient is deteriorating The patient seems to be unstable and may get worse, we need to do something

R	**Recommendation**
	I suggest or request that you <u><say what you would like to see done></u>
	    Transfer the patient to critical care
	    Come to see the patient at this time
	    Talk to the patient or family about code status
	    Ask the on-call family practice resident to see the patient now
	    Ask for a consultant to see the patient now
	Are any tests needed:
	    Do you need any tests like CXR ABG EKG CBC or BMP?
	    Others?
	If a change in treatment is ordered then ask:
	    How often do you want vital signs?
	    How long do you expect this problem will last?
	    If the patient does not get better, when would you want us to call again?

FIGURE 8-2 This SBAR tool was developed by Kaiser Permanente. Used with permission from the Institute for Healthcare Improvement.

meetings where the outgoing and the incoming nurses meet face to face for a review of the pertinent information; (2) tape-recorded reports in which the outgoing nurse "reports" all pertinent information to the incoming nurse; and (3) "walking" reports in which the incoming and the outgoing nurses "walk" to the patient's room and report the pertinent information while observing the patient.

There are advantages and disadvantages to each form of change-of-shift report. The face-to-face meetings and walking reports allow for questions to be exchanged between the nurses. The walking report also has the added advantages of both nurses assessing the patient's situation, and of patient participation. Both of these face-to-face reports, however, can be costly if they are not completed in a timely manner. The taped report can be a more efficient way to impart the necessary information, but there is little opportunity for questioning and sharing of information, which may be important to the plan of care.

Regardless of the type of change-of-shift report, there are some pointers that may assist the incoming nurse.

- Report vital information: allergies, code status, diagnosis, critical laboratory values, and family and medical team information.
- Review current status and therapeutics of the patient: This may be done in a systems approach (head to toe) or using an organization-specific report document.
- Discuss upcoming plans: This is important so the incoming nurse can prepare for events, such as a patient who is going for an examination and needs to have nothing by mouth (NPO).
- Review discharge plan as appropriate.
- Discuss any other information pertinent to the patient's care: this may include family responses to care and results of multidisciplinary team meetings.

The report is a vital link in the communication of patient status and needs. It is a crucial time to communicate accurate information about the patient status and the plan of care. One of the most frequent errors in shift report is the omission of critically important safety information. A change-of-shift report may be given orally in person, by audiotape recording, or during walking-planning rounds at the patient's bedside. Many hospitals are moving toward the use of walking reports (in the patient room) at the end of shifts. This type of change-of-shift reporting allows the incoming nurse to assess the patient situation and to ask questions of the outgoing nurse based on the assessment. It also allows the patient to participate and to confirm the information the outgoing nurse is communicating.

There are several options for organizing the information that one passes on in the handoff to the next shift. Some hospitals have templates for the report that are used by all staff members. SBAR is used in some institutions. Some institutions organize the report according to body systems; the report is presented based on the patient's body systems. Some organize the report on a "head-to-toe" assessment. Some report by exception, focusing solely on variances, or patient problems. No matter what style of report is used, it should be done professionally using the guidelines given in Table 8-3 which compares the do's and don't of change of shift reports. Another example is "I Pass the Baton" for **handoff** reporting. This is part of the Team STEPPS method of team work and communication.

STEP

A tool for monitoring situations in the delivery of health care. The leader of the care delivery team and all members of the team are tasked with situation monitoring. Components of situation monitoring are as follow (AHRQ, 2014):

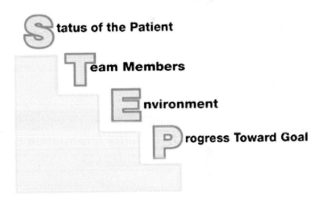

Assess Status of patient
   __ Patient history
   __ Vital signs
   __ Medications
   __ Physical exam
   __ Plan of care
   __ Psychosocial
Assess Team members' levels
   __ Fatigue
   __ Workload
   __ Task performance
   __ Skill
   __ Stress
Assess Environment
   __ Facility information
   __ Administrative information

TABLE 8-3 Comparison of Do's and Don'ts of Change-of-Shift Report

Do's	Don'ts
Provide only essential background information about the client (name, age, sex, physician's diagnosis, medical history, allergies).	Don'ts review all routine care procedures or tasks (e.g., bathing, scheduled changes).
Identify the client's nursing diagnosis or health care problems and their related causes.	Don'ts review all biographical information already available in written form.
Describe objective measurements or observations about client's condition and response to health problem; emphasize recent changes.	Don'ts use critical comments about a client's behavior, such as "Mrs. Willis is so demanding."
Share significant information about family members as it relates to client's problems.	Don'ts make assumptions about relationships between family members.
Continually review ongoing discharge plan (e.g., need for resources, client's level of preparation to go home).	Don'ts engage in idle gossip.
Relay to staff significant changes in the way therapies are given (e.g., different position for pain relief, new medication).	Don'ts describe the basic steps of a procedure.
Describe instructions given in teaching plans and the client's response.	Don'ts explain detailed content unless staff members ask for clarification.
Evaluate results of nursing or medical care measures (e.g., effect of back rub or analgesic administration).	Don'ts simply describe results as "good" or "poor." Be specific.
Be clear about priorities to which incoming shift must attend.	Don'ts force incoming staff to guess what to do first.

Adapted from Potter, P. A., & Perry, A G. (2008). *Fundamentals of nursing* (7th ed). St. Louis: Mosby.

TABLE 8-4 Handoff

Strategy Designed to Enhance Information Exchange During Transitions in Care

	Step	Description
I	Introduction	Introduce yourself and your role/job (include patient).
P	Patient	Identifiers, age, sex, location.
A	Assessment	Presenting chief complaint, vital signs, symptoms, and diagnosis.
S	Situation	Current status/circumstances, including code status, level of uncertainty, recent changes, and response to treatment.
S THE	Safety	Critical lab values/reports, socioeconomic factors, allergies, and alerts (falls, isolation, etc.).
B	Background	Comorbidities, previous episodes, current medications, and family history.
A	Actions	What actions were taken or are required? Provide brief rationale.
T	Timing	Level of urgency and explicit timing and prioritization of actions.
O	Ownership	Who is responsible (person/team), including patient/family?
N	Next	What will happen next? Anticipated changes? What is the plan? Are there contingency plans?

AHRQ. (2014).Team Stepps. www.ahrq.gov/professionals/education/curriculum-tools/teamstepps/instructor/essentials/pocketguide.html.

___ Human resources
___ Triage acuity
___ Equipment
Assess Progress toward goal
___ Status of team's patient(s)?
___ Established goals of team?
___ Tasks/Actions of team?
___ Plan still appropriate?

CONFLICT RESOLUTION

Conflict resolution among staff members, or patients and families is a challenging part of the profession. The resolution process includes using the principles of negotiation, which can result in one group winning, or both groups winning. In situations where the outcome is a win/win result for both sides, collaboration and negotiation are required.

In dealing with conflict resolution, the following communication principles apply (adapted from Jones, 2007, p. 214):

- Identify who is involved in or who is the source of the conflict.
- Identify interests and clarify issues.
- Build mutual trust.
- Separate the individuals from the conflict.
- Stay in the present; avoid dwelling in the past.
- Avoid placing blame.
- Remain focused on the identified issues.
- Discover options.
- Develop outcomes.
- Come to a consensus.

In the Team STEPPS model, the following communication method is used (AHRQ, 2014).

DESC Script. A constructive approach for managing and resolving conflict

D: Describe the specific situation or behavior; provide concrete data.
E: Express how the situation makes you feel/what your concerns are.
S: Suggest other alternatives and seek agreement.
C: Consequences should be stated in terms of impact on established team goals; strive for consensus.

AHRQ. (2014).Team STEPPS. www.ahrq.gov/professionals/ education/curriculum-tools/teamstepps/instructor/essentials/ pocketguide.html.

There are times when staff members need to evaluate the progress of the team as it progresses through the day. One such method is cross-monitoring. This is an error reduction strategy that involves:

- Monitoring actions of other team members.
- Providing a safety net within the team.
- Ensuring mistakes or oversights are caught quickly and easily.
- "Watching each other's back."

Team members also need to advocate for patient safety and at times will need to communicate concerns. Ways of doing this include:

Advocating for the patient.
- Invoking when team members' viewpoints don't coincide with that of the decision maker. Assert a corrective action in a firm and respectful manner
- Making an opening.
- Stating the concern.
- Offering a solution.
- Obtaining an agreement.

Two-Challenge Rule:

When an initial assertion is ignored:
- It is your responsibility to assertively voice concern at least *two times* to ensure it has been heard.
- The team member being challenged must acknowledge.

If the outcome is still not acceptable:
- Take a stronger course of action.
- Use supervisor or chain of command.

Empowers all team members to "stop the line" if they sense or discover an essential safety breach.

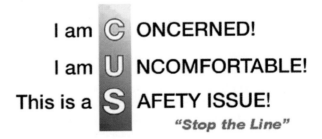

I am C ONCERNED!

I am U NCOMFORTABLE!

This is a S AFETY ISSUE!

"Stop the Line"

Remember that as a nurse you will communicate information about patients to staff and to families so that all team members can make appropriate decisions about patient care. It is important that all forms of communication are timely, accurate, and relevant.

ORGANIZATION-WIDE COMMUNICATION

The last type of communication is organization-wide communication. Organization-wide communication occurs in many formats. Formal communication about changes in practice, policy, and other important institution-wide activities often occurs formally through newsletters, intranet communication, formal education, or other methods of structured communication. Such formal communication usually is governed by the organizational culture and is defined by a specific flow. That is, the communication is directed to the specific individuals and groups that need the communication. A change in nursing policy is communicated from the nursing practice council to the care unit and then to the individual nurses. This top-to-bottom communication often follows defined distribution channels. Formal communication also occurs from the bottom up. Health care organizations have methods of collecting information from point-of-care workers that is delivered up the chain of command. It is important for all employees to know the chain of command. Employees are expected to respect the chain of command. For example, if a staff nurse has a concern, he or she is to communicate it to the person who is next in the chain of command, her the immediate supervisor. The supervisor then brings takes the communication up the chain of command. The chain of command follows the organizational structure of the organization. Some of this formal information may take the form of data collection through the use of employee surveys, customer complaints, budget requests, or strategic planning information. This information is further discussed in Chapters 3 and 18.

Informal communication also occurs in all institutions and in many situations, but it often occurs with individuals who are not part of the organizational hierarchy. Nurses often talk during breaks about patient conditions, suggestions for plans of care, and policies and procedures. The content may be perceived as formal, but the actual communication occurs in a nonstructured setting. Another type of informal communication is the "grapevine." Communication via the grapevine occurs outside of the traditional formal structures. A challenge with grapevine communication is that it is often altered as it moves across the grapevine. Another concern about informal communication is its lack of defined lines of communication. Information communicated via an informal network may not reach all parties. Therefore it is vital that information about the patient, staff policies and rules, and any information that is necessary for practice be communicated via a formal structure so that receipt of the information can be validated.

SUMMARY

Good communication is essential to the operations of all patient care activities. Communication occurs among staff, patients, and families; from staff to staff; and among departments. Professional communication forms the basis for the delivery of patient care from shift to shift and from staff member to staff member. The communication needs to be timely, efficient, correct, and respectful, and it needs to be delivered to all in need of the information, and understood by those who receive it.

CLINICAL CORNER

Team STEPPS (Team Strategies and Tools to Enhance Performance and Patient Safety) is an evidence-based patient safety system that aims to optimize patient outcomes by improving communication and teamwork skills among members of the health care team. This program has been adapted from Crew Resource Management, which has its roots in the aviation industry. A major learning point in Team STEPPS is that the entire health care team is responsible for patient safety, not just the physician in charge, and that every member of the team plays a role. Health care institutions, where Team STEPPS is a part of the culture, encourage and expect all members of the team to "speak up when something is wrong." Through the use of root cause analysis it has been shown that the majority of patient safety issues in health care can be traced back to poor communication. Team STEPPS provides the health care team with the tools and resources they need to foster team work and improve overall patient safety. Using interdisciplinary education facilitates breaking down the hierarchy of medicine. Often Team STEPPS education sessions are the first time that all members of the health care team from all disciplines are learning and training together. There

CLINICAL CORNER—cont'd

are multisite, ongoing research projects to measure the effectiveness of this training.

The Valley Hospital has begun to ingrain Team STEPPS philosophy into its culture. It is part of the larger "Just culture" of the institution. Through the use of simulation, the patient care units have begun to weave Team STEPPS into interdisciplinary education. The main concepts of teamwork, communication and speaking up when you see something that is not right, or "stopping the line" are the concepts that have been embraced at this institution. The expectation is that all members of the health care team

will report and act upon anything that is wrong or concerning. It is hoped that this concerted effort amongst all of us will further increase our already strong safety results. They will continue to adapt these concepts and many others from Team STEPPS to improve patient safety, and optimize communication among the team members.

Beth McGovern, MSN, RNC-OB
Clinical Practice Specialist
Women and Children's Services
The Valley Hospital, Ridgewood, NJ

EVIDENCE-BASED PRACTICE

Rehabilitation Nursing

Laws, D., & Amato, S. (2010). Incorporating bedside reporting into change-of-shift report. *Rehabilitation Nursing, 35*(2), 70–74.

Abstract

Communication failures during shift reports are a leading cause of sentinel events in the United States. Providing adequate information during change-of-shift reporting is essential to promoting patient safety. In addition, patients want to be more involved in decisions regarding their plan of care. The purpose of the article is to discuss how a stroke rehabilitation unit was able to implement bedside change-of-shift reporting to meet both of these goals.

One of the 2007 National Patient Safety Goals for Hospitals established by the Joint Commission (2006) is implementing a standardized approach to hand-off communication. An example is a change-of-shift report. This article discussed how a stroke rehabilitation unit implemented a bedside change-of-shift reporting process.

Shift reports have been done in different ways. One way was to tape the report, and the incoming nurse would listen to the report while the outgoing nurse would still be on the unit. One of the issues with a bedside change-of-shift report is confidentiality; the patient in the next bed, and/or visitors may be in the room.

A benefit to the bedside change-of-shift report is that the incoming nurse can see the patient and any equipment such as a ventilator or an IV pump. Another benefit is better communication between the nurses. The patient has the opportunity to meet the new nurse, and to ask questions when both the outgoing and the incoming nurses are at the bedside together.

Several factors were cited for the need to change change-of-shift reporting to bedside reporting. They were: the audiotape at times would list irrelevant patient information, and there was no format for this reporting; the facility wanted more input from the patient; and the philosophy at the facility was A Nursing Partnership Model of Care.

Preimplementation

True statements According to Nurses-Preimplementation
1. Bedside report can improve patient safety.
2. Bedside report violates patient confidentiality.
3. Bedside report provides an opportunity for patients to discuss their plan of care
4. Bedside report takes longer than taped report.
5. Bedside report holds off-going staff more accountable than a taped report.
6. Bedside report reassures patients that staff work as a team.

The next steps were to build a team and to educate the patients and staff. One week before implementation, there was an in-service education. An educational manual was also developed and placed on the units.

Evaluation

The nurses felt that patient safety was improved. They also thought the new system held the outgoing nurse accountable. Some areas for improvement were confidentiality, as well as full reporting not done for in-coming night nurses because patients were asleep. The patients still needed to be encouraged to speak up if there were any questions or issues.

Dawn Laws, BSN, RN, CRRN
Shelly Amato, MSN, RN, CNS, CRRN

■ NCLEX® EXAMINATION QUESTIONS

1. What is the transfer of information (along with authority and responsibility) during transitions in care across the continuum, to include an opportunity to ask questions, clarify, and confirm?
   A. Communications
   B. Change-of-shift report
   C. Handoff
   D. Physician order entry

2. When working in team situations, which of the following is the most effective tool to use?
   A. Team STEPPS (team strategies and tools to enhance performance and patient safety)
   B. STEP (status of the patient, team members, environment, progress toward goal)
   C. Huddle
   D. Situation monitoring

3. Your patient is coming into the trauma unit and you are the registered nurse for the patient. Example: Leader: "Airway status?"; Resident: "Airway clear"; Leader: "Breath sounds?"; Resident: "Breath sounds decreased on right." Leader: "Blood pressure?"; Nurse: "BP is 90/40." Which strategy is in use?
   A. Call-out
   B. Check-back
   C. SBAR (situation, background, assessment, recommendation)
   D. STEPPS

4. The electronic physician order entry system:
   A. Prevents all medication errors
   B. Provides many online alerts and warnings for clinical care givers
   C. Poses problems when the system is done
   D. Is not the most acceptable type of physician's orders

5. Which of the following is on the list of "don'ts" regarding the change-of-shift report?
   A. Share significant information about family members
   B. Relay to staff significant changes in the way therapies are given
   C. Continually review ongoing discharge plan
   D. Review all routine care procedures

6. When calling the physician and following the SBAR process, which of the following items is included under the Situation criteria?
   A. Identify the patient's ethnicity and religious affiliation
   B. Briefly state the problem, what it is, when it happened or started, and its severity
   C. Inform the physician regarding the patient's roommates
   D. Describe patient's mental status

7. In nursing, clear and precise communication is essential in the care of the patient. As a nurse, you are aware that messages can be:
   A. Native and foreign
   B. Verbal and nonverbal
   C. Coded and encoded
   D. Clear and unclear

8. Regarding the SBAR process, pertinent background information related to the situation includes:
   A. Socioeconomic status of the family
   B. List of current medications allergies, intravenous fluids, and laboratory results
   C. Patient's dietary needs before hospitalization
   D. Family history of disease

9. SBAR stands for:
   A. Situation, Background, Assessment, Recommendation
   B. Situation, Background, Assessment, Reaction
   C. Situation, Background, Assessment, Reply
   D. Situation, Background, Action, Recommendation

10. Which of the following is on the list of "do's" regarding the change-of-shift report?
    A. Provide essential background information about the patient
    B. Identify the patient's discharge plans
    C. Share significant information about family friends
    D. Discuss every routine order for the patient

Answers: 1. C   2. A   3. A   4. B   5. B   6. B   7. B
8. B   9. A   10. A

REFERENCES

Agency for Healthcare Research and Quality (AHRQ). (2014). Team STEPPS. www.ahrq.gov/professionals/education/curriculum-tools/teamstepps/instructor/essentials/pocket guide.html.

Goodnough, K. (2007). Electronic system for physician orders improves patient safety. *UConn Advance, 25*(29). http://advance.uconn.edu/2007/070423/07042311.htm.

Institute for Healthcare Improvement. (2007). *SBAR technique for communication: A situational briefing model.* www.ihi.org/IHI/Topics/PatientSafety/Safety General/Tools/SBARTechniqueforCommunication ASituationalBriefingModel.htm.

Institute of Medicinc. (1999). *To err is human.* Washington, DC: Author.

Jones, R. (2007). *Nursing leadership and management.* Philadelphia F. A. Davis.

Potter, P. A., & Perry, A. G. (2008). *Fundamentals of nursing* (7th ed.). St. Louis: Mosby.

Sullivan, E., & Decker, P. (2009). *Effective management in nursing* (3rd ed.). Redwood City, CA: Addison-Wesley Publishing.

Texas Tech University Health Sciences Center. (2007). *Physician's orders, receiving and noting. Policy No. 3.04.* www.ttuhsc.edu/som/clinic/policies/CPolicy3.04.pdf.

The Joint Commission. (2014). *Comprehensive accreditation manual: The official handbook.* Update 2.

Tschabitscher, H. (2005). *Top ten most important rules of e-mail netiquette.* http://e-mail.about.com/cs/netiquettetips/tp/core_netiquette.htm.

9

Personnel Policies and Programs in the Workplace

OBJECTIVES

- Discuss employment law as it relates to health care.
- Differentiate between workplace safety and patient safety.
- Explain why violence in the workplace is of particular concern for nurses.
- Differentiate between abuse and assault.
- Compare and contrast lateral and vertical violence.
- Identify legal issues concerning workplace violence.
- Identify issues of importance for safety in the workplace.

- Discuss potential safety hazards in the workplace.
- Review measures to protect the employee.
- Identify interventions designed to deal with workplace violence.
- Identify signs and symptoms of impaired practice.
- Discuss the role of the nurse and nurse manager in dealing with impaired colleagues.
- Explain the role of the employee assistance program.

OUTLINE

KEY TERMS

employee assistance program (EAP) confidential, short-term counseling service for employees with personal problems that affect their work performance

equal employment opportunity same employment opportunities must exist in an institution for all individuals regardless of race, color, national origin, religion, sex, age, or disability

horizontal violence co-worker act of assault, verbal abuse, threats, battery, manslaughter, or homicide

impaired practice professional working while under the influence of a mind-altering chemical such as alcohol or drugs

KEY TERMS—cont'd

sexual harassment unwelcomed sexual advances, request for sexual favors, or other verbal or physical conduct of a sexual nature, when this conduct explicitly or implicitly affects an individual's employment, unreasonably interferes with an individual's work performance, or creates an intimidating, hostile, or offensive work environment

workplace violence any violent act, including physical assaults and threats of assault, directed toward persons at work or on duty

This chapter deals with multiple issues of importance within the nursing workplace. The first section deals with the hiring and interviewing processes, and their importance to entering the workplace. The later section deals with the personnel policies and programs that impact the safe working environment for nursing staff.

EMPLOYEE LAW

There are a number of federal and state laws that play a major role in the employment of staff. It is very important to have an understanding of these laws and any local or institution specific regulations affecting the human resource function of your job. Understanding these laws will decrease your exposure to liability in your hiring practices.

Equal Employment Opportunity Laws

Several laws have been implemented to ensure there are equal employment opportunities for all individuals regardless of race, color, national origin, religion, sex, age, or disability. These laws are enforced by the U.S. Equal Employment Opportunity Commission (EEOC).

The federal laws prohibiting job discrimination are as follow (www.eeoc.gov/abouteeo/overview_laws.html):

- Title VII of the Civil Rights Act of 1964 (Title VII), which prohibits employment discrimination based on race, color, religion, sex, or national origin.
- The Equal Pay Act of 1963 (EPA), which protects men and women who perform substantially equal work in the same establishment from sex-based wage discrimination.
- The Age Discrimination in Employment Act of 1967 (ADEA), which protects individuals who are 40 years of age or older.

- Title I and Title V of the Americans with Disabilities Act of 1990 (ADA), which prohibit employment discrimination against qualified individuals with disabilities in the private sector, and in state and local governments.
- Sections 501 and 505 of the Rehabilitation Act of 1973, which prohibit discrimination against qualified individuals with disabilities who work in the federal government.
- The Civil Rights Act of 1991, which among other things, provides monetary damages in cases of intentional employment discrimination.

Included in these laws are laws that prohibit sexual harassment in the workplace. It is the responsibility of the organization to have human resource policies and procedures in place that are in compliance with the requirements of these laws (Table 9-1).

Many of these regulations relate to the hiring process (Chapter 21), whereas some relate to the work environment. In addition to the employment laws and regulations, many institutions are unionized. Some organizations have differing unions for different sets of employees. The nurses may be unionized under a nurses union; the environmental care employees may be represented by another union; and the licensed practical nurses may belong to a different union again. In such a multiunion environment, it is important for you to know the provisions of the union agreement(s). The union agreement(s) will affect everything from the hiring process (Chapter 21) to the delivery of patient care. If you join a unionized environment, as a new employee you will receive orientation materials from the union in addition to its benefits and contract requirements. The new manager in a unionized environment will also receive information regarding all of the union rules that affect the management of the unit.

TABLE 9-1	Selected Federal Labor Legislation	
Year	Legislation	Primary Purpose of the Legislation
1935	Wagner Act; National Labor Act	Unions, National Labor Relations Board established
1947	Taft-Hartley Act	Equal balance of power between unions and management
1962	Executive Order 10988	Public employees could join unions
1963	Equal Pay Act	Became illegal to pay lower wages based on gender
1964	Civil Rights Act	Protected against discrimination based on race, color, creed, national origin, etc.
1967	Age Discrimination	Act protected against discrimination based on age
1970	Occupational Safety and Health Act	Ensured healthy and safe working conditions
1974	Wagner Amendments	Allowed nonprofit organizations to unionize
1990	Americans with Disabilities Act	Barred discrimination against workers with disabilities
1991	Civil Rights Act	Addressed sexual harassment in the workplace
1993	Family and Medical Leave Act	Allowed work leaves based on family and medical needs

WORKPLACE VIOLENCE

In a national survey of registered nurses conducted by American Nurses Association (ANA) in 2001, 88% of working nurses reported that health and safety concerns influence their decisions to continue working in the field of nursing, and also the kind of nursing work they choose to perform. Hospitals are perceived as places of safe haven, but in reality they are potential breeding grounds for many types of incidents, ranging from disruptive staff, patients, and families, to chemical and infection exposure. Nurses have a right to a safe workplace.

Approximately 15% of all nonfatal violence occurs in the workplace (U.S. Department of Justice, 2011). In fact, a safe workplace is necessary for the provision of patient care (American Nurses Association [ANA], 2007). Hazardous material exposure is covered in Chapter 17. This chapter deals with issues of concern for the nurse dealing with potentially explosive workplace situations.

Workplace violence ranges from offensive or threatening language, to homicide. The National Institute for Occupational Safety and Health (NIOSH) defines workplace violence as violent acts (including physical assaults and threats of assaults) directed toward persons at work, or on duty. Workplace violence can be divided into four categories: violence by strangers, clients (patients), co-workers, and personal relations (American Association of Critical Care Nurses [AACN], 2004).

More than 5 million U.S. hospital workers from many occupations perform a wide variety of duties. They are exposed to many safety and health hazards, including violence. Recent data indicate that hospital workers are at high risk for experiencing violence in the workplace.

Statistics for workplace violence in nursing indicate the following:

- In 2009 more than 50% of emergency center nurses experienced violence by patients on the job. There were 2050 assaults and violent acts reported by registered nurses (RNs) requiring an average of 4 days away from work. Of these acts, 1830 were inflicted with injuries by patients or residents (Emergency Nurses Association).
- From 2003 to 2009, eight registered nurses were fatally injured at work (Bureau of Labor Statistics, [BLS], 2011).
- A study of student nurses reported that 53% had been put down by a staff nurse (Longo, 2007); 52% reported having been threatened, or experienced verbal violence at work (ANA, 2004).

Retrieved from www.nursingworld.org/Bullying-Workplace-Violence

Employee assaults may originate from patients, families, and co-workers. Assault can range from minor to major assaults. Outbursts of violence can affect the employee causing disability, psychological trauma, or death. Several risk factors may lead to violence in the health care setting (Tomey, 2004):

- People under the influence of alcohol or drugs.
- Working understaffed.
- Long waiting times.
- Overcrowded waiting rooms.
- Working alone.

BOX 9-1   Warning Signs of Violence

- Attendance problems
- Carelessness at work
- History of physical violence
- Performance problems
- Personality changes
- Poor hygiene
- Substance abuse
- Social isolation

From Tomey, A. M. (2004). *Guide to nursing management and leadership* (7th ed., p. 162). St. Louis: Mosby.

BOX 9-2   Signs of Impending Physical Violence

- Clenched jaws or fists.
- Increased movement.
- Increased respirations.
- Pacing.
- Shouting threats.
- Staring or pointing.
- Use of profanity.

From Gates, D. M., Kroeger, F. (2003). Violence against nurses: the silent epidemic. *ISNA Bulletin, 29,* 25–29; National Institute for Occupational Safety and Health (NIOSH). (2002a). Occupational violence www.cdc.gov/niosh/topics/violence/. DHHS (NIOSH) publication No. 2002-101.

- Unlimited public access.
- Poorly lit corridors, rooms, parking lots.
- Contact with public.
- Exchange of money.
- Working in community-based settings.
- Hospitalized prisoners.
- Isolated work with patients during exams and treatments.

Hospitals are microcosms of society, and as such, are socialized to violence.

Workplace violence is a multifaceted event with the potential to increase in frequency and scope (Ehrmann & Zuzelo, 2007). As a nurse and manager, you need to have a basic understanding of the risk for workplace violence to intervene in effective, efficient, and meaningful ways. You have already learned about potentially violent patients and how to handle them, but you need to be able to transfer some of this knowledge to the potentially violent employee. Boxes 9-1 and 9-2 provide warning signs of physical violence.

Although there is no universal strategy to prevent workplace violence, all hospitals have developed security plans to protect the employee from an unsafe workplace. The risk factors vary from hospital to hospital and from unit to unit. You have learned many ways of assessing individuals for altered levels of dealing with stress, and intervening in such situations. These are important to remember. Maintain behavior that helps diffuse anger.

- Present a calm, caring attitude.
- Do not match the threats.
- Do not give orders.
- Acknowledge the person's feelings (e.g., "I know you are frustrated").
- Avoid any behavior that may be interpreted as aggressive (e.g., moving rapidly, getting too close, touching, or speaking loudly).

Be alert.

- Evaluate each situation for potential violence when you enter a room or begin to relate to a staff member, patient, or visitor.
- Be vigilant throughout the encounter.
- Do not isolate yourself with a potentially violent person.
- Always keep an open path for exiting—do not let the potentially violent person stand between you and the door.

Take these steps if you cannot defuse the situation quickly.

- Remove yourself from the situation.
- Call security for help.
- Report any violent incidents to your management.

When you are dealing with potential staff violence or patient and family violence, it is important to maintain the safety of the patient care situation. If possible, remove the potentially violent individual from the patient care area.

CONFLICT MANAGEMENT

In managing the conflict, you will need to determine the cause of the conflict. First, determine the basis of the conflict. Is there difficulty between two shifts (intergroup), or two individuals (interpersonal)? Often there is conflict between shifts that spills over to stressful situations. Some of these conflicts may relate to perceptions of work left undone by one shift, or other work-related concerns. Second, you will need to analyze the source of the conflict. Conflict management techniques stress the importance of open and honest communication, and assertive dialogue. During conflict situations the nurse manager should view the total situation and use positive communication. Conflict resolution techniques are described in a variety of ways by a variety of authors (Tomey, 2004; Yoder-Wise & Kowalski, 2006). The following is a list of strategies for conflict resolution, the third step of conflict management (Huber, 2013):

- Avoiding: If you avoid the problem, you can trick yourself into believing that there is no problem.
- Withholding or withdrawing: In this situation, parties remove themselves from participation in a solution; this does not resolve a conflict.
- Reassuring: Parties do not withdraw, but try to make everyone feel good. In this situation, reassuring strategies are used to diffuse strong conflicts; this may be a way of hindering open communication.
- Accommodating: This is often used in vertical conflict when there is a power differential. It may also be used when one individual has a vested interest in a solution that may be relatively unimportant to the other individual.
- Competing: This is an assertive strategy in which one individual's needs are satisfied at another's expense.
- Compromising: This strategy is used when both individuals play a part in the decision. It is a basis of conflict management.
- Confronting: Individuals will speak for themselves in a way that the other individual hears the concern.
- Collaborating: Parties work together to find a mutually beneficial solution.
- Bargaining and negotiating: This involves both parties in a back-and-forth discussion to reach a level of agreement.
- Problem solving: The goal is to find a workable solution for all parties.

The following strategies will help the nurse manager resolve conflict before it escalates into a serious situation:

- Recognize conflict early: Recognizing the early warning signs of conflict is the first step toward resolution. Pay attention to body language and be cognizant of the moods of the staff.
- Be proactive: Address the issue of concern at an early stage. Avoiding the conflict may cause frustration and escalate the problem.
- Actively listen: Focus your attention on the speaker. Try to understand, interpret, and evaluate what's being said. The ability to listen actively can improve interpersonal relationships, reduce conflicts, foster understanding, and improve cooperation.

- Remain calm: Keep responses under control and emotions in check. Don't react to volatile comments. Your calmness will help set the tone for the parties involved.
- Define the problem: Clearly identify and define the problem. A clear understanding of the issues will help minimize miscommunication and facilitate resolution.
- Seek a solution: Manage the conflict in a way that successfully meets the goal of reaching an acceptable solution for both parties (Johanson, 2012).

Box 9-3 provides a model for managing conflict.

BOX 9-3   Model for Managing Conflict

Determine the Basis of the Conflict:
Intrapersonal.
Interpersonal.
Group.
Intergroup.
Organizational.

Analyze the Sources of the Conflict:
Cultural differences.
Different facts.
Separate pieces of information.
Different perceptions of the event.
Defining the problem differently.
Divergent views of power and authority.
Role conflicts.
Number of organizational levels.
Degree of association.
Parties dependent on others.
Competition for scarce resources.
Ambiguous jurisdictions.
Need for consensus.
Communication barriers.
Separation in time and space.
Accumulation of unresolved conflict.

Consider Alternative Approaches to Conflict Management:
Avoiding.
Accommodating.
Compromising.
Collaborating.
Competing.

Choose the Most Appropriate Approach.
Implement the Conflict Management Strategy.
Evaluate the Results.

From Tomey, A. M. (2004). *Guide to nursing management and leadership* (7th ed., p. 144). St. Louis: Mosby.

HORIZONTAL VIOLENCE IN THE WORKPLACE

Many of the issues that interfere with workplace safety arise from the interactions routinely occurring between staff members. In times of stress, there is often miscommunication among colleagues. Most of these conflicts can be resolved with open communication. However, there is a growing concern among health employees about horizontal violence between staff members. Horizontal violence is an act of aggression toward another colleague (Box 9-4). It may range from verbal or emotional abuse, or extend to physical abuse. Subtle acts of horizontal abuse may include belittling a fellow staff member, withholding information, or freezing a colleague out of group activities. As a nurse the challenge will be to identify behaviors that could be considered horizontally violent. Some of this behavior occurs between physicians and nurses. Two thirds of nurses say that they have experienced such abuse at the hands of physicians (Cook, 2001; Rosenstein, 2002; The Joint Commission, 2008).

Horizontal conflict is based on differences between colleagues. Vertical conflict relates to differences between managers and staff associates. These differences are often related to inadequate communication, opposing interests, and lack of shared attitudes. If staff members continue with horizontally violent behavior, the outcome is low morale and stress (Rosenstein, 2002). As a new nurse leader, it will be your responsibility to stop such behavior. The following steps are recommended to stop the cycle (Longo, 2007, p. 36):

- Analyze the culture of your work unit: observe for verbal and nonverbal cues in the behavior of your staff.
- Name the problem when you see it, and use the term "horizontal violence."
- Raise the issue at staff meetings and educate your staff about horizontal violence to help break the silence.
- Allow staff members to tell their stories if horizontal violence is part of the culture of the unit.
- Ensure there is a process for dealing with this issue if it occurs in your unit and be responsive when issues are brought to your attention.
- Engage in self-awareness activities and reflective practice to ensure that your leadership style does not support horizontal violence.
- Provide your nursing staff members with training about conflict management skills, and empower them to defend themselves against bullying behavior.

Although there is no federal standard that requires workplace violence protections, effective January 1, 2009, The Joint Commission created a new standard in the "Leadership" chapter (LD.03.01.01) that addresses disruptive and inappropriate behaviors. Some states have sought legislative solutions including mandatory establishment of a comprehensive prevention program for health care employers, in addition to increased penalties for those convicted of assaults of a nurse and/or other health care personnel. These states include AL, AK, AR, AZ, CA, CO, CT, FL, HI, ID, IL, IA, KS, LA, MI, MS, MT, NE, NV, NJ, NM, NY, NC, OH, OK, RI, TN, VT, VA, WV, and WY. Retrieved from www.nursingworld.org/Bullying-Workplace-Violence.

> ### BOX 9-4 Horizontal Violence in the Workplace
>
> Nonverbal behaviors such as the raising of eyebrows or making faces in response to comments by the victim.
>
> Verbal remarks that could be characterized as being snide or abrupt responses to questions raised by the victim.
>
> Activities that undermine the victim's ability to perform professionally, including either refusing or not being available to give assistance.
>
> The withholding of information about a practice or patient that will undermine a victim's ability to perform professionally.
>
> Acts of sabotage that deliberately set up victims for negative situations in their work environment.
>
> Group in-fighting and establishment of cliques designed to exclude some staff members.
>
> Failure to resolve conflicts directly with the individual involved, choosing instead to complain to others about an individual's behavior.
>
> Failure to respect the privacy of others.
>
> Broken confidences.

From Longo, J., Sherman, R. (2007). Leveling horizontal violence. *Nursing Management*, *38*(3), 35.

SEXUAL HARASSMENT

Some instances of abuse may be forms of sexual harassment. Sexual harassment can result from collegial interpersonal conflict. Sexual harassment is a form of sex discrimination that violates Title VII of the Civil Rights Act of 1964. It is defined as unwelcomed sexual advances, request for sexual favors, or other verbal, or physical conduct of a sexual nature, when this conduct explicitly or implicitly affects an individual's employment, unreasonably interferes with an individual's work performance, or creates an intimidating, hostile, or offensive work environment (U.S. Equal Employment Opportunity Commission, 2015).

All employment agencies are required to have sexual harassment policies and reporting procedures. This will be part of your new hire and mandatory annual education. When exposed to an incident of sexual harassment, remember that it needs to be confronted immediately. Confront the harasser with a statement such as, "I need you to know that I do not want you telling me sexual jokes." If the behavior continues, inform your immediate supervisor.

Although incidences of interpersonal conflict are inevitable in any workplace, it is the responsibility of both staff and leadership to recognize concerns and then intervene appropriately if the workplace is to be conducive to a satisfying and professional workplace.

As a nurse and nurse manager, you must do the following (AACN, 2004, p. 2):

- Actively develop a culture where violence is not tolerated, incidents are promptly addressed and managed, and comprehensive support for co-workers who experience violence is provided.
- Advocate for enforceable violence management policies in the workplace, and hold others accountable for their behavior.
- Participate in educational training on violence awareness and prevention.
- Mentor colleagues on how to respond when incidents occur.

VIOLENCE: OCCUPATIONAL HAZARDS IN HOSPITALS

As a nurse manager, you may be involved in the development of a comprehensive violence prevention program. No universal strategy exists to prevent violence. The risk factors vary from hospital to hospital and from unit to unit. The goal of the violence prevention program is to identify risk factors in specific work scenarios, and to develop strategies for reducing them (National Institute for Occupational Safety and Health [NIOSH], 2002).

BOX 9-5   Hospital's Environmental and Administrative Controls for Violence Prevention

Environmental Controls
- Install emergency alarms.
- Install monitoring systems (cameras).
- Install metal detectors.
- Provide security escorts to parking lots/decks.
- Provide adequate waiting areas to prevent overcrowding.
- Provide staff members with secure, lockable bathrooms.
- Provide adequate lighting.
- Replace lights immediately if defective.
- Provide video for high-risk areas.

Administrative Controls
- Establish liaison with local police and fire departments.
- Report incidents of violence.
- Require employees to report assaults and/or threats.
- Provide a trained response team.
- Distribute visitor passes.
- Maintain proper reports of incidents.
- Develop and implement hospital-wide safety plan (see Chapter 7).
- Enforce all safety and security policies and procedures (see Chapter 7).
- Distribute staff identification badges (enforce use of same).

Occupational Safety and Health Administration (OSHA) has identified eight essential components for a violence prevention plan:

1. Management commitment.
2. Employee involvement.
3. Work site analysis.
4. Prevention of hazards.
5. Training and education.
6. Prompt recognition, control, and monitoring.
7. Record keeping.
8. Evaluation.

This follows a model that is similar for the work of the hospital-wide safety committee.

The safety committee has the responsibility for developing and implementing the environmental controls within a hospital setting. This committee is also responsible to document that physical rounds are made in the facility and outside of the facility to maintain the hospital's environmental and administrative controls for violence prevention (Box 9-5).

BOX 9-6 Employee Education

- Workplace violence prevention policy and procedure.
- Early recognition of escalating behavior.
- Early reaction response plan of violent behavior.
- Cultural and ethnic diversity awareness plan.
- Location and activation of emergency alarms.
- Awareness of emergency exits.
- Awareness of employee roles in the event of workplace violence.

All hospitals are required to have a new employee/volunteer/student orientation program and an annual employee/volunteer program that must be clearly documented. The human resources department of the hospital is required to maintain these records. The state board of health and/or The Joint Commission usually requests these documents on an inspection or a survey. Required employee education is documented in Box 9-6.

Precise record keeping is required in the event of an incident. The hospital will have either a policy and procedure for a written incident report or a computer-based program. Whether your hospital uses the written form or the computer-based program, the exact date, time, and occurrence must be properly documented. The follow-up of the event is also clearly documented for future reference. The documents are used for impending court cases, review of types of employee and/or visitor injuries, needlestick injuries, or bodily harm.

WORKPLACE VIOLENCE CHECKLIST

As a new nurse contemplating working within a facility, the checklist in Box 9-7 can serve as an assessment of the personal safety of the facility.

IMPAIRED PRACTICE

Sometimes issues of staff conflict are symptomatic of other personal issues that may be impairing a staff member. Such issues may be stress at home, financial difficulties, or actual impairment from drugs and/or alcohol. Although all staff members will have personal issues that affect the workplace at various times, it is important for you to know when these personal issues interfere with workplace and/or patient safety.

The ANA estimated that 7% to 10% of nurses in the United States are impaired by alcohol or drugs. Some of this addictive behavior is accentuated by the constant availability of mind-altering drugs, and some nurses come to the workplace with addictive difficulties.

Boxes 9-8 and 9-9 provide signs and physical symptoms of alcohol or drug dependency.

Marquis and Huston (2014) discuss the profile of the impaired nurse and group characteristics into three primary areas: personality/behavior changes, job performance changes, and time and attendance changes.

Common Personality/Behavior Changes of the Chemically Impaired Employee

- Increased irritability with patients and colleagues; often followed by extreme calm.
- Social isolation, eats alone, avoids unit social functions.
- Extreme and rapid mood swings.
- Euphoric recall of events or elaborate excuses for behaviors.
- Unusually strong interest in narcotics, or the narcotic cabinet.
- Sudden, dramatic change in personal grooming or any other area.
- Forgetfulness, ranging from simple short-term memory loss to blackouts.
- Change in physical appearance, which may include weight loss, flushed face, red or bleary eyes, unsteady gait, slurred speech, tremors, restlessness, diaphoresis, bruises, cigarette burns, jaundice, and ascites.
- Extreme defensiveness regarding medication errors.

Common Job Performance Changes of the Chemically Impaired Employee

- Difficulty meeting schedules and deadlines.
- Illogical or sloppy charting.
- High frequency of medication errors, or errors in judgment affecting patient care.
- Frequently volunteers to be medication nurse.
- Has a high number of assigned patients who complain that their pain medication is ineffective in relieving their pain.
- Consistently meeting work performance requirements at minimal levels, or doing the minimum amount of work necessary.
- Judgment errors.

BOX 9-7   Workplace Violence Checklist

This checklist helps identify present or potential workplace violence problems. Employers may be aware of other serious hazards not listed here.

Periodic inspections for security hazards include identifying and evaluating potential workplace security hazards and changes in employee work practices which may lead to compromising security. Please use the following checklist to identify and evaluate workplace security hazards. **TRUE** notations indicate a potential risk for serious security hazards:

____T____F This industry frequently confronts violent behavior and assaults of staff.

____T____F Violence has occurred on the premises or in conducting business.

____T____F Customers, clients, or co-workers assault, threaten, yell, push, or verbally abuse employees, or use racial or sexual remarks.

____T____F Employees are NOT required to report incidents or threats of violence to employer, regardless of injury or severity.

____T____F Employees have NOT been trained by the employer to recognize and handle threatening, aggressive, or violent behavior.

____T____F Violence is accepted as "part of the job" by some managers, supervisors, and/or employees.

____T____F Access and freedom of movement within the workplace are NOT restricted to those persons who have a legitimate reason for being there.

____T____F The workplace security system is inadequate (e.g., door locks malfunction, windows are not secure, and there are no physical barriers or containment systems).

____T____F Employees or staff members have been assaulted, threatened, or verbally abused by clients and patients.

____T____F Medical and counseling services have NOT been offered to employees who have been assaulted.

____T____F Alarm systems such as panic alarm buttons, silent alarms, or personal electronic alarm systems are NOT being used for prompt security assistance.

____T____F There is no regular training provided on correct response to alarm sounding.

____T____F Alarm systems are NOT tested on a monthly basis to ensure correct function.

____T____F Security guards are NOT employed at the workplace.

____T____F Closed circuit cameras and mirrors are NOT used to monitor dangerous areas.

____T____F Metal detectors are NOT available or NOT used in the facility.

____T____F Employees have NOT been trained to recognize and control hostile and escalating aggressive behaviors and to manage assaultive behavior.

____T____F Employees CANNOT adjust work schedules to use the "buddy system" for visits to clients in areas where they feel threatened.

____T____F Cellular phones or other communication devices are NOT made available to field staff to enable them to request aid.

____T____F Vehicles are NOT maintained on a regular basis to ensure reliability and safety.

____T____F Employees work in areas where assistance is NOT readily available.

From Occupational Safety and Health Administration (OSHA). (2003). *Guidelines for preventing workplace violence for health care and social service workers* (rev. 2003). Washington, DC: OSHA, U.S. Department of Labor. www.osha.gov/SLTC/etools/hospital/hazards/workplaceviolence/checklist.html; Huber, D. L. (2013). *Leadership and nursing care management* (3rd ed., p. 681). Philadelphia: Elsevier.

BOX 9-8   Signs of Nursing Drug Diversion

- Arriving early, staying late, and coming to work on scheduled days off.
- Excessive wasting of drugs.
- Regularly signing out large quantities of controlled drugs.
- Volunteering often to give medication to other nurses' patients.
- Taking frequent bathroom breaks.
- Patients reporting unrelieved pain despite adequate prescription of pain medication.
- Discrepancies in the documentation of controlled substance administration.
- Medications being signed out for patients who have been discharged or transferred, or who are off the unit for procedures or tests.

From Maher-Brisen. (2001). Addiction: An Occupational Hazard in Nursing. *American Journal of Nursing, 107*(8), 778–779.

BOX 9-9   **Physical Symptoms of Alcohol or Drug Dependency**

- Shakiness, tremors of hands, jitteriness.
- Slurred speech.
- Watery eyes, dilated or constricted pupils.
- Diaphoresis.
- Unsteady gait.
- Runny nose.
- Nausea, vomiting, diarrhea.
- Weight loss or gain.
- Blackouts (memory losses while conscious).
- Wears long-sleeved clothing continuously.

From Sullivan, E., Bissel, L., Williams, E. (1988). *Chemical dependency in nursing: the deadly diversion.* Menlo Park, CA: Addison-Wesley Nursing.

- Sleeping or dozing on duty.
- Complaints from other staff members about the quality and quantity of the employee's work.

Common Time and Attendance Changes of the Chemically Impaired Employee

- Increasingly absent from work without adequate explanation or notification; most frequently absent on a Monday or Friday.
- Long lunch hours.
- Excessive use of sick leave, or requests for sick leave after days off.
- Frequently calling in to request compensatory time.
- Arriving at work early, or staying late for no apparent reason.
- Consistent lateness.
- Frequent disappearances from the unit without explanation.

It is your responsibility as a nurse and nurse manager to report any issues of co-worker behaviors. You should be alert to any signs and symptoms (see Box 9-4) of a co-worker under the influence and be aware of methods of reporting. You should report the health care worker to your immediate supervisor. It is the supervisor's responsibility to take further action. In keeping with the institution's policies and procedures, the human resources department should be alerted to assist the supervisor or nurse manager with confronting the employee. Reporting laws and consequences vary in each state. Clear documentation regarding the employee must be kept. Documentation should include tardiness, absenteeism,

BOX 9-10   **Examples of New Jersey Board of Nursing Level I Mandatory Reporting**

- Suspected drug diversion.
- Misappropriation.
- Theft.
- Physical and verbal abuse.
- Sexual abuse or exploitation.
- Intoxication on duty.
- Failing to account for wastage of controlled medication.

patient or co-worker complaints, records of controlled substances on the unit, and physical signs and symptoms, both observed and reported. (See employee assistance program discussion later in this chapter.)

Health care workers who abuse drugs or alcohol place both the patient and their fellow staff at considerable risk. It is important for you to know your responsibilities when dealing with an impaired nurse. The safety of the patient is paramount. Many state boards of nursing have adopted mandatory reporting of suspected impairment. Look to the rules and regulations in your state to determine your responsibility.

An example is the New Jersey Board of Nursing Level I mandatory reporting, which always requires the following to be reported (Box 9-10):

- Conduct that clearly violates expected standards of care and may result in various degrees of harm.
- Conduct that demonstrates a pattern of poor judgment or skill.

AMERICAN NURSES ASSOCIATION CODE OF ETHICS

The ANA Code of Ethics for nurses does not distinguish the cause from the effect.

In a situation where a nurse suspects another practitioner may be impaired, the nurse's duty is to take action designed both to protect patients and to ensure that the impaired individual receives assistance in regaining optimal function. This advocacy role does not stop once the impairment is identified. Nurses in all roles should advocate for colleagues, whose job performance may be impaired, to ensure they receive appropriate assistance, treatment, and access to fair institutional and legal processes. This includes supporting the return to practice of the individual who has sought assistance and is ready to resume professional duties (American Nurses Association [ANA], 1991).

Many boards of nursing have set up advocacy programs for impaired nurses to provide them with the assistance necessary to overcome the addiction. Information about these programs is available on state board websites.

But what do you do immediately when you suspect a co-worker is coming to work impaired? You call your immediate supervisor. Different hospitals have differing procedures on handling such situations, and it is important to follow the procedure. What you do not do is nothing. Many state boards of nursing have investigatory units that will assist the agency in uncovering suspected drug diversion or unsafe practice. In these situations, the health care agency refers the complaint to the state board, which then investigates and determines final action. In such a situation, if the complaint is found to be valid, the state board will have the nurse surrender his or her license to practice. The nurse is then referred to assistance and is monitored by the state board. Reinstatement of the license can occur depending on the rules and regulations of the state board. Nurses can also voluntarily surrender their license if they think that they are in need of assistance.

In the late 1970s, the ANA began efforts to secure assistance for chemically and mentally impaired nurses (Haack & Yocum, 2002). The assistance is in the form of diversion programs, intervention, or peer assistance programs. It is a voluntary, confidential program for registered nurses whose practice may be impaired because of chemical dependency or mental illness.

EMPLOYEE ASSISTANCE PROGRAMS

All of the issues dealt with in this chapter may be supported by the use of employee assistance programs (EAPs). The majority of health care employers across the United States have created EAPs. An EAP is a confidential, short-term counseling service for employees with personal problems that affect their work performance. EAPs grew out of industrial alcoholism programs of the 1940s. EAPs should be part of a larger company plan to promote wellness that involves written policies, supervisor and employee training, and an approved drug testing program (Canadian Centre for Occupational Health and Safety, 2015).

These programs allow employees to confidentially deal with concerns that may be causing problems in their personal or professional life. As a nurse manager you may refer staff members to this program. An example of an employee issue would be continual patterns of lateness and/or attendance. More serious issues may be for a drug or alcohol abuse problem. A referral can also be a self-referral. EAPs always protect the employee's privacy, and assist employees in getting the help that they need without fear of a break of confidentiality. Family members may also use the EAP in some institutions. Exact steps for the referral process should be in the hospital's policy and procedure manual.

EAP services provide counseling to employees and their families in an attempt to help the employee and his or her family return to a functional unit. EAPs may provide assistance in dealing with the following issues:

- Personal issues
- Job stress
- Relationship issues
- Eldercare, childcare, parenting issues
- Harassment
- Substance abuse
- Separation and loss
- Balancing work and family
- Financial or legal
- Family violence

Some EAP providers are also able to offer other services including retirement or layoff assistance and wellness/health promotion and fitness (e.g., weight control, nutrition, exercise, or smoking). Others may offer advice on long-term illnesses, disability issues, counseling for crisis situations (e.g., death at work), or advice specifically for managers/supervisors in dealing with difficult situations (Canadian Centre for Occupational Health and Safety, 2015).

▌ SUMMARY

The nursing workplace is a complicated environment.

After employment, the nurse needs to be aware of the professional polices and programs that ensure a safe practice workplace. The nurse within a shared governance environment is expected to take a leadership role in the continued development of a safe workplace and to continually advocate for a safe workplace.

CLINICAL CORNER

Lateral Violence: Can She Take It and Can She Make It?

New graduate nurses are among the most vulnerable to becoming a victim of lateral violence. Some experienced nurses seem to believe it is their "duty" to make sure the new grad has what it takes to make it in their unit. Successful assimilation of the new grad into the nursing staff is a key responsibility of the preceptor, charge nurse, and nurse manager, as illustrated by the following vignette.

A new graduate nurse is in the second week of her orientation in the surgical intensive care unit (ICU) of an academic teaching hospital. Because this new grad had successfully worked as a tech on the unit while in nursing school, the nurse manager hired her, knowing that some of the nurses oppose hiring any new grads. The preceptor assigned to orient this new graduate is an experienced ICU nurse and an excellent teacher who is committed to seeing that this new nurse succeeds. However, she has been assigned to teach a basic life support course during the morning today, and the charge nurse has been asked to act as preceptor to the new grad. This charge nurse's opinion that new grads do not belong in the ICU setting is well known, but on this busy day there is no other preceptor available. During the interdisciplinary rounds on a very complex patient assigned to the new grad, the charge nurse grills her about aspects of the patient's medical condition that even experienced nurses may not know. Although embarrassed for the new grad, none of the

nurses, physicians, or other team members speak up to help the new grad. Two of the charge nurse's closest friends are heard in the background laughing and saying, "Get her!"

This is an example of sabotage where the new graduate is set up to fail and to look bad in front of the team. It is also an example of the negative behaviors that often drive new graduates out of a unit—and sometimes out of nursing altogether.

How can this negative situation be reversed for the vulnerable new grad?

1. *Individual intervention* by the preceptor to provide support and encouragement as well as education to the new graduate to repair the damage done to her self-confidence; this includes suggestions of what the new grad can say if a similar situation occurs
2. *Private discussion* between preceptor and charge nurse confronting the negative charge nurse's behavior
3. *Group meeting* with nurse manager, all preceptors, and all charge nurses to develop a plan for teaching new grads and other new staff in a way that is supportive rather than unfair "testing"
4. *Educational offering* about lateral violence in nursing that teaches all staff how to manage episodes of lateral violence and includes them in developing an action plan to eliminate lateral violence from their unit
5. *Intervention with staff* that illustrates how lateral violence behaviors among staff members compromises the care and safety of patients

Karen M. Stanley

EVIDENCE-BASED PRACTICE

Weaver, K., (2013, May/June). The effects of horizontal violence and bullying on new nurse retention. *Journal of Nurses Professional Development 29*(3), *138–142*.

Abstract

"Horizontal violence and bullying are pervasive throughout nursing. New graduate nurses are at higher risk. Challenged with the task of making the transition from student to practitioner, new graduates often lack the confidence and social connectivity that may ward off interpersonal conflict. Continued interpersonal violence directed at new graduates may lead to negative physical and psychological consequences, high turnover rates, or abandonment of the profession. This article describes possible strategies to break the chain of violence."

NCLEX® EXAMINATION QUESTIONS

1. Several laws have been implemented to ensure that there are equal employment opportunities for all individuals regardless of race, color, national origin, religion, sex, age, or disability. Which of the following acts prohibits discrimination against qualified individuals with disabilities who work in the federal government?
   A. Title VII
   B. Title I
   C. Sections 501 and 505
   D. Sections 101 and 2012

2. The list of strategies for conflict resolution according to Huber (2013) includes all of the following except:
   A. Avoiding
   B. Reassuring
   C. Withholding
   D. Commending

3. When individuals speak for themselves in a way that the other individual hears, the concern is called:
   A. Confronting
   B. Collaborating
   C. Problem solving
   D. Competing

4. Which is an assertive strategy in which one individual's needs are satisfied at another's expense?
   A. Compromising
   B. Accommodating
   C. Competing
   D. Bargaining

5. In managing conflict, what is the first step?
   A. Determine the cause of the conflict
   B. Determine who is right and who is wrong
   C. Determine the punishment for the people in conflict
   D. Determine who was the aggressive person

6. Which of the following does not maintain behavior that helps diffuse anger?
   A. Do not match threats

B. Avoid any behavior that may be interpreted as aggressive
   C. Yell louder at the individual who is shouting at you
   D. Do not give orders

7. Which of the following is not considered a risk factor for violence in the health care setting?
   A. Isolated work with patients during exams and treatments
   B. Unlimited public access
   C. Overcrowded waiting rooms
   D. Security guard appointed to walk employee to car

8. The Age Discrimination in Employment Act of 1967 (ADEA), protects individuals age_____ and older.
   A. 30
   B. 40
   C. 50
   D. 60

9. What agency defines workplace violence as violent acts (including physical assaults and threats of assaults) directed toward persons at work or on duty?
   a. U.S. Department of Justice
   b. National Institute for Occupational Safety and Health (NIOSH)
   c. Occupational Safety and Health Administration (OSHA)
   d. American Nurses Association (ANA)

10. Which act provides monetary damages in cases of intentional employment discrimination?
   A. The Civil Rights Act of 1991
   B. Title I and Title V Act of 1990
   C. Title VII of the Civil Rights Act of 1964
   D. The Equal Pay Act (EPA)of 1963

Answers: 1.C   2.B   3.A   4.C   5.A   6.C   7.D   8.B   9. B   10. A

REFERENCES

American Association of Critical Care Nurses [AACN]. (2004). *Position statement: Workplace violence prevention.* Aliso Viejo, CA: Author.

American Nurses Association [ANA]. (2012). *Bullying in the workplace: Reversing a culture.* Silver Spring, MD: Author.

American Nurses Association, Department of Government Affairs. (2007). *Health care worker safety.* www.anapoliticalpower.org.

American Nurses Association [ANA]. (1991). *ANA position statement on abuse of prescription drugs.* www.nursingworld.org/MainMenuCategories/Policy-Advocacy/Positions-and-Resolutions/ANAPosition

Statements/Position-Statements-Alphabetically/
Abuse-of-Prescription-Drugs.html.

Becher, J., & Visovsky, C. (2012). Horizontal violence in nursing. *Med-Surg Nursing, 21*(4), 210–213.

Canadian Centre for Occupational Health and Safety. (2015). *Employee assistance programs (EAP).* www.ccohs. ca/oshanswers/hsprograms/eap.html.

Cook, J., Green, M., & Topp, R. (2001). Exploring the impact of physician verbal abuse on perioperative nurses. *AORN Journal, 74*(3), 317–320, 322-327, 329-331.

Erikson, L., & Williams-Evans, S. (2000). Attitudes of emergency nurses regarding patient assaults. *Journal of Emergency Nursing, 26*(3), 210–215.

Ehrmann, G., & Zuzelo, P. R. (2007). *Conference abstracts: 2007.* Presented at the National Association of Clinical Nurse Specialists (NACNS) National Conference, February 28–March 3, 2007, Phoenix, AZ.

Gates, D. M., & Kroeger, F. (2003). Violence against nurses: The silent epidemic. *ISNA Bulletin, 29*, 25–29.

Haack, M. R., & Yocum, C. J. (2002). State policies and nurses with substance abuse disorders. *Journal of Nursing Scholarship, 34*(1), 89-94.

Huber, D. L. (2013). *Leadership and nursing care management,* (5th ed.). Philadelphia: Elsevier.

Johansen, M. (2012, February). Keeping the peace: Conflict management strategies for nurse managers. *Nursing Management, 43*(2), 50–54.

Jones, R. A. (2007). *Nursing leadership and management: Theories, processes and practice.* Philadelphia: F. A. Davis.

Longo, J. (2007). Horizontal violence among nursing students. *Archives of Psychiatric Nursing, 21*(3), 177–178.

Longo, J., & Sherman, R. (2007). Leveling horizontal violence. *Nursing Management, 38*(3), 34–37 50-51.

Longo, J., Dean, A., Norris, S. D., Wexner, S. W., & Kent, L. N. (2011). It starts with a conversation: A community approach to creating healthy work environments. *Journal of Continuing Education in Nursing, 42*(1), 27–35.

Maher-Brisen, P. (2011). Addiction: An occupational hazard in nursing. *American Journal of Nursing, 107*(8), 778–779.

Marquis, B., & Huston, C. (2014). *Leadership roles and management functions in nursing: Theory and application* (5th ed.). Philadelphia: Lippincott Williams & Wilkins.

National Institute for Occupational Safety and Health [NIOSH]. (2002a). *Occupational violence.* www.cdc.gov/niosh/docs/ 2002-101/. DHHS (NIOSH) publication No. 2002–2101.

National Institute for Occupational Safety and Health [NIOSH]. (2002b). *Workplace violence.* www.cdc.gov/niosh/docs/ 2002-101/. DHHS (NIOSH) publication No. 2002–2101.

Occupational Safety and Health Administration [OSHA], U.S. Department of Labor. (2003). *Guidelines for preventing workplace violence for health care and social service workers.* Washington, DC: Author. OSHA publication 3148 (rev. 2003).

Roche, M., Diers, D., Duffield, C., & Catling-Paull, C. (2010). Violence toward nurses, the work environment, and patient outcomes. *Journal of Nursing Scholarship, 42*(1), 13–22.

Rosenstein, A. (2002). Nurse-physician relationships: Impact on nurse satisfaction and retention. *American Journal of Nursing, 102*, 26–34.

Sullivan, E., Bissel, L., & Williams, E. (1988). *Chemical dependency in nursing: The deadly diversion.* Menlo Park, CA: Addison-Wesley Nursing.

The U.S. Equal Employment Opportunity Commission. (2015). *Sexual harassment.* www.eeoc.gov/laws/types/ sexual_harassment.cfm.

The Joint Commission. (2008). *Sentinel event alert: Behaviors that undermine a culture of safety.* www.joint commission. org/assets/1/18/SEA_40.

Tomey, A. M. (2004). *Guide to nursing management and leadership* (7th ed.). St. Louis: Mosby.

Thomas, C., & Siela, D. (2011). The impaired nurse: Would you know what to do if you suspected substance abuse? *American Nurse Today, 6*(8).

U.S. Department of Justice. (2011). *"State" Bill "The Violence Prevention in Health Care Faciliti Act."* www.nursing world.org/MainMenuCategories/Policy-Advocacy/State/ Legislative-Agenda-Reports/State-WorkplaceViolence/ ModelWorkplaceViolenceBill.pdf.

Yoder-Wise, P. S., & Kowalski, K. E. (2006). *Beyond leading and managing: Nursing administration for the future.* St. Louis: Elsevier.

Exemplary Professional Practice

SECTION OUTLINE

"Exemplary professional practice in Magnet recognized organizations is evidenced by effective and efficient care services, interprofessional collaboration, and high quality patient outcomes. Magnet nurses partner with patients, families, support systems, and interprofessional teams to impact patient care and outcomes. The autonomous nurse provides care based on the unique needs and attributes of a patient and family and support system. The knowledge, skills, and resources that have been identified by the nursing staff as necessary to practice are the foundation for the care delivery system. Competency assessment and peer review ensure that nurses deliver safe, ethical and evidence-based care. Magnet recognized institutions embrace a culture that empowers nurses to identify and bring forth concerns without fear of retribution. The achievement of exemplary professional practice is grounded in a culture of safety, quality monitoring, and quality improvement" (American Nurses Credentialing Center [ANCC], 2013, p. 42).

Professional practice implies much more than the delivery of care. It is the delivery of safe, efficient, effective evidence-based care in an environment where nurses participate in all aspects of care delivery. This section will deal with the structures and processes that exist to assist nurses in the delivery of safe, effective, evidence-based care.

10

Professional Development

OBJECTIVES

- Discuss professional development opportunities of the nurse.
- Analyze the nurse's responsibility in individual professional development.
- Analyze the progression of nursing clinical competence.
- Discuss the importance of professional organizations in professional development.
- Identify the steps and progression of the staff registered nurse in a clinical ladder program.
- Review the various certifications available for the nurse.

OUTLINE

KEY TERMS

certification recognition by a professional organization of nursing knowledge in a particular specialty

competencies areas in which employees are to be determined to be qualified to perform

clinical ladder process whereby the employee is developed for progression within a position category

organizational learning development of new knowledge and skills within an organization. Such learning is achieved through research, development, evaluation, and improvement cycles

professional organizations the commitment to professional development is a hallmark of a Magnet organization and any organization with a focus on excellence. Magnet-recognized organizations use multiple strategies to support a lifelong learning culture that promotes continued role development, academic achievement, and career advancement.

BENNER FIVE STAGES

As the new nurse enters the workforce, it is important to realize that this is just the beginning of the professional journey. Benner (1984) posits that the nurse moves through five stages of clinical competence: novice, advanced beginner, competent, proficient, and expert nurse (Box 10-1).

These different levels reflect changes in three general aspects of skilled performance:
1. One is a movement from reliance on abstract principles to the use of past concrete experience as paradigms.
2. The second is a change in the learner's perception of the demand situation, in which the situation is seen

119

BOX 10-1   **Five Stages of Transition from Novice to Competent Practitioner**

Stage I
The nurse is overwhelmed by the number of potentially relevant details that pertain to a patient's care.

Stage II
The new nurse may suffer exhaustion while trying to manage their patients within the confines of the unit guidelines and protocols.

Stage III
Successfully embracing policy and protocol enables feelings of confidence and serves as a critical marker of readiness.

Stage IV
A period of transition in the preceptee-preceptor relationship. The preceptor serves as a resource, frequently retreating from the forefront of patient care.

Stage V
The "comfort zone" of a preceptor is withdrawn as orientation is successfully completed.

From Reddish, M., & Kaplan, L. (2007). When are new graduates competent in the critical care unit? *Critical Care Quarterly* *30*(3), 199–205.

less and less as a compilation of equally relevant bits, and more and more as a complete whole, in which only certain parts are relevant.

3. The third is a passage from detached observation to involved performer. The performer no longer stands outside the situation, but is now truly engaged in the situation.

As you read this content, think of your own areas of experience in nursing. Decide where you think you fit.

Stage 1: Novice

Beginners have not had experience in any of the situations that they are expected to deal with as professional nurses. Novices are taught rules to help them perform their duties. The rules are context free and independent of specific cases; hence, the rules tend to be applied universally. The rule-governed behavior typical of the novice is extremely limited and inflexible. As such, novices have no "life experience" in the application of rules.

"Just tell me what I need to do and I'll do it."

Stage 2: Advanced Beginner

Advanced beginners are those who can demonstrate marginally acceptable performance of their nursing duties; those who have coped with enough real situations to note, or to have pointed out to them by a mentor, the recurring meaningful situational components. These components require prior experience in actual situations for recognition. Principles to guide actions begin to be formulated. The principles are based on experience.

Stage 3: Competent

Nurses who have been on the job in the same or similar situations for 2 or 3 years develop competence, and begin to see their actions in terms of long-range goals or plans of which they are consciously aware. For the competent nurse, a plan establishes a perspective, and the plan is based on considerable conscious, abstract, analytic contemplation of the problem. The conscious, deliberate planning that is characteristic of this skill level helps achieve efficiency and organization. The competent nurse lacks the speed and flexibility of the proficient nurse, but does have a feeling of mastery and the ability to cope with and manage the many contingencies of clinical nursing. The competent person does not yet have enough experience to recognize a situation in terms of an overall picture or in terms of which aspects are most salient, and most important.

Stage 4: Proficient

The proficient performer perceives situations as wholes rather than in terms of chopped-up parts or aspects, and performance is guided by maxims. Proficient nurses understand a situation as a whole because they perceive its meaning in terms of long-term goals. The proficient nurse learns from experience what typical events to expect in a given situation, and how plans need to be modified in response to these events. The proficient nurse can now recognize when the expected normal picture does not materialize. This holistic understanding improves the proficient nurse's decision making; it becomes less labored because the nurse now has a perspective about which of the many existing attributes and aspects in the present situation are the important ones. The proficient nurse uses maxims as guides, which reflect what would appear to the competent or novice performer as unintelligible nuances of the situation; they can mean one thing at one time, and quite another thing later. Once one has a deep understanding of the situation overall; however, the maxim provides direction as to what must be taken into account. Maxims reflect nuances of the situation.

Stage 5: The Expert

The expert performer no longer relies on an analytic principle (rule, guideline, and maxim) to connect their understanding of the situation to an appropriate action. The expert nurse, with an enormous background of experience, now has an intuitive grasp of each situation, and zeroes in on the accurate region of the problem without wasteful consideration of a large range of unfruitful, alternative diagnoses and solutions. The expert operates from a deep understanding of the total situation. For instance the chess master, when asked why they made a particularly masterful move, will just say, "Because it felt right; it looked good." The performer is no longer aware of features and rules; his or her performance becomes fluid and flexible and highly proficient. This is not to say that the expert never uses analytic tools. Highly skilled analytic ability is necessary for those situations with which the nurse has had no previous experience. Analytic tools are also necessary for those times when the expert gets a wrong grasp of the situation, and then finds that events and behaviors are not occurring as expected. When alternative perspectives are not available to the clinician, the only way out of a wrong grasp of the problem is by using analytic problem solving (Benner, 1984, pp. 13 to 34).

You do progress in professional competence as you work. Self-assessment to your current level of performance is an important function in nursing. Much of your progression will also greatly depend on the work environment. The organization provides the environment for the clinical progression of all staff, both for organizational needs and for the personal development of the nurse. Such professional work environments are evidenced in the various health care organizations that have achieved Magnet status (American Nurse Credentialing Center [ANCC], 2013).

STAFF COMPETENCY

The Joint Commission states that a hospital must provide the right number of competent staff to meet the needs of the patients (2014). Competent staff are qualified and

> ### BOX 10-2 New Employee Orientation: Mandatory Content
>
> - Mission and governance
> - Service excellence requirements
> - Code of conduct
> - Fire safety
> - Safe environment
> - Culture of safety
> - Age-specific patient content
> - Infection control
> - Blood borne pathogens
> - Process improvement
> - Corporate compliance
> - Just workplace
> - Health Insurance Portability and Accountability Act (HIPAA)
> - Benefits

able to perform the work according to professional standards. Staffing is discussed in Chapter 12. To meet the goal of providing adequate competent staff, the hospital must carry out the following processes and activities:

- Providing competent staff either through traditional employer-employee arrangements, or through contractual arrangements with other entities or persons.
- Orienting, training, and educating staff (Box 10-2).
- Providing ongoing in-service and other education and training to increase staff knowledge of specific work-related issues.
- Assessing, maintaining, and improving staff competence.
- Ongoing, periodic assessing of competence to evaluate staff members' continuing abilities to perform throughout their association with the organization.
- Promoting self-development and learning. Staff is encouraged to pursue ongoing professional development goals, and provide feedback about the work environment (The Joint Commission, 2014).

The American Nurse Credentialing Center (ANCC) (2013) in the Magnet model calls for the continuous professional development of the nurse as evidenced by advancing degree completion and professional certification. They also call for nurses to participate in professional development activities designed to improve their knowledge, skills, and practice in the workplace. These professional practice activities are designed to improve the practice of nursing and patient outcomes. Both the

ANCC (2013) and the Institute of Medicine (IOM) (2010) in the Future of Nursing report, call for the facilitation of the effective transition of nurses, and advanced practice nurses into the work environment. This occurs through residency programs at all levels (new graduates, experienced nurses moving to a new specialty, new Advance Practice Nurse (APN) graduates, and APNs moving to new areas of practice).

The nurse's initial step in professional development occurs through an organizational orientation, which is discussed in Chapter 14.

CONTINUED EMPLOYEE DEVELOPMENT

As nurses progress from novice to expert, many health care facilities have a system that allows for promotion of nurses along clinical ladders. Education and benefits for progression in clinical competence form the basis for such ladders.

CLINICAL LADDERS

Clinical ladders are programs that reward nurses for their advancement in nursing. It permits horizontal advancement, allowing excellent clinicians to remain in their role at the bedside. Nurses advance through a determined number of levels within a position category based on predetermined criteria. When a level is reached, there are additional advantages for the nurse. When the highest level for a particular position has been reached, advancement requires additional education in nursing.

Clinical ladders were developed in organizations in reaction to Benner's concept of *From Novice to Expert* (1984). They were developed as a means to promote an individual's growth as a professional nurse on the path to expert status. Using organizationally established criteria in conjunction with an interview, health care organizations decide on the merits of individual clinical advancement. The process for Professional Clinical Career Ladder progression is usually both clinically and academically based.

Rockingham Memorial Hospital (RMH) supports an environment that promotes professionalism and excellence in nursing care. The following are some areas of clinical practice and professional excellence that are recognized in this clinical ladder program:

- Professional nursing service
- Clinical nursing competence
- Leadership skills

- Continuing education
- Evidence-based practice in nursing
- Nursing career plans
- Volunteer nursing/health service outside of hospital
- Customer service and hospital-wide initiatives for excellence
- National certification in nursing specialty area
- Shared governance participation on hospital or unit committees
- Health education for staff, patients, and others

Objectives

- Promote, recognize, and reward excellence in clinical practice and professionalism of RMH nursing staff
- Promote exceptional bedside nursing patient care and clinical performance by participation in the areas of leadership, continuing education, and through evidence-based practice participation
- Provide clear delineation of nursing competence levels;
- Use nurses who have been educationally prepared for a variety of levels of practice
- Encourage excellence in practice to ensure quality care of patients
- Champion recruitment and retention of qualified registered nurses
- Commitm to customer service and RMH excellence standards
- Promote participation in volunteer community and health nursing service

Automatic Advancement Levels I and II:

- Clinical Nurse I: Clinical ladder entry level for a new graduate bedside registered nurse. After successful completion of department orientation, a nurse will automatically advance to a Clinical Nurse I.
- Description: A new bedside registered nurse developing nursing skills, expanding knowledge, and assuming job responsibilities.
- Clinical Nurse II: After completion of a year of employment, and receiving a satisfactory evaluation, a bedside registered nurse will automatically advance to Clinical Nurse II level. A newly hired, experienced registered nurse (with at least 1 year of recent nursing experience) will be placed at a Clinical Nurse II level. After successful completion of department orientation and first successful evaluation, may advance to higher clinical ladder levels following all program requirements. All registered nurses (RNs) will remain at Clinical Nurse II level if they do not choose to advance to higher levels.

- Description: An experienced bedside registered nurse capable of independent patient care. Actively developing more advanced nursing skills and knowledge through education and involvement in nursing activities beyond basic job requirements and responsibilities.

Automatic Advancement Levels III, IV, and V:

- Clinical Nurse III: Requires annual portfolio submission and complying with all clinical ladder program requirements. Advancement to this level requires self-paced and self-motivated participation.
- Description: A bedside registered nurse highly skilled in patient care. Demonstrates leadership and mentorship abilities. Active involvement in continuing education and in nursing activities beyond the basic job requirements and responsibilities.
- Clinical Nurse IV: Requires annual portfolio submission and compliance with all clinical ladder program requirements. Advancement to this level requires highly self-paced and self-motivated participation.
- Description: A bedside registered nurse who has a broad base of advanced nursing experience. Recognized for professional nursing leadership and knowledge. Leadership extends to education and development of others. Involvement in multiple nursing activities beyond basic job requirements and responsibilities. Acquiring research skills by participating in evaluation of clinical outcomes to improve nursing through evidence-based practice.
- Clinical Nurse V: Requires annual portfolio submission and compliance with all clinical ladder program requirements. Advancement to this highest level on the clinical ladders requires extraordinary and exceptional self-paced and self-motivated participation. (Must be nationally certified in nursing specialty.)
- Description: A bedside registered nurse who has exceptional advanced nursing experience. Recognized for expert professional nursing leadership and knowledge. Leadership is recognized at a role-model level. Involvement in multiple nursing activities beyond the basic job requirements and responsibilities. Active and ongoing professional involvement in improving nursing through evidenced-based practice, such as research activities, writing a published nursing article, etc. All submitted evidence-based practice submissions and research materials must be presented in a professional format with extensive information such as charts, graphs, studies, stats, outcomes, etc.

(Clinical Ladders developed by Rockingham Memorial Hospital. www.rmhonline.org/rmh_human_resources/pages/RMH_clinical_ladders.html.)

As nurses move up the clinical ladder, the educational progression of the nurse becomes more specific. The organization-wide specific education goes beyond the requirements mandated by regulators to those that are specific to the needs and current performance of the organization. Organizations are required to perform annual needs assessments to determine the educational needs of the staff. These assessments need to go beyond what the staff "wants" to learn but needs to move toward an outcomes-based model, where the "needs to know" education is planned (Figure 10-1).

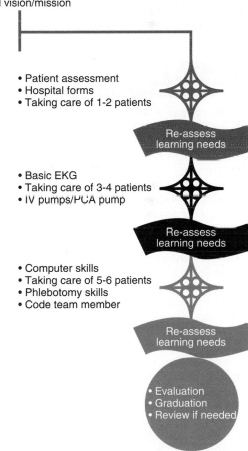

- Start orientation
- Review policy/procedures
- Hospital vision/mission

- Patient assessment
- Hospital forms
- Taking care of 1-2 patients

Re-assess learning needs

- Basic EKG
- Taking care of 3-4 patients
- IV pumps/PCA pump

Re-assess learning needs

- Computer skills
- Taking care of 5-6 patients
- Phlebotomy skills
- Code team member

Re-assess learning needs

- Evaluation
- Graduation
- Review if needed

FIGURE 10-1 A sample training roadmap. (Lee, V., & Harris, T. [2007]. Mentoring new nursing graduates. www.minoritynurse.com/features/other/080207d.html.)

Such an educational needs assessment needs to occur at all levels of the organization, so that the educational needs of all levels of nurses (administrators, advanced practice nurses, staff nurses, managers, etc.) can be planned. The nurses' role here is to be self-aware of the current levels of performance outcomes in their area and the educational needs based on current evidence based practice changes.

Not all continuing professional development will be provided by the organization. It is the nurses' responsibility to search out continuing education opportunities and match them to their professional goals. Nurses are expected to set practice and professional goals that align with those of the organization on an annual basis. These goals are set during the Annual Performance review process (Chapter 15). They most always include professional growth goals.

Large amounts of professional continuing education occur through the professional organizations and certifying organizations within nursing. Box 10-3 lists the varying professional organizations within nursing.

BOX 10-3 List of Professional Nursing Organizations

- Academy of Medical-Surgical-Nurses
- Academy of Neonatal Nursing
- Air & Surface Transport Nurses Association
- American Academy of Ambulatory Care Nursing
- American Academy of Nurse Practitioners
- American Assembly for Men in Nursing
- American Assisted Living Nurses Association
- American Association of Colleges of Nursing
- American Association of Critical-Care Nurses
- American Association of Diabetes Educators
- American Association of Heart Failure Nurses
- American Association of the History of Nursing
- American Association of Legal Nurse Consultants
- American Association of Managed Care Nurses
- American Association of Neuroscience Nurses
- American Association of Nurse Anesthetists
- American Association of Nurse Assessment Coordinators
- The American Association of Nurse Attorneys
- American Association of Nurse Life Care Planners
- American Association of Occupational Health Nurses
- American College of Cardiovascular Nurses
- American College of Nurse-Midwives
- American College of Nurse Practitioners
- American Holistic Nurses Association
- American Nephrology Nurses' Association
- American Nurses Association
- American Nursing Informatics Association
- American Organization of Nurse Executives
- American Pediatric Surgical Nurses Association
- American Psychiatric Nurses Association
- American Society of Ophthalmic Registered Nurses
- American Society for Pain Management Nursing
- American Society of PeriAnesthesia Nurses
- American Society of Plastic Surgical Nurses
- Army Nurse Corps Association
- Asian American/Pacific Islander Nurses Association
- Association of Camp Nurses
- Association of Child and Adolescent Psychiatric Nurses
- Association of Child Neurology Nurses
- Association of Community Health Nursing Educators
- Association of Faculties of Pediatric Nurse Practitioners
- Association of Nurses in AIDS Care
- Association of periOperative Registered Nurses
- Association of Rehabilitation Nurses
- Association of Women's Health, Obstetric and Neonatal Nurses
- Dermatology Nurses' Association
- Emergency Nurses Association
- Endocrine Nurses Society
- Federal Nurses Association
- Home Healthcare Nurses Association
- Hospice and Palliative Nurses Association
- Infusion Nurses Society
- International Association of Forensic Nurses
- International Council of Nurses
- International Nurses Society on Addictions
- International Society of Nurses in Genetics
- International Society of Psychiatric–Mental Health Nurses
- National Alaska Native American Indian Nurses Association
- National Association of Bariatric Nurses
- National Association Directors of Nursing Administration/Long Term Care
- National Association of Clinical Nurse Specialists
- National Association of Hispanic Nurses
- National Association of Indian Nurses of America
- National Association of Neonatal Nurses
- National Association of Nurse Massage Therapists
- National Association of Nurse Practitioners in Women's Health
- National Association of Orthopaedic Nurses
- National Association of Pediatric Nurse Practitioners
- National Association for Practical Nurse Education and Service
- National Association of Registered Nurse First Assistants

- National Association of School Nurses
- National Association of State School Nurse Consultants
- National Black Nurses Association
- National Federation of Licensed Practical Nurses
- National Gerontological Nursing Association
- National League for Nursing
- National Nurses in Business Association
- National Nursing Staff Development Organization
- National Organization for Associate Degree Nursing
- National Organization of Nurse Practitioner Faculties
- National Private Duty Association
- National Student Nurses' Association
- Navy Nurse Corps Association
- Nurses Organization of Veterans Affairs
- Oncology Nursing Society
- Pediatric Endocrinology Nursing Society
- Respiratory Nursing Society
- Rural Nurse Organization
- Philippine Nurses Association of America
- Sigma Theta Tau International, The Honor Society of Nursing
- Society of Gastroenterology Nurses and Associates
- Society of Otorhinolaryngology and Head-Neck Nurses
- Society of Pediatric Nursing
- Society of Trauma Nurses
- Society of Urologic Nurses and Associates
- Society for Vascular Nursing
- Transcultural Nursing Society
- Visiting Nurse Associations of America
- Wound, Ostomy and Continence Nurses Society

(The Ultimate List of Professional Associations for Nurses [2014]. http://nursinglink.monster.com/education/articles/11850-the-ultimate-list-of-professional-associations-for-nurses?page=2.)

Nursing membership in a professional organization is of vital importance to the future of nursing. Membership in such an organization will assist you in keeping current with up-to-date evidence-based practice and research in addition to providing you a networking base with fellow nursing professionals. It will also allow you access to some of the most current conferences and education within your specialty.

One of the first questions the nurse just ending the second year of employment needs to ask is "Do I need to pursue a professional practice certification?" The answer is "yes" especially if you work in a Magnet institution.

Certification signifies that the nurse possesses expert knowledge in a practice area. Magnet organizations are expected to have increasing numbers of certified nurses in the future. According to the American Association of Colleges of Nursing (AACN), in 2013 there were 62,818 nurses certified at the specialty (not advanced practice) level; health care organizations are strategically planning to increase these numbers. These certifications only reflect those certifications from the AACN, not other specialty organizations. There are 310 recognized certifications in nursing. Box 10-4 provides a complete list.

BOX 10-4 Titles of Various Nursing Certifications

Accredited Case Manager
Acute Care Nurse Practitioner
Adult Clinical Nurse Specialist
Adult Nurse Practitioner
Adult Psychiatric & Mental Health Clinical Nurse Specialist
Adult Psychiatric & Mental Health Nurse Practitioner
Adult-Gerontology Acute Care Nurse Practitioner
Adult-Gerontology Primary Care Nurse Practitioner
Advance Certified Hospice and Palliative Nurse
Advanced Certified Hyperbaric Registered Nurse
Advanced Critical Care Clinical Nurse Specialist: Adult-Gerontology
Advanced Diabetes Management for Clinical Nurse Specialist & Nurse Practitioner
Advanced Health & Fitness Specialist
Advanced Holistic Nurse Board Certified
Advanced Neurovascular Practitioner
Advanced Oncology Certified Clinical Nurse Specialist
Advanced Oncology Certified Nurse
Advanced Oncology Certified Nurse Practitioner
Advanced Practice Nurse in Genetics
Advanced Public Health Nurse (Public/Community Health Clinical Nurse Specialist: PHCNS-BC (before 2008)
Advanced Public Health Nursing
AIDS Certified Registered Nurse
Ambulatory Care Nursing
Bone Marrow Transplant Certified Nurse
Cardiac Medicine (Subspecialty) Certification
Cardiac Rehabilitation Nurse
Cardiac Surgery (Subspecialty) Certification
Cardiac/Vascular Nurse
Cardiovascular (Cath Lab, Intervention IF RCIS-certified)
Cardiovascular (CCU/CVICU and Cath lab)
Cardiovascular (Ed, telemetry, & stepdown)

Cardiovascular Educator
Cardiovascular Nurse Practitioner
Cardiovascular Nurse Specialist
Care Manager Certified
Case Management Nurse
Certificate for OASIS Specialist - Clinical
Certification in Hyperbaric Technology
Certification in Transcultural Nursing - Advanced
Certification Specialist in Healthcare Accreditation
Certified Addictions Registered Nurse
Certified Administrator Surgery Center
Certified Aesthetic Nurse Specialist
Certified Alcohol & Drug Counselor
Certified Ambulatory Perianesthesia Nurse
Certified Anesthesia Technician
Certified Anesthesia Technologist
Certified Anticoagulation Care Provider
Certified Assisted Living Administrator
Certified Asthma Educator
Certified Athletic Trainer
Certified Bariatric Nurse
Certified Brain Injury Specialist
Certified Brain Injury Specialist Trainer
Certified Breast Care Nurse
Certified Breast Patient Navigator - Cancer
Certified Breast Patient Navigator - Imaging
Certified Breastfeeding Counselor
Certified Cardiac Device Specialist
Certified Cardiographic Technician
Certified Cardiothoracic Nurse (within Cardiac Surgery Subspecialty)
Certified Case Manager
Certified Chemical Dependency Counselor
Certified Childbirth Educator
Certified Clinical Documentation Specialist
Certified Clinical Hemodialysis Technician
Certified Clinical Research Coordinator
Certified Clinical Research Professional
Certified Clinical Transplant Coordinator
Certified Clinical Transplant Nurse
Certified Coding Associate
Certified Coding Specialist
Certified Continence Care Nurse
Certified Correctional Health Professional
Certified Corrections Nurse
Certified Diabetes Educator
Certified Diabetes Educator Certification
Certified Dialysis Nurse
Certified Director of Nursing in Long Term Care
Certified Disability Management Specialist
Certified Emergency Nurse

Certified Enterostomal Therapy Nurse (C) Canada
Certified EP Specialist
Certified Flight Registered Nurse
Certified Foot Care Nurse (new)
Certified Forensic Nurse
Certified Gastrointestinal Registered Nurse
Certified General Nursing Practice
Certified Health Care Compliance
Certified Health Care Recruiter
Certified Health Education Specialist
Certified Healthcare Emergency Professionals
Certified Healthcare Executive
Certified Healthcare Quality Management
Certified Healthcare Simulation Educator
Certified Heart Failure Nurse
Certified Hematopoetic Transport Coordinator
Certified Hemodialysis Nurse
Certified Home/Hospice Care Executive
Certified Hospice and Palliative Nurse
Certified Hospice and Palliative Pediatric Nurse
Certified Hyperbaric Registered Nurse
Certified Hyperbaric Registered Nurse Clinician
Certified in Cardiovascular Nursing (C) Canada
Certified in Cardiovascular Perfusion
Certified in Community Health Nursing (C) Canada
Certified in Executive Nursing Practice
Certified in Gastroenterology Nursing (C) Canada
Certified in Healthcare Research Compliance
Certified in Hospice Palliative Care Nursing (C) Canada
Certified in Infection Control
Certified in Medical-Surgical Nursing (C) Canada
Certified in Nephrology (C) Canada
Certified in Neuroscience Nursing (C) Canada
Certified in Occupational Health Nursing (C) Canada
Certified in Oncology Nursing (C) Canada
Certified in Perinatal Loss Care
Certified in Perioperative Nursing (C) Canada
Certified in Psychiatric and Mental Health Nursing (C) Canada
Certified in Rehabilitation Nursing (C) Canada
Certified in Thanatology: Death, Dying and Bereavement
Certified Infant Massage Instructor/Educator
Certified Institutional Review Board (IRB) Professional
Certified Joint Commission Professional
Certified Labor Support Doula
Certified Managed Care Nurse
Certified Materials & Resource Professional
Certified Medical Audit Specialist
Certified Medical Office Manager
Certified Medical-Surgical Registered Nurse
Certified Nephrology Nurse – Nurse Practitioner

Certified Nephrology Nurse
Certified Neuroscience Registered Nurse
Certified Nurse Educator
Certified Nurse in Critical Care (C) Canada
Certified Nurse in Critical Care Pediatrics (C) Canada
Certified Nurse Life Care Planner
Certified Nurse Manager and Leader
Certified Nurse Manager and Leader
Certified Nurse Midwife
Certified Nurse Operating Room
Certified Nursing Home Administrators
Certified Nutrition Support Clinician
Certified Nutrition Support Nurse
Certified Occupational Health Nurse
Certified Occupational Health Nurse, Case Management
Certified Occupational Health Nurse, Safety Manager
Certified Occupational Health Nurse, Safety Manager with CM
Certified Occupational Health Nurse-Specialist
Certified Ostomy Care Nurse
Certified Otorhinolaryngology Nurse
Certified Pediatric Emergency Nurse
Certified Pediatric Emergency Nurse
Certified Pediatric Hematology Oncology Nurse
Certified Pediatric Nurse
Certified Pediatric Nurse Practitioner – Acute Care
Certified Pediatric Nurse Practitioner – Primary Care
Certified Pediatric Oncology Nurse
Certified Peritoneal Dialysis Nurse
Certified Personal Trainer; Exercise Specialist; Clinical Exercise Specialist; Health/Fitness Instructor; Registered Clinical Exercise Physiologist
Certified Plastic Surgery Nurse
Certified Post Anesthesia Nurse
Certified Prenatal/Postnatal Fitness Instructor
Certified Procurement Transplant Coordinator
Certified Professional Coder-Hospital
Certified Professional in Healthcare Information and Management Systems
Certified Professional in Healthcare Management
Certified Professional in Healthcare Quality
Certified Professional in Healthcare Risk Management
Certified Professional in Learning and Performance
Certified Professional in Patient Safety
Certified Radiology Nurse
Certified Registered Nurse Anesthetist
Certified Registered Nurse First Assistant
Certified Registered Nurse Infusion
Certified Registered Nurse Ophthalmology
Certified Rehabilitation Registered Nurse
Certified Renal Lithotripsy Specialist

Certified Respiratory Therapist
Certified Safe Patient Handling Professional
Certified Specialist in Poison Information
Certified Stroke Registered Nurse
Certified Surgical First Assistant
Certified Surgical Technologist
Certified Transcultural Nurse – Basic
Certified Transplant Preservationist
Certified Transport Emergency Nurse
Certified Urologic Clinical Nurse Specialist
Certified Urologic Nurse Practitioner
Certified Urology Registered Nurse
Certified Vascular Nurse
Certified Wound Associate
Certified Wound Care Nurse
Certified Wound Ostomy Continence Nurse Advance Practice
Certified Wound Ostomy Nurse
Certified Wound Specialist
Certified Wound, Ostomy, Continence Nurse
Certified Addictions Registered Nurse – Advance Practice
Child & Adolescent Clinical Nurse Specialist
Clinical Breast Examiner
Clinical Documentation Improvement Professional
Clinical Genetic Nurse
Clinical Nurse Leader
Clinical Nurse Specialist Child & Adolescent
Clinical Nurse Specialist in Home Health Nursing
Clinical Nurse Specialist Public Community Health
Clinical Nurse Specialist, Core
Clinical Research Associate
College Health Nurse
Community Health Nurse
Credentialed member, American Academy of Medical Administrators
Critical Care Clinical Nurse Specialist (Adult, Neonatal, Pediatric Acute)
Critical Care Paramedic – Certified
Critical Care Registered Nurse (Adult, Neonatal, and Pediatric Acute)
Critical Care RN with Cardiac Medicine Subspecialty
Critical Care RN with Cardiac Surgery Subspecialty
Critical Care RN with Tele-ICU specialty
Dermatology Certified Nurse Practitioner
Dermatology Nurse Certified
Developmental Disabilities Nursing Certification
Dietetic Technician, Registered
Diplomate of Acupuncture
Diplomate of Asian Bodywork Therapy
Diplomate of Chinese Herbology
Diplomate of Oriental Medicine

Electronic Fetal Monitoring
Emergency Nurse Certified (C) Canada
Evidence-Based Design Accreditation and Certification
Family Nurse Practitioner
Family Psychiatric & Mental Health Nurse Practitioner
Flight Paramedic – Certified
Gerontological Clinical Nurse Specialist
Gerontological Nurse
Gerontological Nurse Certified (C) Canada
Gerontological Nurse Practitioner
Global Professional in Human Resources
Group Fitness Instructor Certification
Health and Wellness Nurse Coach Board Certified
Healthcare Accreditation Certification Program
Hemapheresis Practitioner Certification
High-Risk Perinatal Nurse
Holistic Baccalaureate Nurse, Board Certified
Holistic Nurse Board Certified
Home Care Clinical Specialist: OASIS
Home Care Coding Specialist: Diagnosis
Home Health Nurse
Informatics Nurse
Inpatient Obstetric Nursing
International Board Certified Lactation Consultant
Lamaze Certified Childbirth Educator
Legal Nurse Consultant Certified
Lifestyle & Weight Management Consultant
Low Risk Neonatal Nursing
Master Addiction Counselor
Master Certified Health Education Specialist
Maternal Child Nursing
Maternal Newborn Nursing
Medical-Surgical Registered Nurse
MS Nurse
National Certified Addictions Counselor
National Certified Counselor
National Certified School Nurse
National Registry of Emergency Medical Technicians-First
    Responder
National Registry of Emergency Medical Technicians-
    Intermediate
National Registry of Emergency Medical Technicians-
    Paramedic
National Registry of Emergency Medical Technicians-
    Basic (Med Tech) (EMT)
Neonatal Intensive Care Nursing
Neonatal Nurse Practitioner
Neonatal Pediatric Transport
Neurovascular Nurse (RN)
Nurse Coach Board Certified

Nurse Executive (Certified Nurse Administration -
    CNA,BC before 2008)
Nurse Executive, Advanced (Certified Nurse
    Administration - CNAA,BC before 2008)
Nursing Professional Development
Obstetric, Gynecologic, and Neonatal Nursing
Oncology Certified Nurse
Orthopaedic Nurse Practitioner - Certified
Orthopaedic Nursing Certified (C) Canada
Orthopedic Clinical Nurse Specialist - Certified
Orthopedic Nurse Certified
Pain Management Nurse
Pediatric Clinical Nurse Specialist
Pediatric Nurse
Pediatric Nurse Practitioner
Pediatric Primary Care Mental Health Specialist
PeriAnesthesia Nurse Certified (C) Canada
Perinatal Nurse
Perinatal Nurse Certified (C) Canada
Personal Trainer Certification
Physician Assistant
Professional in Human Resources
Progressive Care Certified Nurse
Progressive Care Certified Nurse with Cardiac Medicine
    Subspecialty
Psychiatric & Mental Health Nurse
Qualified Professional Case Manager
Quality Auditor
Registered Cardiac Electrophysiology Specialist
Registered Cardiac Sonographer
Registered Cardiovascular Invasive Specialist
Registered Diagnostic Cardiac Sonographer
Registered Diagnostic Medical Sonographer
Registered Dietician
Registered Radiology Assistant
Registered Respiratory Therapist
Registered Vascular Specialist
Registered Vascular Technologist
Reproductive Endocrinology/Infertility Nurse
RN-Coder
School Nurse
School Nurse Practitioner
Senior Professional in Human Resources
Sexual Assault Nurse Examiner: Adult
Sexual Assault Nurse Examiner: Pediatric
Six Sigma Black Belt
Telephone Nursing Practice
Vascular Access-Board Certified
Women's Health Care Nurse Practitioner
Wound Care Certified

As you can see, there is a professional organization and certification for all levels of nurses. There is no excuse for a lack of professional growth.

Another decision for the continued professional development of the nurse is whether or not to continue academic education. The IOM (2010), in the Future of Nursing, called for 80% of all nurses in the United States to have a Bachelor of Science in Nursing (BSN) by 2020. There are a number of state-wide initiatives working to move the nursing workforce in this direction. Magnet organizations are also calling for organizations to have plans in place to meet this goal. So if you do not have the BSN, the time is now!

Other degrees in nursing include the Master of Science in Nursing (MSN), which focuses on advanced preparation in nursing. A master's degree in nursing is required to become an advanced practice nurse (APN or APRN), and

to qualify for an advanced practice certification. The Nurse Practitioner (NP) tracks (Adult Nurse Practitioner, Family Nurse Practitioner, Midwifery, Certified Nurse Anesthetist, etc.) require a minimum of an MSN. Some states are moving toward a Doctorate in Nursing Practice (DNP) as the minimum requirement to practice as an NP

There are three types of doctorates in nursing: a Doctor of Nursing Practice (DNP), which focuses on the clinical aspects of nursing; a Doctor of Nursing Science (DNSc, also a DSN or DNS); and the PhD and EdD, which focus on nursing theory, and research and education. The latter two types are the more common choice for those who wish to be professors at nursing programs, or researchers. It is not uncommon to see some doctoral-prepared nurses remaining at the bedside at Magnet organizations.

SUMMARY

Nurses progress on a continuum of competency from novice to expert during their careers according to the work of Benner (1984). This continuum forms the basis for many career development opportunities available to the nurse. The strategic plan of the organization will

have Human Resource objectives with outcomes specifying the academic and professional role progression of its staff. As a nurse, it is your personal and professional responsibility to continually advance your professional knowledge and expertise.

CLINICAL CORNER

The Role of the Doctor of Nursing Practice in Clinical Practice

The changing demands of this nation's health care environment require the highest level of scientific knowledge and practice expertise to ensure quality patient outcomes. The Doctor of Nursing Practice (DNP) is the terminal degree that prepares the graduate in both leadership and clinical roles to provide the most advanced level of nursing care for individuals, families, and communities. Some of the many factors supporting the momentum for change in nursing education at the doctoral level include the rapid expansion of knowledge underlining practice; increased complexity of patient care; and national concerns about the quality of care and patient safety.

I was practicing as an autonomous advanced practice nurse for 3 years before I returned to school for my DNP. I developed confidence in my ability to manage acute and chronic illnesses. I had seen many patients in many different settings and was able to build upon each experience. However, I was growing increasingly frustrated with the dysfunctions in the health care system, and at the end of the day, I just wanted to be able to provide the absolute

best care for the patients I served, and felt that I was not using the latest proven evidence in my care. This became the impetus for my return to school to attain the terminal DNP degree. Practicing as a DNP for 7 years, I am a more adaptive clinician and view my patients, their health concerns, and the health system from a different perspective. I still see the same patients with their acute and chronic illnesses, but what has changed is my management and treatment modalities that are evidence based and patient centered. It would be easy to just take care of patients' health issues and ignore the rest, because patients are multidimensional and never just present as an illness or a disease. In addition to differences in pathophysiology, patients do bring their own cultural, societal, and health beliefs to each and every encounter with a provider. The key is being able to navigate these complex intertwined systems and design the best care for that patient in a given situation.

I am using the expert leadership skills from my advanced education in my administrative role in my organization as vice president for advanced practice professionals, in academia as faculty for medical students, and coordinator for the graduate APN students. My clinical expertise is used as not only the administrative director but also a practicing partner in the first full nurse practitioner–run adult primary care practice in Bergen County.

I would like to share a story I call "The Road Less Traveled" depicting a typical day at the office in my life as a DNP:

I worry that the primary care provider is a dying breed. Though it was once considered the noblest profession, U.S. medical students today believe the work is too hard, the hours too long, and the pay too low. So I have observed they are choosing to hit the ROAD…the high-paying specialties of radiology, ophthalmology, anesthesiology, and dermatology.

But if you think being a primary care provider is hard, I would like to introduce you to Ethel. Not many people have it harder than Ethel. She is the one patient that always leaps to mind when I consider how our health care system can at times, fail our patients, and why I chose to stay in primary care. I am Ethel's primary care provider, and though I care deeply about her, seeing her name on my schedule evokes mixed feelings: irritation that I'll be at least 45 minutes behind schedule the rest of the day; trepidation over the 50-50 chance she'll need admission over uncontrolled hypertension as a result of confusion over medication regimen; and fear about her intractable social problems.

Ethel is a 76-year-old African American with mischievous brown eyes; she's feisty, funny, and utterly determined. Her old New York Bronx neighborhood has seen generations of immigrants, and streets lined with brick apartments and corner markets. Ethel remembers her youth as plagued by illness, yet she graduated from high school, worked, married, divorced because of physical abuse, and still managed to raise two daughters.

Ethel has a calcified mitral valve and enlarged heart, hypertension, and newly rising alkaline phosphatase and liver function enzymes. Testing uncovered a devastating neoplastic tumor behind the pancreas. The existing conditions were overwhelming enough to manage with little resources because of minimal insurance coverage, but where do I go from here to get Ethel the services she now needs to hopefully survive? Tirelessly pursuing phone call after phone call, I found a lucky break at a New York hospital where a specialist was willing to take Ethel for admission to perform an operative procedure known as a "Whipple" to remove the tumor. With this great news, I still had to discuss the options with Ethel and inform her of the risks and benefits of undergoing this procedure.

Adding to this mix, Ethel is estranged from her children, takes 14 medications daily, and now has to get into New York for admission and surgery. With no real family

support system, my concern for Ethel was posthospitalization, providing she survived the procedure and the endless follow-up visits to the surgeon, and me. She had a rocky perioperative course, but ultimately a good outcome. Somehow Ethel did it; her tenacity was astounding.

Ethel's pharmacy is one of the few that still has the personal touch. Through my perseverance in making sure Ethel's medications stay organized, her pharmacy is able to provide her pills in blister packs weekly by mail. There is a real pharmacist I can speak to on the phone; he knows Ethel well and all her medications, and is there every day so when I need to adjust medications he will send them to her by the next day. It all seems like a gift from above.

Traveling with the assistance of a walker chair down the sidewalk of her Ridgefield Park neighborhood, is just part of Ethel's daily routine. Draped over the bar to her walker, she keeps a bag containing all her medications with a book of all her physician phone numbers and upcoming appointments. One day, a desperate stranger found Ethel an easy target, and in a moment her bag was gone. Ethel felt like her world was gone as well. Soon after this event, Ethel called me at the office begging for my help to replace her medications.

To urgently replace her medications, I had to get authorization from Medicaid, her insurance company. The following is an excerpt of my conversation: "I understand she is not due for her medications yet, but as I just explained to you, her medications were stolen." I don't know how many people I spoke to, but no one seemed to be able to fix the problem. Without her medications, Ethel would probably be back in the hospital within 48 hours. Finding someone who understood the seriousness of the situation and could help seemed impossible. Even her pharmacist was willing to give her only a few days' supply until Ethel sorted things out with her insurance company: our government. Somehow, miraculously, I persuaded someone to replace Ethel's medications.

But for Ethel, such miracles are rare. She arrives at the office for a routine follow-up visit, clearly distraught. She struggles through frustration and tears to try to tell me what's wrong, as she hands me the phone. I ask, "Do you want me to call someone?" She nods. "Who?" "A relative?" "Your surgeon?" "Do you need a refill on your medications?" She lurches forward. I think, I may be on the right track, but for which question? Ethel begins to frown; now I think, I'm off track. "What do you need?" I ask. Of course I know Ethel isn't sure, and I'm now frustrated too. I finally figure out that she needs me to call her pharmacist. Without knowing why, I dial the phone. "I was expecting your call," he says. "There is a problem

CLINICAL CORNER—cont'd

with Ethel's treatment. She's been dropped from Medicaid and is no longer eligible for her medications." My heart sinks. Ethel's eyes are filled with fear, and it is as bad as she thinks. Again the pharmacist offers a few days' supply until Ethel can straighten things out. At this point, I just want to scream!

I call Medicaid, and talk to the social workers. I was connected to every department in the vast Medicaid bureaucracy, repeating the story over and over again, getting variations on a standard response: "That shouldn't have happened, Dr. Kutzleb, but I'm not sure how to reverse the problem." Luckily, Ethel's pharmacist is flexible about a few days' supply of meds, and after about a month, Ethel is back on the Medicaid logs. It was a fluke, I'm told; a simple error that could send a life into a tailspin.

Ethel's life is filled with such stories, but she musters awe-inspiring strength and determination for each challenge. At times, it does feel too hard to be Ethel's provider. But it has priceless rewards those medical students on the ROAD may never have the opportunity to experience. If Ethel comes into the office that is not my office day, I get a call and head on over to see her. As I knock and open the exam room door, a huge smile comes over her face. She can relax; she knows I care. It is at times like this, I recognize my deep satisfaction with the road I've chosen to travel.

Judith Kutzleb, DNP, RN, CCRN, CCA, NP-C
Holy Name Medical Center
Teaneck, NJ

EVIDENCE-BASED PRACTICE

In an article published in the March 2013 issue of *Health Affairs*, nurse researcher Ann Kutney-Lee and colleagues found that a 10-point increase in the percentage of nurses holding a Bachelor of Science in Nursing (BSN) within a hospital was associated with an average reduction of 2.12 deaths for every 1000 patients; and for a subset of patients with complications, an average reduction of 7.47 deaths per 1000 patients.

In the February, 2013 issue of the *Journal of Nursing Administration*, Mary Blegen and colleagues published findings from a cross-sectional study of 21 university health system consortium hospitals, which found that hospitals with a higher percentage of registered nurses (RNs) with baccalaureate or higher degrees had lower congestive heart failure mortality, decubitus ulcers, failure to rescue, and postoperative deep vein thrombosis or pulmonary embolism, and shorter length of stay.

NCLEX® EXAMINATION QUESTIONS

1. In an institution that encourages clinical ladder programs, the number of ladder positions is usually:
   A. three
   B. four
   C. five
   D. six

2. A bedside registered nurse who has exceptional advanced nursing experience and is recognized for expert professional nursing leadership and knowledge, is the automatic advancement level:
   A. II
   B. III
   C. IV
   D. V

3. A bedside nurse highly skilled in patient care and provides leadership and mentorship abilities is the automatic advancement level:
   A. I
   B. II
   C. III
   D. IV

4. An experienced bedside registered nurse capable of independent patient care is the automatic advancement level:
   A. I
   B. II
   C. III
   D. IV

5. _____are programs that reward nurses for their advancement in nursing. It permits horizontal advancement, allowing excellent clinicians to remain in their role at the bedside.
   1. Clinical ladders
   2. Self-assessments
   3. Annual competencies
   4. Performance appraisals
6. Which two agencies call for the facilitation of the effective transition of nurses and advanced practice nurses into the work environment?
   1. American Nurses Credentialing Center (ANCC) and Institute of Medicine(IOM)
   2. ANCC and American Nurses Association (ANA)
   3. IOM and State Boards of Nursing
   4. ANA and State Boards of Nursing
7. _____states that a hospital must provide the right number of competent staff to meet the needs of the patient.
   A. The Joint Commission
   B. The American Nurses Association
   C. The National League for Nursing
   D. The State Boards of Nursing
8. Benner states that the nurse who has been on the job in the same or similar situations for 2 to 3 years, when the nurse begins to see his or her actions in terms of long-range goals, or plans of which he or she is consciously aware is the:
   A. novice
   B. advanced beginner
   C. competent
   D. expert
9. Nurses who are those who can demonstrate marginally acceptable performance, those who have coped with enough real situations to note or to have pointed out to them by a mentor, the recurring meaningful situational components, according to Benner are in what stage?
   A. Novice
   B. Advanced beginner
   C. Competent
   D. Proficient
10. Competencies are usually completed by every employee at the institution:
    A. annually
    B. biannually
    C. every 6 months
    D. every 18 months

Answers: 1. C   2. D   3. C   4. B   5. A   6. A   7. A   8. C   9. B   10. A

REFERENCES

American Nurses Credentialing Center [ANCC]. (2013). *2014 Magnet application manual.* Silver Spring, MD: ANCC.

American Nurses Credentialing Center [ANCC]. (2013). *2013 Certification Data.* www.nursecredentialing.org/Certification/FacultyEducators/FacultyCategory/Statistics/2013-ANCC-Certification-Statistics-pdf.pdf.

American Nurses Credentialing Center [ANCC]. (2014). *National Certifications Currently Included in the DDCT.* www.nursecredentialing.org/Magnet/Magnet-CertificationForms.

Benner, P. (1984). *From novice to expert: Excellence and power in clinical nursing practice.* Menlo Park, CA: Addison-Wesley.

Ferguson, L., Day, R., Anderson, C., & Rohatnsky, N. (2007). The process for mentoring new nurses into professional practice. *Conference presentation at the National Healthcare Leadership Conference, 2007.* www.healthcareleadershipconference.ca/assets/PDFs/Presentation%20PDFs/June%2012/Pier%209/The%20Process%2020of%2020Mentoring%2020New%2020Nurses%2020into%2020Professional%2020Practice.pdf.

Goode, C. J., Lynn, M. R., Krsek, C., et al. (2009). Nurse residency programs: an essential requirement for nursing. *Nursing Economics, 27*(3), 142–159.

Hardy, R., & Smith, R. (2001). Enhancing staff development with a structured preceptor program. *Journal of Nursing Care Quality, 15*(2), 9–17.

Krugman, M., Bretscneider, J., Horn, P. B., et al. (2006). The National Post-Baccalaureate Graduate Nurse Residency Program. *Journal for Nurses in Staff Development, 22*(4), 196–205.

Lee, V., & Harris, T. (2007). *Mentoring new nursing graduates.* Retrieved July 8, 2014, from www.minoritynurse.com/features/other/080207d.html.

Neuman, J., Brady-Schluttner, K., McKay, A., Roslien, J., Tweedell, D., & James, K. (2004). Centralizing a registered nurse preceptor program at the institutional level. *Journal for Nurses in Staff Development, 20*(1), 17–24.

Reddish, M., & Kaplan, L. (2007). When are new graduates competent in the critical care unit? *Critical Care Quarterly, 30*(3), 199–205.

Speers, A., Strzyzewski, N., & Ziololkowski, L. (2004). Preceptor preparation: an investment in the future. *Journal for Nurses in Staff Development, 20*(3), 127–133.

Sullivan, E. J., & Decker, F. J. (2013). *Effective leadership and management in nursing* (5th ed.). Upper Saddle River, NJ: Prentice-Hall.

The Joint Commission. (2014). *Hospital accreditation standards.* Oakbrook Terrace, IL: Author.

Williams, C. A., Goode, C. J., Krsek, C., et al. (2007). Post-baccalaureate nurse residency 1-year outcomes. *Journal of Nursing Administration, 37*(7/8), 357–365.

11

Professional Practice and Care Delivery Models and Emerging Practice Models

OBJECTIVES

- Differentiate between the traditional function care delivery models and professional care delivery models.
- Discuss the pros and cons of each of the delivery systems.
- Determine the responsibility of the nurse in the professional practice model.

- Identify outcome measures of professional practice and care delivery models.
- Differentiate between a professional practice model and a care delivery system.
- Identify the opportunities for nurses related to the emerging models of practice and care delivery.

OUTLINE

KEY TERMS

accountable care organization a collaboration among primary care clinicians, a hospital, specialists, and other health professionals who accept joint responsibility for the quality and cost of care provided to its patients

care delivery system a system for the delivery of care that delineates the nurses' authority and accountability for clinical decision making and outcomes; it is integrated with the professional practice model and promotes continuous, consistent, efficient, and accountable nursing care

medical home a mechanism to provide patients with a central primary care practice or provider who coordinates the patients' care across settings and providers

nurse-managed clinics nurse-run facilities that provide comprehensive primary care

professional practice model a schematic description of a theory, phenomenon, or system that depicts how nurses practice, collaborate, communicate, and develop professionally to provide the highest quality care for those served by the organization (American Nurses Credentialing Center [ANCC], 2013)

PROFESSIONAL PRACTICE MODELS

The **professional practice model** is the driving force of nursing care (American Nurses Credentialing Center [ANCC], 2013, p. 74). The professional practice model of an organization illustrates the alignment and integration of nursing practice with the mission, vision, and values of the organization and the nursing department. It is the overarching conceptual framework for nurses, nursing care, and interprofessional patient care. It is usually presented as a schematic that describes how nurses practice, collaborate, and develop professionally to deliver care that meets the three aims of effectiveness, efficiency, and patient experience. At the center or forefront of such models is the patient and family. Figure 11-1 represents the professional practice model of Massachusetts General Patient Care Services.

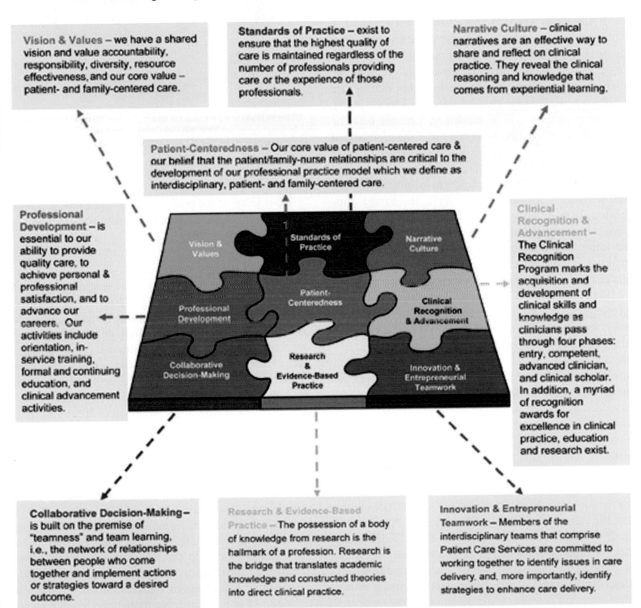

Vision & Values – we have a shared vision and value accountability, responsibility, diversity, resource effectiveness, and our core value – patient- and family-centered care.

Standards of Practice – exist to ensure that the highest quality of care is maintained regardless of the number of professionals providing care or the experience of those professionals.

Narrative Culture – clinical narratives are an effective way to share and reflect on clinical practice. They reveal the clinical reasoning and knowledge that comes from experiential learning.

Patient-Centeredness – Our core value of patient-centered care & our belief that the patient/family-nurse relationships are critical to the development of our professional practice model which we define as interdisciplinary, patient- and family-centered care.

Professional Development – is essential to our ability to provide quality care, to achieve personal & professional satisfaction, and to advance our careers. Our activities include orientation, in-service training, formal and continuing education, and clinical advancement activities.

Clinical Recognition & Advancement – The Clinical Recognition Program marks the acquisition and development of clinical skills and knowledge as clinicians pass through four phases: entry, competent, advanced clinician, and clinical scholar. In addition, a myriad of recognition awards for excellence in clinical practice, education and research exist.

Collaborative Decision-Making – is built on the premise of "teamness" and team learning, i.e., the network of relationships between people who come together and implement actions or strategies toward a desired outcome.

Research & Evidence-Based Practice – The possession of a body of knowledge from research is the hallmark of a profession. Research is the bridge that translates academic knowledge and constructed theories into direct clinical practice.

Innovation & Entrepreneurial Teamwork – Members of the interdisciplinary teams that comprise Patient Care Services are committed to working together to identify issues in care delivery, and, more importantly, identify strategies to enhance care delivery.

FIGURE 11-1 The Massachusetts General Hospital professional practice model.

This professional practice model represents the interconnected pieces of the "puzzle" that forms nursing practice at Massachusetts General Hospital. Nursing is delivered through the many pieces of the puzzle, and the expectation of how each nurse in the institution practices is defined in this model. This goes beyond the care delivery models described in Chapter 2. Those models—team nursing, functional nursing, and primary nursing—describe how the actual delivery of care is organized. The professional practice model describes the environment in which the professional nurse practices. This professional nurse practice environment empowers nurses by providing them with opportunities for autonomy, accountability, and control over the care that they provide and the environment in which they deliver care (Zelauskas & Howes, 1992 as cited in ANCC, 2013). Shared governance, as discussed in Chapter 6 is the vehicle by which the decision making of the professional practice model occurs. In this model the patient remains at the center of all care decisions. The nursing vision and values, as well as the standards of practice, guide the activities of the professional nurse. The nurse is supported through professional development and clinical recognition and achievement. Practice is continually advanced and delivered through collaborative decision making, the narrative culture, research, evidence-based practice, and innovation and entrepreneurial teamwork.

The University of California–Los Angeles (UCLA) professional practice model (Figure 11-2) is philosophically similar in many respects, but the schematic reflects the culture of the larger organization. The patient, family, and community are at the center of care. The overall mission of UCLA and the mission and values form the next circle of the model. This professional practice model is guided by the O'Rourke Model of the professional role, the Watson Theory of Human Caring, and the Swanson Five Caring Processes. Relationship-based care is the care delivery model. This schematic includes the theoretical models upon which the professional practice model is based. The professional nurse as decision maker is guided by the American Nurses Association (ANA) Code of Ethics, the ANA Standards, the State Nursing Practice Act, and State Titles. Lastly, the nurse has roles as leader, scientist, transferor of knowledge, and practitioner.

Both of the above professional practice models clearly describe the professional environment of nursing within the institution as well as the expectations of the nurse and the nursing department.

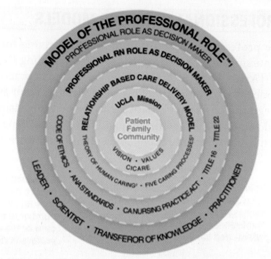

[1]O'Rourke Model of the Professional Role™ [2]Watson Theory of Human Caring [3]Swanson Five Caring Processes

FIGURE 11-2 The University of California Los Angeles Professional Practice Model.

Knowledge of the professional practice model can be an important determinant in a nurse's decision to join a particular organization.

CARE DELIVERY SYSTEM

The **care delivery system** is integrated into the professional practice model. It is continually improved to adjust to national patient safety goals, value-based outcomes, regulatory requirements, and current best evidence. It describes the manner in which care is delivered, the context of care, and the expected outcomes of care. Nurses create care delivery systems that describe the nurses' accountability and shared authority for evidence-based practice, clinical decision making and outcomes, performance improvement initiatives, and staffing and scheduling processes (ANCC, 2013, p. 42).

Limitations of the more traditional definitions of care delivery (team, functional, primary care, etc.) have been documented, and many consider them inadequate for depicting the multiplicity of actual nursing work organization models in practice (O'Connor et al. 2006; Tiedman & Lookinland, 2004). The care delivery models described by Massachusetts General and UCLA reflect a taxonomy of nursing care organization models that incorporate a broader range of attributes than found in the traditional care delivery models. Dubois et al. (2013) proposed that a nursing care delivery model should consist of the following five key dimensions:

1. Staffing intensity
2. Skill and nursing education mix
3. Professional scope of practice in six domains of practice: assessment and planning, teaching, communication, supervision, quality of care, and knowledge updating
4. Nursing practice environment (nurse participation in hospital affairs, nursing foundations for quality, nurse manager leadership and support, resource adequacy and nurse–physician relations)
5. Unit-level capacity for innovation measured on five criteria: expanded RN roles, sharpened focus of care on the patient, attention to patient transitions, leveraging of technologies, and performance monitoring and feedback

In a study comparing outcomes of such professional models and the more traditional functional models (Dubois et al. 2013) more positive patient outcomes were seen with the more innovative professional care delivery models. This supports the notion that patient safety results from more than just staffing models. The lowest rates of negative outcomes were seen in the professional models characterized by richer skill and education mix, higher staffing intensity, and a practice environment more supportive of professional practice and with greater investments in innovation. These associations are consistent with findings reported for Magnet hospitals, known for the excellence of their conditions for both nurses and patients.

Frameworks for the Delivery of Patient Care

In recognition of the unique characteristics of patients and their needs, each organization/unit/service/clinic develops a method of delivering care. Information provided in the development and improvement of the care delivery model should include the following:

- Populations served/patient characteristics
- Age, ethnic, cultural, and spiritual patient characteristics
- Scope and complexity of patients
- Admission characteristics
- Assessment/reassessment practices and standards
- Staffing ratios and staff mix
- Educational mix of the nursing staff
- Standards for assignment of patients
- Required competencies of the unit staff to meet patient needs

- The nursing philosophy, mission, vision, and values
- Interprofessionals who support care delivery
- Standards to ensure continuity of care
- Professional nursing standards that guide care delivery
- Use of evidence to drive innovation
- Performance improvement indicators to measure the effectiveness and efficiency of the care delivery system for the unit.

It is imperative that the delivery of care is continually evaluated. Outcomes need to be evaluated throughout the shift as acuity changes, as well as daily, weekly, monthly, quarterly, and annually.

The professional practice model and care delivery models are evaluated and revised based on new evidence and/or research and on outcome data such as the following:

- Accreditation standards and National Patient Safety Goals
- Patient satisfaction survey results
- National Database of Nursing Quality Indicators (NDNQI) nursing sensitive indicator outcomes
- Unit scorecards (quality and financial data)
- The NDNQI staff registered nurse satisfaction survey
- Centers for Medicare & Medicaid Services (CMS) core measures
- Hospital Consumer Assessment of Healthcare Providers and Systems (HCAHPS) results
- Unit-based surveys

(Adapted from Jupiter Medical Center *Description of JMC Care Delivery System*. www.jupitermed.com/care-delivery-system.)

EMERGING CARE DELIVERY MODELS

Many of these care delivery models can be adjusted to meet the needs of various populations, such as ambulatory centers, nurse-managed clinics, medical homes, and the wide variety of organizations that provide health care. But the role of nurses in emerging care delivery models will be a true test of the patient advocacy role of the professional nurse in the delivery of safe, efficient, and effective care. RNs are fundamental to the success of emerging patient-centered care delivery models.

The Patient Protection and Affordable Care Act of 2010 (PPACA) directs renewed attention and substantially more resources and incentives to promote those elements of care that are also the backbone of nursing practice. These essentials of nursing practice include patient-centered or "holistic" care, including family and community; care continuity; coordination and integration across settings and providers; chronic disease management; patient education; prevention and wellness care; and information management (American Nurses Association [ANA], 2010, pp. 1–2).

In addition, PPACA recognizes the advance practice registered nurse (APRN) as a valuable provider of primary care services, as well as a potential leader in new integrated care systems. The Institute of Medicine defines primary care as "the provision of integrated, accessible health care services by clinicians who are accountable for addressing a large majority of personal health care needs, developing a sustained partnership with patients, and practicing in the context of family and community" (ANA, 2010, pp. 1–2).

Three emerging care delivery models in particular, are addressed in PPACA. These are the accountable care organization, the medical or health home, and the nurse-managed health center. Nurses and APRNs will play a major role in the planning, implementation, and success of these emerging care delivery models.

In an accountable care organization a set of health care providers (including primary care physicians, nurses, specialists, and hospitals) work together collaboratively and accept collective accountability for the cost and quality of care delivered to a population of patients. Care is delivered across the transitions of care and includes primary care practices, hospitals, home health agencies, rehabilitation facilities, and other areas where health care is delivered.

The Patient-Centered Medical Home model was first proposed in 2007. It is, in essence, an enhanced primary care delivery model that strives to achieve better access, coordination of care, prevention, quality, and safety within the primary care practice, and to create a strong partnership between the patient and the primary care practitioner. Accountable Care Organizations (ACOs) are also based around a strong primary care core. However, ACOs are comprised of many "medical homes"; in other words, many primary care providers and/or practices that work together. Some have even dubbed ACOs the "medical neighborhood."

Nurse-Managed Health Clinics (NMHCs) (authorized under Title III of the Public Health Service Act) are health care delivery sites operated by APRNs, primarily nurse practitioners. These clinics are often associated with a school, college, university, department of nursing, federally qualified health center, or independent nonprofit health care agency. Although managed by APRNs, NMHCs are staffed by an interdisciplinary team of health care providers that includes physicians, social workers, and public health nurses. NMHCs provide primary care, health promotion, and disease prevention to individuals with limited access to care, regardless of their ability to pay. Services available at these clinics include physical exams, cardiovascular checks, diabetes and osteoporosis screenings, smoking cessation programs, immunizations, and other prevention-focused services. These clinics provide care to vulnerable populations in America's rural, urban, and suburban communities. For many patients in medically underserved areas, NMHCs and nurse practitioners are the area's only primary care providers. NMHCs serve as critical access points to keep patients out of the emergency room, saving the health care system millions of dollars annually.

One example of an emerging care delivery model is the Transitional Care Model (TCM) (Naylor, 2013). This nursing-developed model focuses on the care delivered through the varied transitions of care of those individuals with chronic illness.

Ten Essential Elements of Traditional Care Models

TCMs target older adults with two or more risk factors, including a history of recent hospitalizations, multiple chronic conditions, and poor self-health ratings.

1. The transitional care nurse (TCN), a master's-prepared nurse with advanced knowledge and skills in the care of this population, acts as the primary coordinator of care to ensure continuity throughout acute episodes of care.
2. In-hospital assessment, collaboration with team members to reduce adverse events and prevent functional decline, and preparation and development of a streamlined, evidenced-based plan of care.
3. Regular home visits by the TCN with ongoing telephone support (7 days per week) through an average of 2 months post-discharge.
4. Continuity of medical care between hospital and primary care providers facilitated by the TCN accompanying patients to first follow-up visit(s).
5. Comprehensive, holistic focus on each patient's goals and needs, including the reason for the primary hospitalization as well as other complicating or coexisting health problems and risks.
6. Active engagement of patients and family caregivers with a focus on meeting their goals.

7. Emphasis on patients' early identification and response to health care risks and symptoms to achieve longer-term positive outcomes and avoid adverse and untoward events that lead to readmissions.

8. Multidisciplinary approach that includes the patient, family care givers and health care providers as members of a team.

9. Physician-nurse collaboration across episodes of acute care.

10. Communication to, between, and among the patient, family care givers and health care providers.

Outcomes of this model of care include the following:

- Reductions in preventable hospital readmissions for both primary and co-existing health conditions.
- Improvements in health outcomes. Short-term improvements in physical health, functional status, and quality of life were reported by patients who received TCM.
- **Enha**ncement of patient satisfaction.
- Reductions in total health care costs. Both total and average reimbursements per patient have been reduced in TCM 3.

SUMMARY

Nurses are accountable for the delivery of safe, efficient, and effective patient/family care. The professional practice model and care delivery system and model serve as the vehicles for the delivery of such care. The decisions are based on a variety of information and current evidence and research. With the advent of the PPACA of 2010, nurses will be at the forefront of the development and implementation of evidence-based models of care delivery to meet the needs of the population.

CLINICAL CORNER

Professional Practice Model Development

According to the American Nursing Credentialing Center, a professional practice model (PPM) is a schematic depiction of a theory, phenomenon, or system that depicts how nurses practice, collaborate, communicate, and develop professionally. It is the conceptual framework and philosophy of nursing at a specific organization. The creation of a schematic depiction of a theory or phenomenon of how nurses see themselves practicing nursing in an organization can be challenging. This challenge was accepted by the Professional Practice Council in collaboration with the Nurse Executive Council. One of the goals behind this challenge was that nurses at every level in the organization would participate in this endeavor. Making this model with front-line nurse involvement was essential for the enculturation. A task force was developed and a literature review begun. The Professional Practice Model was to be grounded in theory, utilizing a qualitative methodology to discover the embedded phenomenon that was in existence.

An invitation was sent out to all nurses in the organization requesting volunteers to participate in establishing a PPM for the organization. The response rate captured nurses at all levels in the organization. A focus group was created and the moderator and assistant moderator were assigned. Characteristics that the moderator needed to possess were the ability to exercise unobtrusive behavior, adequate knowledge of the PPM concept, and to identify as one of the participants. The assistant moderator would need to be able to handle the logistics, take careful notes, and use flip charts. In this case the Chair of the Professional Practice Council was selected for the moderator, and the Magnet Coordinator was selected for the assistant moderator. Data analysis was undertaken using the Colaizzi method; collecting and transcribing, extracting significant statements, collapsing into like categories, and clustering themes into categories, those categories reflecting the elements of the PPM.

The first item on the agenda was education regarding the explanation of a PPM and its relationship to nursing theory as it pertains to the patient, nurse, environment, and health. Education about our Nursing Theorist, Jean Watson, was instrumental in capturing the true essences of the PPM and providing the groundwork for the philosophy of nursing in the organization. The organization's mission and vision statement were also presented during the education session. Identifying a nursing philosophy and depicting what is important to nursing within an organization is imperative and must be aligned with the organizational mission and vision. Giving examples of existing PPMs was the last step in the education part of the session.

Everyone then broke into different teams to brainstorm and describe how nursing practice could be depicted in a schematic model representing the organization and its vision: "Pursuing Excellence in Health Care." The statement

Continued

Professional Practice Model Development

"Pursuing Excellence in Nursing Practice" was the starting point for the development of the PPM. The elements that were important to the PPM were recorded on flip charts: practice, collaboration, communication, and professional development. A fifth element, "caring," as in the Jean Watson Theory of Caring, was added to incorporate our nursing theory. Every element was a driving force for delivering high-quality health care with the nurse in the lead. Everyday nursing practice deals with communication, collaboration, professional development, and caring.

Nursing practice in our PPM encompasses many components including but not limited to patient-centered care, high-quality care, shared governance, evidence-based practice, and research in the delivery of care. When shared governance is strong and nurses have a voice, many changes based on evidence and research will occur. The philosophy of shared governance implies that nurses at every level play a role in the decisions that affect nursing, and it requires nurses to be accountable for their decisions (Porter-O'Grady, 1989). These decisions should be based on evidence. Evidence-based practice is the "conscientious, explicit, and judicious use of the current best evidence in making decisions about the care of individuals" (Sackett et al., 1996, p. 71). It encompasses clinical and administrative practices that have been proven to consistently produce specific intended results. Research is vital to evidence-based practices. By definition, research is an organized study with methodical investigation into a subject to discover facts, to establish or revise a theory, or to develop a plan of action based on the facts discovered. It is the discovery of new knowledge. It is no longer the norm to say we do it that way because we have always done it that way. Nurses are educated and knowledgeable and can apply evidence to their practice. When research is applied and evidence is presented, high-quality care will be delivered.

Another element in our PPM is collaboration, as evidenced by the statement in our model: "Nurses act as facilitators and advocates. We develop a partnership in care with our patients, their families and with fellow health care professionals." This is demonstrated through our Care Delivery Model in which the nurse is considered to be the coordinator of care for patients as they navigate through a complex health care system. Our Care Delivery Model needed to be updated to align with our PPM. This was done after the PPM was developed and disseminated. Our multidisciplinary rounds are nurse-led and the collaboration between all disciplines is essential to providing high-quality care and establishing a strong discharge plan that will empower our patients and

families to care for themselves at home. Our rounds include patient and family goals, projected length of stay, and any barriers that will hinder that length of stay. At present, our Nursing Informatics Council is working on a "rounding tool" that incorporates all aspects of our rounds including the disease-specific certification requirements of The Joint Commission. It is a proactive tool that will keep the patients' goals obtainable. This tool will be embedded in the electronic medical record.

Our communication element addresses our goal to promote the professional image of nursing through active engagement in patient education, quality initiatives, and innovation to promote continuity of care for patients and their families, including local and global outreach. There is a strong relationship between the communication and collaboration elements. The communication element has enhanced our nurses' ability to reach out to our communities, both local and global. Our Nursing Leadership meetings provide nurses with the opportunity to present their global and local outreach endeavors to other nurses within the organization. This forum also promotes nurses taking the lead in promoting the image of nursing and encourages nurses to give back to the community, at both the local and global level.

The promotion of professional development has blossomed within our organization and continues to grow since the implementation of our PPM. Certification is taken seriously and we have celebrated Certification Day every year for the past 6 years. Our celebration includes having nurses within the organization set up booths to promote their professional organizations and has stirred up competition about which units have the largest increases in certified nurses for the past year. Every year follows a different theme, and money is raised to help buy appropriate tools to encourage nurses to join their organization and go for their certification. We are fortunate enough to have a certification champion who speaks to all nurses when they begin their orientation to the medical center. This sends a strong message that certification means you are an expert in your specialty. It is also incorporated into our Clinical Ladder Program. In the past couple of years we have also partnered with area colleges to have the schools come to our campus to encourage nurses who have been nursing for years to return to school for their Bachelor of Science in Nursing degree. An educational assistant program has also been implemented to streamline the reimbursement process and provide counseling for those returning to school.

The caring element is what connects all the components. As our model states: "Our Professional Practice Model

CLINICAL CORNER—cont'd

Professional Practice Model Development

is based on Jean Watson's Theory of Caring, which is a convergence of the art, theory, and science of nursing." According to Gallup polls, nurses are historically the most trusted profession, having always looked after the patients and families entrusted to their care. There is now an awareness of the importance of caring for each other. We are now working hard to encourage nurses to care for themselves. Our Nurses' Day celebrations encompass caring modalities, such as providing the nurses with reiki and massages. We have also established a Caritas Committee, which has educated all of the practice, peer, and unit-based councils about the importance of the Jean Watson Theory of Caring. All the council meetings begin with an inspirational reading and deep breathing and relaxation techniques before starting the meeting. The effect has been contagious. In the past year we have offered reiki certification classes to staff at all levels and are in the process of instituting a policy to offer reiki to our patients. The Caritas Committee has also

been instrumental in obtaining a Care Channel for our patients to help them heal in a healing environment.

The nurses at our organization are constantly improving the care they render to patients and their families at our medical center, and our PPM has empowered our nurses to be at the forefront of change. This change includes, and is not limited to, creating a healing environment, creating a healthy work environment, and establishing practices based on evidence and research.

References

Sackett, D. L., Rosenberg, W. M. C., Gray, J. A. M., Haynes, R. B., & Richardson, W. S. (1996). Evidence based medicine: what it is and what it isn't. *BMJ, 312*(71).

Porter-O'Grady, T. (1989). Shared governance: reality or sham? *American Journal of Nursing, 89*(3), 350–351.

Catherine Herrmann, BSN, RN, CCRN
Hackensack UMC

EVIDENCE-BASED PRACTICE

O'Rourke, M.W. (2003). Rebuilding a professional practice model. The return of role-based practice accountability. *Nursing Administration Quarterly, 27*(2), 95–105.

Abstract

There is no patient care without clinical practice. To improve the quality of health care, organizations must build a finely tuned and resilient clinical enterprise, one founded on clear role accountability and decision authority within the team. The author views scope of practice and professional standards as the foundation for practice accountability and decision authority. A case is made that an interdisciplinary professional practice model is an appropriate delivery model in today's health care environment, a model that places the professional role in its rightful place as decision maker and supports the role's inherent accountability to evaluate and monitor practice performance. The importance of measuring professional practice performance is seen as a key link toward better understanding ways to reduce error and ensure patient safety.

In 1990 the Institute of Medicine study, "To Err is Human," brought to the nation's attention the ills of our health care system. The study reported alarming rates of errors in hospitals. There was a national response by consumers, employers, and purchasers of services. They demanded reform to improve patient safety.

The articles discussed three kinds of practice: organizational, team, and individual. In organizational practice they were looking at cost-cutting. Roles were redesigned. The organizational plan incorporated patient care models. The patient care models determined roles and clear standards of practice, evaluation of practice performance, and improved outcome. An interdisciplinary professional practice model provided clear messages about professional, technical, and assistive roles.

The professional practice model and decision-making authority is important. There must be role accountability and role authority. The core competencies of the members of a profession are supported and include the following:

- Self-directed role authority based on substantial knowledge and technical skill with a rigorous professional practice process guided by science and theory.
- Using theory to direct practice, including modifying new theory to practical application and generating new theory.
- Transferring knowledge—explaining and predicting discipline-specific and interdisciplinary outcomes of care through science-based practice.
- Introducing new learning in the interest and service of the public and apply one's unique goal and practice by providing care.

In the 1990s team nursing was popular. In this model, scope of practice must be taken into consideration when

EVIDENCE-BASED PRACTICE—cont'd

team assignments are made. Each team member must know their roles and scope of practice. Boards of nursing mandated that all name tags should clearly designate the person's role. The registered nurse played a key role, addressing the hard questions of education and error rates in hospitals.

A patient care model based on an interdisciplinary professional practice approach is divided into three components. They are:

1. Organizational performance standard.
   * Reestablish the professional clinical process as the core operating system, the foundation for our business, and build from there.
   * Create practice environments that uphold legal, professional, and regulatory expectations.
   * Take direct action to ensure the rigorous application of the professional process tasks under which staff function and manage the patient condition.

2. Performance standard.
   * Demonstrate the value of each profession's contribution to improving patient care.
   * Tie organizations and clinical practice competence with performance outcomes.

3. Clinical practice standard.
   1. Deliberately shift to process-versus task-based thinking and work.
   2. Capture the intellectual capacity of the interdisciplinary team members.
   3. Involve medical staff in establishing and upholding the practice standard of all professional disciplines.
   4. Demonstrate the value of each profession's contributions to improving patient care.

NCLEX® EXAMINATION QUESTIONS

1. What is a collaboration among primary care clinicians, a hospital, specialists, and other health professionals who accept joint responsibility for the quality and cost of care provided to its patients?
   A. Medical home
   B. Accountable care organization
   C. Professional practice model
   D. Care delivery system

2. What are the emerging care delivery models addressed by the Patient Protection and Affordable Care Act (PPACA) of 2010?
   A. Accountable care organization
   B. Medical or home health
   C. Nurse-managed health center
   D. All of the above

3. Who is the fundamental health care provider to meet the success of emerging patient-centered care delivery models?
   A. The registered nurse
   B. The physician
   C. The physician's assistant
   D. The nurse practitioner

4. Which authors propose that the nursing care delivery model should consist of five key dimensions, including staffing intensity; skill and nursing education mix; professional scope of practice in six domains of practice (assessment and planning, teaching, communication, supervision, quality of care, and knowledge updating); nursing practice environment; and unit-level capacity for innovation?
   A. Dubois, D'Amour, Tchouaket, Clarke, Rivard, & Blais (2013)
   B. O'Connor, Bennett, Crawford, & Korfiatis (2006)
   C. ANCC (2013)
   D. Zelauskas & Howes (1992) as cited in ANCC (2013)

5. The care delivery system continually improved to do what?
   A. Adjust to national patient safety goals
   B. Value-based outcomes
   C. Meet regulatory requirements
   D. All of the above

6. The professional nurse as decision maker is guided by which of the following?
   A. The American Nurses Association (ANA) Code of Ethics
   B. The ANA Standards of the State Nursing Practice Act
   C. State Titles
   D. All of the above

7. In the University of California Los Angeles model, who is at the center of care?
   A. The nurse
   B. The patient, family, and community
   C. The patient and family
   D. The nurse and patient

8. Who is at the center or forefront of a professional practice model?
   A. The nurse
   B. The physician
   C. The health care team
   D. The patient and family

9. Which of the following is a system for the delivery of care that delineates a nurse's authority and accountability for clinical decision making and outcomes?
   A. Medical home
   B. Accountable care organization
   C. Professional practice model
   D. Care delivery system

10. Which of the following is a schematic description of a theory, phenomenon, or system that depicts how nurses practice, collaborate, communicate, and develop professionally to provide the highest quality care for those by the organization (American Nurses Credentialing Center [ANCC], 2013)?
    A. Medical home
    B. Accountable care organization
    C. Professional practice model
    D. Care delivery system

Answers: 1. B   2. D   3. A   4. A   5. D   6. D   7. B
8. D   9. D   10. C

REFERENCES

American Association of Critical-Care Nurses [AACN]. (2013). Policy Brief: *Nurse-managed health clinics: increasing access to primary care and educating the healthcare workforce.* www.aacn.nche.edu/government-affairs/FY13NMHCs.pdf.

Accountable Care Facts. (2014). www.accountablecarefacts.org/topten/what-is-the-difference-between-a-medical-home-and-an-aco-1.

American Nurses Association [ANA] Issue Brief. (2010). *New care delivery models in health system reform: opportunities for nurses and their patient.* www.nursingworld.org/MainMenuCategories/Policy-Advocacy/Positions-and-Resolutions/Issue-Briefs/Care-Delivery-Models.pdf.

American Nurses Credentialing Center [ANCC]. (2013). *2014 Magnet Application Manual.* Silver Spring, MD: Author.

Brannon, R. L. (1994). *Intensifying care: The hospital industry, professionalization, and the reorganization of the nursing labor process.* Amityville, NY: Baywood Publishing Company.

D'Amour, D., Dubois, C.-A., Déry, J., Clarke, S., Tchouaket, E., Blais, R., et al. (2012). Measuring actual scope of hospital nursing practice: a new tool for nurse managers and researchers. *Journal of Nursing Administration, 42*(5), 248–255.

Dubois, C., D'Amour, D., Tchouaket, E., Clarke, S., Rivard, M., & Blais, R. (2013). Associations of patient safety outcomes with models of nursing care organization at unit level in hospitals. *International Journal Quality Health Care, 25*(2), 110–117.

Gardner, K. (1991). A summary of findings of a five-year comparison study of primary and team nursing. *Nursing Research, 40*(2), 113–117.

Jupiter Medical Center. *Description of JMC Care Delivery System.* www.jupitermed.com/care-delivery-system

Kimball, B., Joynt, J., & Cherner, D. (2007). The quest for new innovative care delivery models. *Journal of Nursing Administration, 37*(9), 392–398.

Lake, E. T. (2002). Development of the practice environment scale of the Nursing Work Index. *Res Nurs Health, 25*(3), 176–188.

Massachusetts General Hospital. (2014). *Professional Practice Model.* www.google.com/search?q=professional+practice+model+magnet&rlz=1T4MXGB_enUS598US598&tbm=isch&tbo=u&source=univ&sa=X&ei=HyfVU8ePEoHyATb14CICw&ved=0CDAQsAQ&biw=1366&bih=612.

Naylor, M. (2013). *Transitional Care Model.* www.nursing.upenn.edu/media/transitionalcare/Documents/Information%20on%20the%20Model.pdf.

O'Connor, S. E. (1994). A re-organization that improves patient care: An evaluation of team nursing in acute clinical setting. *Professional Nurse, 9*, 808–811.

O'Connor, B., Bennett, M., Crawford, S., & Korfiatis, V. (2006). The trials and tribulations of team nursing. *Collegian, 13*(3), 11–17.

Sjetne, I. S., Helgeland, J., & Stavem, K. (2010). Classifying nursing organization in wards in Norwegian hospitals: Self-identification versus observation. *BMC Nurs, 9*(3).

Tiedman, M., & Lookinland, S. (2004). Traditional models of care delivery: what have we learned? *Journal of Nursing Administration, 34*(6), 291–297.

University of California–Los Angeles (UCLA). (2014). *Professional Practice Model.* www.google.com/search?q=professional+practice+model+magnet&rlz=1T4MXGB_enUS598US598&tbm=isch&tbo=u&source=univ&sa=X&ei=HyfVU8ePEo-HyATb14CICw&ved=0C-DAQsAQ&biw=1366&bih=612.

Yoder-Wise, P. S. (2011). *Leading and managing in nursing* (4th ed.). St. Louis: Mosby.

12

Staffing and Scheduling

OBJECTIVES

- Discuss the information required for the determination of staffing needs.
- Review the different types of assignment systems.
- Identify the difference between centralized and decentralized staffing.

- Differentiate between the various types of staffing patterns.
- Discuss activities used by the nurse manager to support fluctuating staffing needs.

OUTLINE

KEY TERMS

average daily census (ADC) average number of patients cared for per day for the reporting period

average length of stay (ALOS) average number of days that a patient remained in an occupied bed

block scheduling using the same schedule repeatedly

centralized scheduling scheduling done in one location

decentralized scheduling scheduling done in local areas

FTE full-time equivalent; equal to the equivalent of a full-time employee

nursing hours per patient total paid hours for nursing personnel for a specific time period divided by the number of patient days in the same period

patient acuity measure of nursing workload that is generated for each patient

permanent shifts personnel working the same hours repeatedly

rotating work shifts alternating work hours among days, evening, and nights

self-scheduling staff coordinating their own work schedules

staffing pattern plan that articulates how many and what kind of staff are needed by shift and day to staff a unit or department

staffing ratios number of nursing staff per patient

staffing schedules work schedules for personnel

variable staffing determining the number and mix of staff based on patient needs

variance reports noting differences in budgeted or planned staffing and costs

STAFFING

One of the most time-consuming concerns of most nurse managers is the staffing of the unit. Staffing requires having enough staff to deliver care, and that the staff present are qualified to deliver that care. Hospital nurse staffing has an important relationship to patient safety and quality of care. The available evidence indicates that there is a statistically and clinically significant association between registered nurse (RN) staffing and the adjusted odds ratio of hospital-related mortality, failure to rescue, and other patient outcomes (Kane et al., 2007). **Staffing schedules** are also a major concern of nurses as they enter a health care environment. Issues with schedules are often cited as a major job dissatisfier by nurses leaving the workplace (Halm, Peterson, & Kandelis, 2005).

There have been multiple studies in recent literature supporting the importance of safe staffing and its relation to patient safety (Aiken et al., 2002; Hugonnet, Chevrolet, & Pittet, 2007; Stone, Mooney Kane, & Larsen, 2007; Weissman, Rothschild, & Bendavid, 2007). Higher numbers of hours of nursing care provided by registered nurses and a greater number of hours of care by registered nurses per day are associated with better care for hospitalized patients (Needleman et al., 2002; Needleman et al., 2006).

Health care staffing is a complicated issue, requiring knowledge of patient acuity, nursing productivity, nursing competence, organization finance, and health care regulations.

The Joint Commission

The Joint Commission (TJC) and other accrediting agencies survey hospitals on the quality of care provided. They do not mandate staffing levels, but they do assess an organization's ability to provide the right number of competent staff to meet the needs of patients served by the hospital (The Joint Commission [TJC], 2014).

The American Nurses Association *Principles for Nurse Staffing*

In 2012, the American Nurses Association (ANA) published *Principles for Nurse Staffing* (2nd ed.), which emphasized the importance of the nursing work environment in providing safe patient care (Box 12-1). Appropriate nurse staffing is the match of registered nurse expertise with the needs of the recipient of nursing care services in the context of the practice setting and situation. The provision of appropriate nurse staffing is necessary to reach safe quality outcomes; it is achieved by dynamic, multifaceted decision-making processes that must take into account a wide range of variables (American Nurses Association [ANA], 2012). The ANA *Principles for Nurse Staffing* are organized into five sets according to the following topics (note the relationship with the data required for care delivery decisions [Chapter 11]:

- The characteristics and considerations of the health care consumer.
- The characteristics and considerations of the registered nurses and other
- Interprofessional team members and staff.
- The context of the entire organization in which the nursing services are delivered.
- The overall practice environment that influences the delivery of care.
- The evaluation of staffing plans.

After the first edition of *Principles of Safe Staffing* in 1999, the ANA advocated a work environment that supports nurses in providing the best possible patient care by budgeting enough positions, administrative support, good nurse-physician relations, career advancement options, work flexibility, and personal choice in scheduling (ANA, 2012). This advocacy continues today.

BOX 12-1 The American Nurses Association Principles for Nurse Staffing

Core components of nurse staffing.

- Appropriate nurse staffing is critical to the delivery of quality, cost-effective health care.
- All settings should have well-developed staffing guidelines with measurable nurse sensitive outcomes specific to that setting and health care consumer population that are used as evidence to guide daily staffing.
- Registered nurses are full partners working with other health care professionals in collaborative, interdisciplinary partnerships.
- Registered nurses, including direct care nurses, must have a substantive and active role in staffing decisions to ensure the necessary time with patients to meet care needs and overall nursing responsibilities.
- Staffing needs must be determined based on an analysis of health care consumer status (e.g., degree of stability, intensity, and acuity), and the environment in which the care is provided. Other considerations to be included are professional characteristics, skill set and mix of the staff, and previous staffing patterns that have been shown to improve outcomes.
- Appropriate nurse staffing should be based on allocating the appropriate number of competent practitioners to a care situation; pursuing quality of care indices; meeting consumer-centered and organizational outcomes; meeting federal and state laws and regulations; and attending to a safe, quality work environment.
- Cost effectiveness is an important consideration in delivery of safe, quality care.
- Reimbursement structure should not influence nurse staffing patterns or the level of care provided.

Principles Related to the Health Care Consumer

Staffing decisions should be based on the number and needs of the individual health care consumers, families, and population served. These include the following:

- Age and functional ability.
- Communication skills.
- Cultural and linguistic diversities.
- Severity, intensity, acuity, complexity, and stability of condition.
- Existence and severity of multi-morbid conditions.
- Scheduled procedure(s).
- Ability to meet health care requisites.
- Availability of social supports.
- Transitional care, within or beyond the health care setting.
- Continuity of care.
- Complexity of care needs.
- Environmental turbulence (i.e., rapid admissions, turnovers, and/or discharges).

- Other specific needs identified by the health care consumer, the family, and the registered nurse.

The following elements are to be considered when making the determination:

- Governance within the setting (i.e., shared governance).
- Involvement in quality measurement activities.
- Quality of the work environment of the nurses.
- Development of comprehensive plans of care.
- Practice environment.
- Architectural geography of the unit and institution.
- Evaluation of practice outcomes that include both quality and safety.
- Available technology.
- Evolving evidence.

Principles Related to Registered Nurses and Other Staff

The following nurse characteristics should be taken into account when determining staffing:

- Licensure.
- Experience with the population being served.
- Level of experience (i.e., novice to expert).
- Competency with technology and clinical interventions.
- Professional certification.
- Educational preparation.
- Language capabilities.

Principles Related to Organization and Workplace Culture

These include at a minimum:

- Effective and efficient support services (e.g., transport, clerical, housekeeping, and laboratory).
- Timely coordination, supervision, and delegation as needed to maximize safety.
- Access to timely, accurate, relevant information provided by communication technology that links clinical, administrative, and outcome data.
- Sufficient orientation and preparation, including nurse preceptors and nurse experts to ensure registered nurse competency.
- Preparation and ongoing training for competency in technology or other tools.
- Sufficient time for patient documentation.
- Necessary time to collaborate with and supervise other staff.
- Necessary time to accommodate increased documentation demands created by integration of technology, electronic records, surveillance systems, and regulatory requirements.
- Support in ethical decision making.

BOX 12-1   **The American Nurses Association Principles for Nurse Staffing—cont'd**

Principles Related to Organization and Workplace Culture—cont'd

- Resources and pathways for care coordination and health care consumer/client and/or family education.
- Adequate time for coordination and supervision of nursing assistive personnel by registered nurses.
- Processes to facilitate transitions during work redesign, mergers, and other major changes in work life.
- Supporting the registered nurse's professional responsibility to maintain continuing education and engagement in lifelong learning.

Principles Related to the Practice Environment

Staffing is a structure and process that affects the safety of patients, as well as others in the environment and nurses themselves. Institutions employing a culture of safety must recognize appropriate nurse staffing as integral to achieving goals for patient safety and quality.

Registered nurses have a professional obligation to report unsafe conditions or inappropriate staffing that adversely impacts safe quality care, and the right to do so without reprisal.

Registered nurses should be provided a professional nursing practice environment in which they have control over nursing practice and autonomy in their workplace.

Appropriate preparation, resources, and information should be provided for those involved at all levels of decision making. Opportunities must be provided for individuals to be involved in decision making related to nursing practice.

Routine mandatory overtime is an unacceptable solution to achieve appropriate nurse staffing. Policies on length of shifts; management of meal and rest periods; and overtime should be in place to ensure the health and stamina of nurses and prevent fatigue-related errors.

Principles Related to Staffing Evaluation

Organizations should evaluate staffing plans based on factors including but not limited to the following:

- Outcomes, especially as measured by nurse-sensitive indicators.
- Time needed for direct and indirect patient care.
- Work-related staff illness and injury rates.
- Turnover/vacancy rates.
- Overtime rates.
- Rate of use of supplemental staffing.
- Flexibility of human resource policies and benefit packages.
- Evidence of compliance with applicable federal, state, and local regulations.
- Levels of health care consumer satisfaction and nurse satisfaction.

American Nurses Association [ANA]. (2012). *Principles for nurse staffing* (2nd ed.). Silver Spring, MD: Author.

State departments of health have staffing regulations for health care institutions; these regulations are often broad. Additionally, California has mandatory staffing guidelines. These guidelines have provoked court challenges and much discussion and review in other states. On October 10, 1999, California became the first state in the country to require mandatory, safe licensed nurse/patient ratios in all units in acute-care facilities. The legislation (AB 394) requires that additional nurses be added to a minimum ratio in accordance with a patient classification system based on the severity of the patient's condition. As mandated by state law, the California Department of Health Services requires acute-care hospitals to maintain minimum nurse-to-patient **staffing ratios**. Required ratios vary by unit, from 1:1 in operating rooms to 1:6 on psychiatric units (Agency for Healthcare Research and Quality [AHRQ], 2014). Lawmakers in D.C., New York, Texas, Florida, New Jersey, Iowa, and Minnesota are also considering legislation.

Some states have regulations about specialty unit ratios enforced by Departments of Health.

PROCESS OF STAFFING

A staffing plan addresses the requirements of the unit or organization over a defined period of time. Daily staffing plans outline what is necessary to meet the needs of the patients over a 24-hour period. An annual staffing plan is created to determine the budgetary needs of an organization. "Daily staffing" refers to filling in open shifts on the current work schedule.

"Scheduling" refers to making work assignments for the next work period. It is done from 4 to 8 weeks in advance depending on the institution (Figure 12-1).

Process of Daily Staffing

The process of daily staffing begins with an assessment of the current staffing situation. The assessment includes

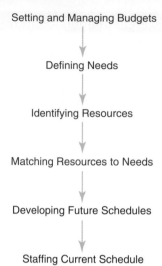

Setting and Managing Budgets

↓

Defining Needs

↓

Identifying Resources

↓

Matching Resources to Needs

↓

Developing Future Schedules

↓

Staffing Current Schedule

FIGURE 12-1 Nurse scheduling and staffing. (From California Health Care Foundation [2005]. *Adopting online nurse scheduling and staffing systems*. Oakland, CA. Used with permission.)

the qualifications and competence of the staff needed and available to meet the needs of the current patients (ANA, 2004). The next step is to formulate a plan to meet future needs. The staffing process culminates in a schedule (organized plan) of personnel to provide patient care services. Scheduling variables are defined as (adapted from Jones, 2007, p. 280):

1. The number of patients, complexity of patients' condition, and nursing care required.
2. The physical environment in which nursing care is to be provided.
3. The nursing staff members' competency levels, qualifications, skill range, knowledge or ability, and experience level.
4. The level of supervision required.
5. Availability of nursing staff members for the assignment of responsibilities.
6. Availability of staff needed for participation in shared governance activities.

The Staffing Plan

The staffing plan consists of four different elements that must be addressed:

1. The health care setting.
2. The care delivery model.
3. Patient acuity.
4. Nursing staff.

These are then incorporated into the next step in the process—the scheduling and staffing system. A staffing plan can also be referred to as the "staffing matrix."

Staffing and Scheduling Systems

There are various types of staffing systems in place in health care. The four major types are:

1. **Centralized scheduling**: Decision making occurs in a "centralized" location for the entire institution.
2. **Decentralized scheduling**: Decision making occurs with the nurse manager on the unit.
3. Mixed scheduling: Blends aspects of items 1 and 2. Individual units may manage staffing, but if they cannot fill open shifts, they might forward their needs to a centralized office.
4. **Self-scheduling**: Individual staff members schedule themselves. The nurse manager then works with staff members to fill empty slots.

Many organizations are moving toward computer-assisted staffing.

Centralized Scheduling

There are two major advantages of centralized scheduling: fairness to employees through consistent, objective, and impartial application of policies and opportunities for cost containment through better use of resources (Tomey, 2008, p. 387).

Decentralized Scheduling

When managers are given authority and assume responsibility, they can staff their own units through decentralized scheduling (Tomey, 2008).

Scheduling staff, which is very time consuming, takes managers away from other duties or forces them to do the scheduling while off duty. Decentralized scheduling may use resources less effectively and consequently make cost containment more difficult (Tomey, 2008).

Mixed Scheduling

An individual may manage staffing, but with the option of consulting a centralized office to help fill open shifts.

Self-Scheduling

Staff nurses coordinate the scheduling. This saves the manager considerable scheduling time. It also increases

TABLE 12-1	**Pros and Cons of Centralized and Decentralized Scheduling**	
Scheduling method	**Pros**	**Cons**
Centralized	Fairness Cost containment	Lack of individualized treatment
Decentralized	Managers have authority Staff get personalized attention Staffing is easier Staffing is less complicated	Schedule used to punish and reward Time consuming for managers Cost containment is more difficult

BOX 12-2   Types of Pattern Scheduling

- Alternating or rotating work shifts: Work schedule is based on a predefined pattern, such as alternate weekends off, or rotating from days to evenings every 3 weeks. Sometimes, however, the rotating of shifts may only occur as needed, such as when the night nurse is off.
- Permanent shifts: Individuals are hired to work specific shifts, such as nights only.
- Block, or cyclical, scheduling: This type of scheduling system uses the same schedule repeatedly. It may be similar to alternating or rotating shifts, but may also include a pattern of days on and days off (4 on; 2 off). It is often used as part of another type of scheduling pattern (see below).

Eight-hour shift, 5-day workweek: This method uses the traditional 5-day, 40-hour workweek. This does not mean that weekends are not covered; the nurse works 5 days a week with 2 days off, and the nurse may work alternating weekends.

Ten-hour day, 4-day workweek: This method requires careful block scheduling to cover all shifts.

Twelve-hour shifts: 3 days on and 4 days off. Some studies demonstrate that this method allows for better use of nursing personnel, increased continuity of care, and improved job satisfaction and morale (Garret, 2008).

Baylor plan—weekend alternative: Baylor University Medical Center in Dallas, Texas, started a 2-day alternative plan. Nurses have the option to work two 12-hour days on the weekends and be paid for 36 hours for day shifts, or 40 hours for night shifts, or to work five 8-hour shifts Monday through Friday. This plan requires a larger nursing staff, filled weekend positions, and reduced turnover. Some hospitals have implemented the Baylor plan, indicating that the extra pay on weekends compensated for vacations, holidays, and sick time (Tomey, 2008, p. 393).

Variable staffing: This type of staffing is dependent on the patient acuity and needs of the unit. If acuity is higher than budgeted, extra staff may be called in on overtime, or additional staff, such as agency or float staff, may be used.

staff members' ability to negotiate with each other and has been associated with perceptions of increased nursing autonomy and satisfaction.

Table 12-1 provides pros and cons of centralized and decentralized scheduling.

Health care organizations must have a system in place to track available personnel. To match personnel with staffing needs, the organization must be able to determine an individual's skills, competencies, license, certifications, etc. Most scheduling is done in advance, therefore future scheduling is used. Institutions use one or more of the following four types of future scheduling in their planning:

1. Pattern scheduling: Staff commit to work a set number of shift types in a given timeframe. At the end of the time period, the pattern repeats (such as 3 weeks of day shift followed by 1 week of night shift, repeated every 4 weeks). Pattern scheduling can also include permanent shifts, block shifts, and rotating shifts (Box 12-2).
2. Preference scheduling: Staff define their preferences for shift type, days of the week, and unit. Defined rules can override preferences.
3. Rules scheduling: This is based on an organization's scheduling policies. Because it does not take pattern or preference into account, it is rarely used alone.
4. Self-scheduling: Scheduling needs are defined, and then staff sign up for available shifts on a rotating, first-come, first-served basis.

Table 12-2 provides pros and cons of scheduling types.

Table 12-3 lists advantages and disadvantages of the types of pattern scheduling.

TABLE 12-2   Pros and Cons of Scheduling Types

Scheduling type	Pros	Cons
Rules based	Incorporates regulatory issues (hours of work, time off overtime, staffing ratios)	Does not take preferences into account Does not take staffing patterns into account Scheduling can be erratic
Pattern	Predictable schedules	Little flexibility Impairs recruitment
Preference	Considers staff needs	Preferences may not match rules
Self	Enables more creativity in covering shifts Increased staff satisfaction Saves time for nurse managers	Less organization and manager control of staffing

From California Health Care Foundation. (2005). *Adopting online nurse scheduling and staffing systems* (p. 13). Oakland, CA: Author. Used with permission.

TABLE 12-3   Advantages and Disadvantages of Types of Pattern Scheduling

Type	Advantages	Disadvantages
Rotating work shifts	Can rotate teams	Rotates among shifts Increases stress Affects health Affects quality of work Disrupts development of work groups High turnover
Permanent shifts	Can participate in social activities Job satisfaction Commitment to the organization Few health problems Less tardiness Less absenteeism Less turnover	Most people want day shifts New graduates predominantly staff evenings and nights Difficulty of evaluating evening and night staff Nurses may not appreciate the workload or problems of other shifts Rigidity
Block, or cyclical, scheduling	Same schedule repeatedly Nurses not so exhausted Sick time reduced Personnel know schedule in advance Personnel can schedule social events Decreased time spent on scheduling Staff treated fairly Helps establish stable work groups Decreases floating Promotes team spirit Promotes continuity of care	
Variable staffing	Use census to determine number and mix of staff Little need to call in unscheduled staff Efficient	

From Tomey, A.M., (2008). *Guide to nursing management and leadership* (8th ed.). St. Louis: Mosby.

FULL-TIME EQUIVALENT

No matter what the shift, the needs of the patient, unit, and organization must be accommodated. There is no end to the creative ways that staffing can be accomplished, but the basic number that is used in staffing is the full-time equivalent (FTE). An FTE is a measure of the work commitment of a full-time employee. A full-time employee works to qualify for full-time employment. In institutions with a 40-hour full-time workweek, this works out to 2080 hours of work time per year (40 hours per week for 52 weeks a year equals 2080 hours of work time). In organizations with a 37.5-hour workweek, this would work out to (37.5 × 52 weeks) 1950 hours of work time per year. Most institutions use a 40-hour workweek for the definition of an FTE (Table 12-4).

Therefore, if the nurse manager needed to cover 40 hours of work per week, it could be done by one full-time employee or two half-time employees, etc. For budget purposes, it would be important to know the state rules and regulations covering benefits. When does an employee receive benefits (health care, vacation time, etc.)? Staff benefits are a costly expense to health care institutions. Benefits are presently estimated as up to 50% beyond actual pay in some institutions.

Another variable in the staffing decision will be the amount of productive versus nonproductive hours. Not all of the 2080 hours of the FTE are productive. Benefit time, such as vacation, sick time, and education time are considered nonproductive time. To determine the amount of productive time of an employee, you would subtract the hours of benefit time from the FTE of 2080 hours. So if an employee had:

5 sick days (5 days × 8 hours/day) = 40 hours
20 vacation days (20 × 8 hours/day) = 160 hours
Holidays (5 days × 8 hours/day) = 40 hours
Education time (3 days × 8 hours/day) = 24 hours

This all adds up to 264 hours of nonproductive time, thus 2080 hours per year - 264 hours = 1816 hours of productive time. When calculating the number of FTEs needed to staff the unit, you would count only the number of productive hours available.

To determine staffing needs, the nurse manager needs to know the number of FTE employees and the amount of nursing hours per patient day. Nursing care hours per patient day are the number of hours worked by nursing staff that have direct patient-care responsibilities. To calculate nursing care hours per patient day, use only productive hours.

Calculation of nursing care hours per patient day (Bernat, 2003):

20 patients on the unit
5 staff on each of three shifts = 15 staff
15 staff each working 8 productive hours = 120 hours ÷ 24 hours
120 nursing care hours ÷ 20 patients = 6.0 nursing care hours per patient

DEVELOPMENT OF A STAFFING PATTERN

One cannot assume that the number of nursing care hours is a permanent number. This number will change based on patient acuity. Patient acuity data are used to predict the amount of nursing care required by a group of patients. The higher the acuity level, the more nursing care is needed by the patient.

To develop a staffing pattern using nursing hours per patient day (NHPPD), you would start with a goal nursing-care hours. If your goal was 5 and you had 35 patients on your 40-bed unit, you would multiply 5 NHPPD × 35 patients to get 175 productive hours needed every day. Dividing 175 by 8-hour shifts worked by a FTE gives you 21.8 FTEs needed per day (adapted from Kelly-Heidenthal, 2003).

The staffing number calculated for the unit is 21.8, but that does not account for nonproductive hours. The manager must provide for the additional staff that will be needed for days off and benefit time. Each 8-hour shift for an FTE is equal to 0.2 FTE; therefore, to provide

TABLE 12-4 **FTE Calculation for Varying Levels of Work Commitment**
1.0 FTE = 40 hours per week or five 8-hour shifts per week
0.8 FTE = 32 hour per week or four 8-hour shifts per week
0.6 FTE = 24 hours per week or three 8-hour shifts per week
0.4 FTE = 16 hours per week or two 8-hour shifts per week
0.2 FTE = 8 hours per week or one 8-hour shift per week

From Kelly-Heidenthal, P. (2003). *Nursing leadership and management* (p. 240). Clifton Park, NY: Thomson Delmar Learning.

coverage for 2 days off a week, multiply the number of staff needed per day by 0.4 FTE. The 21.8 FTEs multiplied by 0.4 would be an additional 8.7 FTEs to cover 2 days off per week for a total of 30.5 FTEs (adapted from Kelly-Heidenthal, 2003).

The next step is to provide coverage for vacation time and other time away from work. If every employee receives 2 weeks of vacation and 2 educational days, this would equate to 1984 hours of productive time (2 weeks = 10 days × 8 hours + 2 days = 16 hours = 96 hours subtracted from the FTE 2080 hours = 1984 productive hours per FTE). Previously, it was decided that a total of 30.5 FTEs were needed to cover the unit. This was based on 2080 productive hours, but you have now found that there are only 1984 productive hours per FTE: 30.5 FTEs × 2080 = 63,440 hours and 63,440 hours ÷ 1984 = 31.9 FTEs needed to cover this unit (adapted from Kelly-Heidenthal, 2003).

The spread of staff across the 24-hour period depends on the type of patients. Typically, intensive care units have a relatively equal spread across the shifts with the spread of FTEs across the 24-hour period falling into the following pattern: days, 33% to 50%; evenings, 30% to 40%; nights, 20% to 33% (adapted from Kelly-Heidenthal, 2003).

Part-Time Staff

Part-time staff are used to decrease staffing shortages in an institution.

Part-time employment has the following benefits for nurses. It can:
- Broaden horizons beyond home;
- Increase income;
- Provide ego satisfaction;
- Help maintain nursing skills; and
- Continue education.

Benefits for the institution include:
- Having a flexible work pool; and
- Decreased benefit costs.

Another option is for two nurses to share one full-time position. The disadvantages to an institution of position sharing are that educational and administrative expenses are higher proportionately for part-time than for full-time help because it costs as much to orient a part-time nurse as it does a full-time nurse, thereby costing more per hours worked. Also, maintaining continuity of care is complicated if two or more part-time people fill budgeted full-time positions. The disadvantages for the nurses are that there are not full-time benefits, such as vacation and sick time.

External Temporary Agencies

Usually as a last resort, an institution may use temporary agency nurses. The staffing agency is a business that has a registry of nurses who have highly flexible schedules. Matching of nurses' credentials with the position is sometimes daunting. Replacement staff from agency pools are usually an expensive means of maintaining staffing. Most hospitals prefer to minimize the use of agency nurses because of the extra cost to the institution. The extra costs arise from the mandated orientations, evaluation of competencies, and the agency fee.

Travel Nurses

"Travelers" are per diem nurses working for a business that places them in contracted hospitals. Unlike agency nurses, travelers usually sign longer-term contracts with hospitals (3 to 6 months or longer).

There are many options used by health care institutions to deal with staffing and daily absences because of sick calls (Box 12-3).

Overtime

In a staffing emergency, institutions may ask nurses to work overtime. Overtime pay is usually at a higher rate than regular pay, and many nurses depend on the extra money provided by overtime. There are a number of issues with overtime that need concern the nurse and nurse manager.
- Length of time the nurse will be working. In a normal shift, the nurse will have already worked up to

---

BOX 12-3   Options Used for Sick Calls

- Use a float, per diem, or agency nurse.
- Ask a nurse to work for the sick person and cancel a shift for that person later in the week.
- Ask a part-time person to work an extra shift, substituting one type of classification for another, such as a licensed practical nurse (LPN) for a registered nurse (RN).
- Ask one staff member to work a few hours of overtime and another to come in a few hours early.
- Do without a substitute.
- Manager covers the shift.

12 hours and an additional shift could have them working a full 24 hours! This can be ameliorated by only allowing 4 hours of overtime in such a situation.

- The nurse manager must be careful to evaluate the exhaustion level of the staff.
- There are documented instances of increased errors when the staff members are exhausted (Garrett, 2008).
- With regard to budget, overtime may increase the dollars spent on care provided. This budget variance will need to be documented.
- State labor law will need to be reviewed as well as union guidelines. These may define the number of hours required between shifts.

Mandatory overtime is never a solution to staffing concerns.

Automated Staffing Systems

Many health care institutions are moving toward the use of computerized staffing and scheduling systems. These systems greatly enhance the manager's ability to properly schedule staff. They also free up much of the time that the manager spends on the creation of the schedule. Integrated online scheduling and staffing products are available for purchase under license.

Evaluation of Staffing Measures

As discussed in the ANA *Principles for Nurse Staffing* (2012), the evaluation of the effectiveness of nurse staffing is of utmost importance. As a nurse manager, you will be evaluated in areas of patient outcomes and budget performance. The ever-evolving management of daily staffing with the patient outcomes and budget requirements is a daunting challenge for nurse administrators. The patient outcomes that are reviewed on a daily/weekly/monthly/quarterly basis are also related to nurse staffing. They include the following:

- Accreditation standards and National Patient Safety Goals.
- Patient Satisfaction survey results.
- National Database of Nursing Quality Indicators (NDNQI) nursing sensitive indicator outcomes.
- Unit scorecards.
- The NDNQI Staff RN Satisfaction Survey.

- Centers for Medicare and Medicaid Services (CMS) core measures.
- Hospital Consumer Assessment of Healthcare Providers and Systems (HCAHPS) results.
- Unit based surveys.

They also relate to the organizational budget performance and expected productivity. Typical Unit Productivity Report Indicators include:

Variance reports for areas of alteration (be they good or negative!) must be shared with the key stakeholders. Performance is an ever-changing and evolving science.

BOX 12-4 Typical Unit Activities Productivity Report Indicators

- Volume statistic: number of units of service for the reporting period
- Capacity statistic: number of beds or blocks of time available for providing services
- Percentage of occupancy: number of occupied beds for the reporting period
- Average daily census (ADC): average number of patients cared for per day for the reporting period
- Average length of stay (ALOS): average number of days that a patient remained in an occupied bed

Formulas for Calculating Volume Statistics
Assume that a 20-bed medical-surgical unit *(capacity statistic)* accrued 566 patient days in June *(volume statistic)*. Ninety-eight of these patients were discharged during the month.

Average Daily Census (ADC) on this unit is 18.9
Formula: patient days for a given time period divided by the number of days in the time period
a. 30 days in June
b. 566 patient days/30 days = ADC of 18.9

Percentage of Occupancy for June is 95%
Formula: daily patient census (rounded) divided by the number of beds in the unit
19 patients in a 20-bed unit =
19 patients/20 beds = 95% occupancy

Average Length of Stay for June is 5.8
Formula: number of patient days divided by the number of discharges
566 patient days/98 patient discharges = 5.8 (rounded)

SUMMARY

Staffing and scheduling represents one of the most challenging of the nurse manager's responsibilities. It requires an accurate sense of the day-to-day workings of the unit as well as a keen awareness of the staff's abilities and personalities. It also requires evaluation of the care delivered and the flexibility to create staffing levels that best meet patient needs.

CLINICAL CORNER

Work Environment: The Context of Nursing Practice

The nursing work environment is complex and its characteristics may vary from setting to setting. A systematic review of the literature on nursing work environments conducted by Schalk et al. (2010) resulted in the identification of elements that are common to most settings, and known to affect the work of nurses. These include teamwork and shared decision making, leadership, autonomy, workload, professional recognition, role clarity, respect and recognition, workplace layout, design and availability of material resources, work scheduling, organizational policies and culture, and opportunities for professional development. Research conducted by Laschinger & Leiter (2006), Aiken et al. (2008), Duffield et al. (2011) and others has consistently demonstrated the effects of the nursing work environment on patient satisfaction and outcomes such as falls, pulmonary failure, failure to rescue, health care–acquired infections and medication errors, and on nurse outcomes including nurse satisfaction, turnover, and workplace injuries (Kalisch & Lee, 2014).

In 2004, an Institute of Medicine (IOM) report examining the nursing work environment relayed serious concerns about the overall deterioration of the nursing work environment as a result of hospital restructuring and re-engineering. The authors highlighted the critical role of the nurse in ensuring patient safety, and identified threats within the four basic components of health care organizations that influence organizational structure, process and outcomes: strength of management and leadership, adequate and appropriate deployment of labor and workforce, effective and efficient work design, and culture. Recommendations included an organizational shift to transformational leadership and evidence-based management, with an emphasis on building trust, as well as involving nurses at all levels of practice in the development of strategies and processes to improve the work environment. The second recommendation included maximizing workforce capability by ensuring adequate and appropriate nurse staffing to provide safe patient care. Additional recommendations focused on creating and sustaining a culture of safety, and on workplace and workspace redesign to promote efficiency and reduce the potential for error and injury. Best scheduling practices and elimination of mandatory overtime to mitigate or eliminate nurse fatigue were also recommended.

Healthy Work Environment

A healthy work environment is one that supports the health, safety, and well-being of nurses and other health care workers, and promotes the provision of quality patient care. As the only full-service professional nursing association representing the interests of all registered nurses, the American Nurses Association (ANA) has emphasized the critical importance of a healthy work environment for nurses for many years through its programmatic work, health policy initiatives and position statements, and legislative activities.

The recently revised *Code of Ethics for Nurses* (American Nurses Association [ANA], 2015) includes nine provisions that establish the framework for ethical nursing practice. Provisions 5, 6, and 7 are pertinent to the development and maintenance of a healthy work environment as they outline the responsibilities of the nurse to maintain competence and continue learning, to improve the health care environment and conditions of employment on an ongoing basis, and to advance the profession. The ANA also maintains a number of position statements focused on improving the work environment including the mitigation and elimination of nurse fatigue (ANA, 2014), elimination of manual patient handling (ANA, 2008), establishing a just culture (ANA, 2010), and the rights of the registered nurse when considering a patient assignment (ANA, 2009). In addition, current legislative activities include the introduction of a safe staffing bill to Congress in the spring of 2015 and the support of a Safe Patient Handling and Mobility bill.

ANA's *Nursing: Scope and Standards of Practice* (2nd ed.) (2010) includes descriptions of several conceptual models that are foundational to a healthy work environment for nurses. The Magnet Recognition Program outlines standards that are required to create and sustain a healthy work environment for nurses (American Nurses Credentialing Center [ANCC], 2013). These include structures

Work Environment: The Context of Nursing Practice

and processes that promote transformational leadership, nurse autonomy, shared decision making, professional development and lifelong learning, optimal staffing for safe patient care, and a safe work environment. The American Association of Critical-Care Nurses (AACN) created an evidence-based body of work resulting in a formal model that defines six standards that are essential to establishing and sustaining a healthy work environment for nurses. The standards focus on communication, collaboration, effective decision making, staffing, professional recognition, and leadership (American Association of Critical-Care Nurses [AACN], 2005). ANCC has also developed a number of tools related to a healthy work environment initiative, including a gap-assessment tool that can be used by organizations to assess the work environment and identify organizational strengths and opportunities for improvement (AACN, n.d.).

Although research and evidence support the importance of a healthy work environment as a necessary component of quality patient and nursing outcomes, clinical nurses, nurse leaders, and health care administrators find it increasingly difficult to achieve and maintain healthy work environments caused by the rapidly changing health care environment. Limiting factors include shrinking health care dollars, increased demand for health care services, and changing demographics associated with the aging patient population and the aging nurse workforce (Hill et al., 2015). Although all of the elements of the work environment discussed thus far can affect patient and nurse outcomes, none are as compelling to nurses at all levels of practice as staffing.

The Issue of Nurse Staffing

Safe and appropriate nurse staffing continues to be a top concern of the nation's 2.8 million nurses, 58% of whom work in acute care settings (ANA, 2013). Although there is a robust body of research demonstrating the positive effects of appropriate and sufficient staffing on clinical outcomes (Kane et al., 2007; Minnesota Department of Health, 2015), increasing demand for health care services coupled with reduced financial resources has resulted in significant gaps and barriers preventing achievement of this goal (Hill et al., 2015). Nurses are very aware of the potential negative consequences of inadequate staffing, which include increased falls, pressure ulcers, medication errors, and failure to rescue. A work environment with chronic understaffing poses additional mental and emotional stress on an already burdened nursing workforce resulting in fatigue, burnout, and increased turnover (Aiken et al., 2008).

Although the majority of nurses currently work in acute care settings, recent events related to the introduction and implementation of the Affordable Care Act (ACA) are creating a shift in care delivery for sicker, complex patients from hospitals to the outpatient setting (Martinez et al., 2015). Staffing models in ambulatory care and long-term care, which typically rely heavily on licensed practical nurses (LPNs) and medical technicians, will need to evolve to include more registered nurses with the education and preparation to care for these patients in the community setting.

A Solution-Oriented Approach

The changing health care environment requires nurse clinicians and leaders to rethink our traditional approach to achieving optimal staffing for safe patient care by considering new staffing and care delivery models, environmental enhancements, and other innovations and interventions to reach this goal. The ANA recognizes that nurse staffing is among the top concerns for nurses today and has developed a significant body of work around this issue. ANA's *Principles of Nurse Staffing* (2nd ed.) defines appropriate nurse staffing as "a match of registered nurse expertise with the needs of the recipient of nursing care services in the context of the practice setting and situation (2012, p. 8). Five principles are identified that must be considered when developing staffing plans and guidelines, including the needs of the health care consumer, the role of the registered nurses and other members of the health care, organization and workplace culture, the practice environment, and staffing evaluation.

Key components of the ANA-supported nurse staffing bill mentioned previously include a requirement that hospitals establish unit-based staffing committees and staffing plans that include clinical nurses as full partners in decision making. Staffing plans will take into account multiple factors, such as unit census, patient acuity, skill level of registered nurses (RNs), skill mix, and other resources. This bill would also require hospitals that participate in CMS to publicly report their staffing plans. From a health policy perspective, a comprehensive white paper on nurse staffing has been commissioned by the ANA in collaboration with a panel of nurse experts from across the country. This work is scheduled for release in that second half of 2015. Lastly, ANA has consistently articulated the need for transparency in reporting with respect to public reporting of nurse staffing. Nurse staffing measures are currently under evaluation for inclusion in the Centers for Medicare & Medicaid Services' Hospital Compare report.

Continued

Work Environment: The Context of Nursing Practice

Anderson et al. (2014) developed a "data driven model of excellence" in staffing. This model provides an organizing framework for staffing across the continuum of care that encompasses five core concepts: (1) Users of health care; (2) Providers of health care; (3) Environment of care; (4) Delivery of health care; and (5) Quality, safety, and outcomes of care. Key components of the model emphasize the role of the health care consumer (the patient) as the owner and driver of their comprehensive plan of health care with the role of the nurse focusing more intently on education and health care coaching. As providers of health care, nurses should practice to the full scope of their education, preparation, and licensure, and leadership skills should be developed and expected of all professional nurses. In addition, advanced education beyond the baccalaureate level is recommended for those in formal leadership positions.

Also emphasized is the importance of the environment of care because research has demonstrated that increased staffing on a unit that has a poor work environment does not necessarily have a significant impact on improving quality care outcomes (Aiken et al., 2011). Delivery of health care is a critical factor that describes how, when, and by whom direct patient care is provided. For example, numerous studies conducted over the past 10 years suggest that a team skill mix with a higher proportion of RNs has a positive impact on patient outcomes such as functional status and effective management of pain (Needleman et al., 2006; Hall et al., 2003).

Lastly, this model highlights the importance of quality, safety and outcomes of care. As nurses work collaboratively within the profession, and with other health care team members and consumers to address the persistent and complex issues related to nurse staffing, innovative staffing models should be developed and implemented using the current and best research and evidence, and revised as needed based on ongoing review of nurse and patient outcomes. Research agendas that further the goal of establishing cause and effect relationships between staffing and healthy work environments and exemplary outcomes will continue to build the business case for safe staffing.

References

Aiken, L., Clarke, S., Sloane, D., Lake, E., & Cheney, T. (2008). Effects of hospital care environment on patient mortality and patient outcomes. *Journal of Nursing Administration, 38*(5), 223–229.

Aiken, L. H., Sloane, D. M., Clarke, S., Poghosyan, L., Cho, E., You, L., et al. (2011). Importance of work environments on hospital outcomes in nine countries. *International Journal for Quality in Health Care, 23*(4), 357–364.

American Association of Critical-Care Nurses [AACN]. (2005). *AACN's standards for establishing and sustaining healthy work environments: Executive summary.* www.aacn.org/wd/hwe/docs/execsum.pdf.

American Association of Critical-Care Nurses (n.d.). Healthy work environment: Resources. www.aacn.org/wd/hwe/content/resources.content?lastmenu=.

American Nurses Association [ANA]. (2010). *Nursing: Scope and standards of practice* (2nd ed.). Silver Spring, MD: Nursebooks.

American Nurses Association [ANA]. (2015). *Code of ethics for nurses.* Silver Spring, MD: Nursebooks.

American Nurses Association [ANA]. (2014). *Addressing nurse fatigue to promote safety and health: Joint responsibilities of registered nurses and employers to reduce risks.* http://nursingworld.org/MainMenuCategories/WorkplaceSafety/Healthy-Work-Environment/Work-Environment/NurseFatigue/Addressing-Nurse-Fatigue-ANA-Position-Statement.pdf.

American Nurses Association [ANA]. (2008). *Elimination of manual patient handling to prevent work-related musculoskeletal disorders.* http://nursingworld.org/position/practice/handling.aspx.

American Nurses Association [ANA]. (2009). *Patient safety: Rights of registered nurses when considering a patient assignment.* http://www.nursingworld.org/MainMenuCategories/Policy-Advocacy/Positions-and-Resolutions/ANAPositionStatements/Position-Statements-Alphabetically/Patient-Safety-Rights-of-Registered-Nurses-When-Considering-a-Patient-Assignment.html.

American Nurses Association [ANA]. (2010). *Just culture.* http://nursingworld.org/psjustculture.

American Nurses Association [ANA]. (2013). *Distribution of RN Employment.* www.nursingworld.org/MainMenuCategories/ThePracticeofProfessionalNursing/workforce/Charts-and-Tables-of-RN-and-APRN-Employment-Data.pdf.

American Nurses Association (ANA). (2012). *Principles of nurse staffing* (2nd ed.). www.nursingworld.org/MainMenuCategories/ThePracticeofProfessionalNursing/NursingStandards/ANAPrinciples/ANAsPrinciplesofNurseStaffing.pdf.

American Nurses Credentialing Center (ANCC). (2013). *2014 Magnet application manual.* Silver Spring, MD: Nursebooks.

Anderson, R., Ellerbe, S., Haas, S., Kerfoot, K., Kirby, K., & Nickitas, D. (2014). Excellence and evidence in staffing: A data-driven model for excellence in staffing. *Nursing Economics, 32*(3, Suppl.), 1–48.

Duffield, C., Diers, D., O'Brien-Pallas, L., Aisbett, C., Roche, M., King, M., & Aisbett, K. (2011). Nursing staffing, nursing workload, the work environment and patient outcomes. *Applied Nursing Research, 24*(4), 244–255.

Hall, L. M., Doran, D., Baker, G. R., Pink, G. H., Sidani, S., O'Brien-Pallas, L., et al. (2003). Nurse staffing models as predictors of patient outcomes. *Medical Care, 41*(9), 1096–1109.

Hill, K. S., Higdon, K., Porter, B. W., Rutland, M. D., & Vela, D. K. (2015). Preserving staffing resources as a system: Nurses leading operations and efficiency initiatives. *Nursing Economics, 33*(1), 26–35.

CLINICAL CORNER—cont'd

Work Environment: The Context of Nursing Practice

Institute of Medicine [IOM]. (2004). *Keeping patients safe: Transforming the work environment of nurses.* www.nap.edu/openbook.php?isbn=0309090679.

Kalisch, B., & Lee, K. H. (2014). Staffing and job satisfaction: Nurses and nursing assistants. *Journal of Nursing Management, 22*(4), 465–471.

Kane, R. L., Shamliyan, T., Mueller, C., Duval, S., & Wilt, T. (2007). *Nursing staffing and quality of patient care.* Rockville, MD: AHRQ Publication No. 07-E005. Agency for Healthcare Research and Quality.

Laschinger, H. K. S., & Leiter, M. P. (2006). The impact of nursing work environments on patient safety outcomes: The mediating role of burnout engagement. *Journal of Nursing Administration, 36*(5), 259–267.

Martinez, K., Battaglia, R., Mastal, M. F., & Matlock, A. M. (2015). Perspectives in ambulatory care. *Nursing Economics, 33*(1), 60.

Minnesota Department of Health. (2015, January). *Hospital nurse staffing and patient outcomes: A report to the Minnesota Legislature Minnesota Department of Health.* www.health.state.mn.us/divs/hpsc/hep/publications/legislative/nursestudy012015.pdf.

Needleman, J., Buerhaus, P. I., Stewart, M., Zelevinsky, K., & Mattke, S. (2006). Nurse staffing in hospitals: Is there a business case for quality? *Health Affairs, 25,* 204–211.

Schalk, D. M., Bijl, M. L., Halfens, R. J., Hollands, L., & Cummings, G. G. (2010). Interventions aimed at improving the nursing work environment: A systematic review. *Implementation Science, 5*(34), 1–11.

Mary Jo Assi, DNP, RN, NEA-BC, FNP-BC
Director of Nursing Practice and Work Environment,
American Nurses Association

EVIDENCE-BASED PRACTICE

Aiken, L. H., Sloane, D. M., Cimiotti, J. P., Clarke, S. P., Flynn, L., Seago, J. A., Spetz, J. & Smith, H. L. (2010). *Implications of the California Nurse Staffing Mandate for other states. Health Services Research, 45*(4):904–921.

This article notes the following:

- Past research has demonstrated a positive link between nurse staffing levels and measures of patient outcomes and nurse retention.
- In 2004, California implemented minimum nurse-to-patient staffing requirements in acute care hospitals in an effort to improve the quality of patient care and nurse job satisfaction.
- This study compared patient and nurse outcomes from hospitals in California versus two states without legislatively mandated staffing ratios, Pennsylvania and New Jersey. The study used data obtained in 2006 from over 22,000 staff nurses from among the three states, as well as hospital discharge databases.
- Among the study findings, the researchers reported that hospital nurses on medical and surgical units in California cared for fewer patients on average than nurses in the other two states. These lower patient-to-nurse ratios were associated with significantly lower patient mortality.
- The study also found that nurses in California reported higher job satisfaction, less burnout, and better ability to care for patients.
- The authors estimated that had patient-to-nurse ratios in Pennsylvania and New Jersey been consistent with those in California during the period of the study, 486 fewer surgical deaths would have occurred in those two states combined.
- The study presents important policy implications for policymakers in other states that are currently considering health care workforce legislation.

NCLEX® EXAMINATION QUESTIONS

1. What is one advantage of centralized scheduling?
   A. Better use of resources
   B. Lack of cost containment
   C. Decreased use of resources
   D. Increase in cost

2. What is the type of scheduling whereby the staff commit to work a set number of shift types in a given time frame called?
   A. Pattern scheduling
   B. Preference scheduling
   C. Rules scheduling
   D. Self-scheduling

3. What is the type of scheduling that blends aspects of centralized and decentralized scheduling whereby individual units may manage staffing?
   A. Mixed
   B. Centralized
   C. Decentralized
   D. Self

4. What is the term used for decision making that occurs with the nurse manager on the unit?
   A. Centralized scheduling
   B. Decentralized scheduling
   C. Self-scheduling
   D. Mixed scheduling

5. The staffing plan consists of four different elements that must be addressed. What do they include?
   A. The health care setting
   B. A care delivery model
   C. Patient acuity and nursing staff
   D. All of the above

6. Which of the following requires knowledge of patient acuity, nursing productivity, nursing competence, organization finance, and health care regulations?
   A. Health care staffing
   B. Health care scheduling
   C. Staff mix
   D. Self-scheduling

7. According to the American Nurses Association (ANA, 2004), the process of daily staffing begins with an assessment of the current staffing situation. The assessment include which of the following?
   A. The qualifications of the staff needed
   B. The competence of the staff needed
   C. The supervisor input
   D. All of the above

8. External temporary agencies are:
   A. Used as first line to replace sick calls
   B. Used usually as a last resort
   C. Not very expensive
   D. No longer used because of high costs

9. What is the average number of days that a patient remained in an occupied bed referred to as?
   A. The average daily census
   B. The average length of stay
   C. Nursing hours per patient
   D. Direct care hours

10. What is the average number of patients cared for per day for the reporting period referred to as?
    A. The average daily census
    B. The average length of stay
    C. Nursing hours per patient
    D. Direct care hours

Answers: 1. A   2. A   3. A   4. B   5. D   6. A   7. D   8. B   9. B   10. A

REFERENCES

Agency for Healthcare Research and Quality [AHRQ]. (2004). *Hospital nurse staffing and quality of care: research in action, Issue 14. March 2004*. Rockville, MD: Agency for Healthcare Research and Quality. www.ahrq.gov/research/findings/factsheets/services/nursestaffing/index.html.

Agency for Healthcare Research and Quality [AHRQ]. (2014). *State-mandated nurse staffing levels alleviate workloads, leading to lower patient mortality and higher nurse satisfaction*. www.innovations.ahrq.gov/content.aspx?id=3708.

Aiken, L., Clarke, S., Sloan, D., Sochalski, J., & Silber, J. (2002). Hospital nurse staffing and patient mortality, nurse burnout, and job dissatisfaction. *Journal of the American Medical Association, 288*(16), 1987–1993.

American Nurses Association [ANA]. (2012). *Principles for nurse staffing*. Silver Spring, MD: Author.

American Nurses Association [ANA]. (2004). *Scope and standards for nurse administrators* (2nd ed.). Silver Spring, MD: author.

Bernat, A. (2003). Effective staffing. In P. Kelly-Heidenthal (Ed.), *Nursing leadership and management* (pp. 238–265). Clifton Park, NY: Thomson Delmar Learning.

California Health Care Foundation. (2005). *Adopting online nurse scheduling and staffing systems.* Oakland, CA: Author.

Garrett, C. (2008). The effect of nurse staffing patterns on medical errors and nurse burnout. *AORN Journal, 87,* 1191–1192, 1194, 1196–1200, 1202–1204.

Halm, M., Peterson, M., & Kandelis, M. (2005). Hospital nurse staffing and patient mortality, emotional exhaustion, and job dissatisfaction. *Clinical Nurse Specialist, 19*(5), 241–251.

Hugonnet, S., Chevrolet, J., & Pittet, D. (2007). The effect of workload on infection risk in critically ill patients. *Critical Care Medicine, 35*(1), 76–81.

Kane, R. L., Shamliyan, T. A., Mueller, C., Duval, S., & Wilt, T. J. (2007). The association of registered nurse staffing levels and patient outcomes. *Systematic Review and Meta-analysis Medical Care, 45*(12), 1195–1204.

Kelly-Heidenthal, P. (2003). *Nursing leadership and management.* Clifton Park, NY: Thomson Delmar Learning.

Needleman, J., Buerhaus, P., Stewart, M., Zelevinsky, K., & Mattke, S. (2006). Nurse staffing in hospitals: Is there a business case for quality? *Health Affairs, 25*(1), 204–211.

Needleman, J., Buerhaus, P., Mattke, S., Stewart, M., & Zelevinsky, K. (2002). Nurse staffing levels and the quality of care in hospitals. *New England Journal of Medicine, 346,* 1715–1722.

Stone, P., Mooney-Kane, C., & Larson, E. (2007). Nurse working conditions and patient safety outcomes. *Medical Care, 45*(6), 571–578.

The Joint Commission [TJC]. (2014). *Comprehensive accreditation manual for hospitals.* Oakbrook Terrace, IL: Author.

Tomey, A. M. (2008). *Guide to nursing management and leadership* (8th ed.). St. Louis: Mosby.

Weissman, J., Rothschild, J., & Bendavid, E. (2007). Hospital workload and adverse events. *Medical Care, 45*(5), 448–455.

Yoder-Wise, P. (2011). *Leading and managing in nursing* (5th ed.). St Louis: Elsevier.

13

Delegation of Nursing Tasks

OBJECTIVES

- Define delegation.
- Identify the five rights of delegation.
- Review the circumstances where delegation is appropriate.
- Identify tasks appropriate for delegation.
- Discuss the role of unlicensed personnel in the delivery of health care.
- Identify the role of the nurse in the delegation of health care.
- Review the legal ramifications of delegation of care.

OUTLINE

KEY TERMS

accountability acknowledgment and assumption of responsibility for actions, decisions, and policies within the scope of the role or employment position and encompassing the obligation to report, explain, and be answerable for resulting consequences

assignment delegation of work to a selected group of patient care givers. The downward or lateral transfer of the responsibility of an activity from one individual to another while retaining accountability for the outcome

delegation transferring the authority to perform a selected nursing task in a selected situation to a competent individual

direct patient care activities activities such as hygienic care, feeding patients, taking vital signs, and so on that are performed on the patient

indirect patient care activities routine activities of the patient unit that deal with the day-to-day functioning of the unit, such as restocking supplies

supervision active process of directing, guiding, and influencing the outcome of an individual's performance of an activity

unlicensed assistive personnel individuals who are not licensed by the state but are trained to assist

nurses by performing patient care tasks as allowed by the organization. There are many job titles for such employees, such as nursing assistant (NA), patient care associate (PCA), and unlicensed assistive personnel (UAP)

DELEGATION

Delegation is defined as the "transfer of responsibility for the performance of an activity from one individual to another while retaining accountability for the outcome. Example: the nurse, in delegating an activity to an unlicensed individual, transfers the responsibility for the performance of the activity, but retains professional accountability for the overall care" (American Nurses Association [ANA], 1992). It is the entrusting of a selected nursing task to an individual who is qualified, competent, and able to perform such a task.

The following principles provide guidance and inform the registered nurse's (RN's) decision making about delegation:

- The nursing profession determines the scope and standards of nursing practice.
- The RN takes responsibility and accountability for the provision of nursing practice.
- The RN directs care and determines the appropriate use of resources when providing care.
- The RN may delegate tasks or elements of care, but does not delegate the nursing process itself.
- The RN considers facility/agency policies and procedures and the knowledge and skills, training, diversity awareness, and experience of any individual to whom the RN may delegate elements of care.
- The decision to delegate is based upon the RN's judgment concerning the care complexity of the patient, the availability and competence of the individual accepting the delegation, and the type and intensity of supervision required.
- The RN acknowledges that delegation involves the relational concept of mutual respect.
- Nurse leaders are accountable for establishing systems to assess, monitor, verify, and communicate ongoing competence requirements in areas related to delegation.
- The organization/agency is accountable to provide sufficient resources to enable appropriate delegation.

- The organization/agency is accountable for ensuring that the RN has access to documented competency information for staff to whom the RN is delegating tasks.
- Organizational/agency policies on delegation are developed with the active participation of registered nurses (ANA and National Council of State Boards of Nursing [NCSBN], 2008).

The majority of health care institutions have care delivery systems that include various levels of caregivers. The acuity of patients within hospitals has increased during the past 10 years, and many hospitals have moved from total patient care, primary care, and other care delivery systems that require an all–registered nurse staff. To meet the needs of the higher-acuity patients, nurses must delegate aspects of care to nonregistered nurse team members. Delegation changes as the health care environment changes. Since the advent of the nursing shortage, unlicensed assistive personnel (UAP) have been used to help fill the workforce gaps. The role of these assistive personnel is set by the institution that employs them and defines their practice. They may be called **noncredentialed assistive personnel**, as well as unlicensed assistive personnel (UAP). Individuals hired into these jobs are trained and evaluated by the facility. They may use a variety of titles, such as nursing assistant (NA), patient care associate (PCA), nursing technician, unit technician, and others (Carroll, 1998). They cannot practice nursing, and they must be directed, supervised, and evaluated by a registered nurse, who is ultimately responsible for all patient care (see Box 13-1 for the nurse's responsibility in delegation). One form of licensed personnel, the licensed practical nurse (LPN), is used by many facilities. The LPN works under the direction and supervision of the registered nurse. Licensed personnel work according to the state board regulations (see **Chapter 11**), but the job descriptions will vary from institution to institution. Various patient care roles are listed in Table 13-1.

There are two types of nursing activities that may be delegated: direct and indirect patient care activities. Direct patient care activities include assisting with

BOX 13-1   Nurse's Responsibility in Delegation

1. Before delegating a nursing task, the nurse shall determine the nursing care needs of the patient. The nurse shall retain responsibility and accountability for the nursing care of the patient, including nursing assessment, planning, evaluation, and nursing documentation.
2. Before the delegation of the nursing task to unlicensed assistive personnel, the nurse shall determine that the unlicensed person has been trained in the task and deemed to be competent.

Criteria for Delegation

1. The delegated nursing task shall be a task that a reasonable and prudent nurse would find within the scope of sound nursing judgment and practice to delegate.
2. The delegated nursing task shall be a task that can be competently and safely performed by the unlicensed personnel without compromising the patient's safety.
3. The nursing task shall not require the unlicensed personnel to exercise independent nursing judgment or intervention.
4. The nurse shall be responsible for ensuring that the delegated task is performed in a competent manner by the unlicensed personnel.

Supervision

1. The nurse shall provide supervision of the delegated nursing task.
2. The degree of supervision required shall be determined by the nurse after an evaluation of the following factors:
   a. Stability and acuity of the patient's condition.
   b. Training and competency of the unlicensed personnel.
   c. Complexity of the nursing task being delegated.
   d. Proximity and availability of the nurse to the unlicensed personnel when the nursing task is being performed.

Adapted from State of Kentucky (1999). *Delegation of nursing tasks.* KRS 311A.170, 314.011, 201 KAR 20:400. www.lrc.state.ky.us/kar/201/020/400.htm.

feeding, grooming, hygienic care, taking vital signs, ambulation, electrocardiogram tracing, and measuring blood sugar levels. Indirect patient care activities are those routinely done to support the functioning of the patient care unit. Such activities include the restocking of supplies, the transport of patients, and clerical activities.

TABLE 13-1   Roles of Patient Team Members

Patient Care Team Members and Their Roles

Registered nurses (RNs)
- Determine the scope of nursing practice.
- Are responsible and accountable for the provision of nursing services.
- Supervise and determine the appropriate use of any UAP involved in patient care.
- Define and supervise the education, training, and use of any unlicensed assistive personnel (UAP).

Licensed Vocational Nurse/Licensed Practical Nurse (LVN/LPN)
- Complete a 1-year to 18-month educational program.
- Provide basic patient care that includes, but is not limited to, taking vital signs, changing dressings, performing phlebotomy, and assisting with activities of daily living, under the supervision of the RN.

UAP
- Work under the direct supervision of an RN to implement the delegated aspects of nursing care.
- Assist the RN in providing patient care.
- Enable the RN to provide nursing care for the patient.
- May include but are not limited to the following titles:
  - Patient care assistant
  - Nurse's aide
  - Technician
  - Multi-skilled worker
  - Practice partner
  - Nursing assistant
  - Nurse extender
  - Orderly
  - Support personnel
  - Practice partner

American Association of Critical-Care Nurses. (2004). http://www.aacn.org/wd/practice/docs/aacndelegationhandbook.pdf

THE FIVE RIGHTS OF DELEGATION

The National Council of State Boards of Nursing (1997) has defined the Five Rights of Delegation, as follows:
1. Right task.
2. Right circumstance.
3. Right person.
4. Right direction/communication.
5. Right supervision.

To assist you in reviewing these five rights, Box 13-2 will help you to determine if you are following these rights in your delegation (ANA and NCSBN, 2008).

BOX 13-2   The Five Rights of Delegation

Right Task

- Has the nursing department established policies and standards consistent with the nurse practice act of the state and professional nursing standards?
- Are you aware of the specific polices and standards of your institution?
- Do you know to whom you can delegate what?
- Can this task be delegated to any staff, or only to certain staff?

Right Circumstance

- Are the setting and resources conducive to safe care?
- Do the job description and competency of the care giver match the patient requirements?
- Do staff members understand how to do the task safely?
- Do staff members have the appropriate resources and equipment to carry out the task safely?
- Do staff members have the appropriate supervision to carry out the task safely?

Right Person

- Is the right person delegating the task, and is the right person being delegated to?
- Is the patient condition appropriate for the level of delegation?
- Do hospital policy and the nurse practice act of the state allow the delegation of this activity?
- Can you verify the knowledge and competency of the staff member to whom you are delegating a specific task?

Right Direction/Communication

- Have you clearly communicated the task with directions, limits, and expected outcomes?
- Are times for feedback specified in your assignment?
- Does the staff member understand what is to be done?
- Can the staff member ask questions as needed?

Right Supervision

- Will you be able to appropriately monitor and evaluate patient response to the delegated task?
- Will you be able to give feedback to the staff member if needed?

Right Task

State boards of nursing regulate nursing practice within each state. It is important for you to know the nurse practice act of the state in which you are practicing and to be aware of the delegation regulation within your state. In addition, most hospitals have policies that very carefully describe what nursing tasks can be delegated to whom; there are differing standards of delegation depending on the type of health care facility in which you practice. Many long-term care facilities assign LPNs as charge nurses, with RNs supervising that care. In ambulatory care settings, medical assistants play a major role in the delivery of care. Just because your institution uses patient care technicians to measure all vital signs and blood sugar levels and to make blood draws, it does not mean that all facilities can or do use such personnel. It is vital to know your institution's standard on delegation and the specific job descriptions and competencies of each level of personnel with whom you will be working. A sample hospital policy on delegation is shown in Figure 13-1. The scope of practice will vary from state to state, so this will vary across the country.

Generally, appropriate tasks for consideration in delegation decision making include those:

- That frequently reoccur in the daily care of a client or group of clients.
- That do not require the UAP to exercise nursing judgment.
- That do not require complex and/or multi-dimensional application of the nursing process.
- For which the results are predictable and the potential risk is minimal.
- That use a standard and unchanging procedure.

(The Five Rights of Delegation. www.ncsbn.org/fiverights.pdf.)

Right Circumstance

The right circumstance refers to the workplace. The circumstance is the context in which the delegation takes place. As stated earlier, an LPN will be performing different tasks under different circumstances. In a long-term facility, it is not unusual to have an LPN as "charge nurse" with an RN covering multiple units for supervision. However, it would be unusual to have an LPN assigned as a "charge nurse" in an acute care facility with a high acuity of patients. There may be differences in extreme circumstances, such as disasters, but in such a situation, the right communication/direction needs to occur.

Right Person

The requirement of the right person means that you must know the competency level, job description, individual

THE VALLEY HOSPITAL
Ridgewood, New Jersey

PATIENT CARE SERVICES (PCS) POLICY AND PROCEDURE

SUBJECT: Delegation – Nursing Tasks

POLICY:

1. In delegating selected nursing tasks to licensed practice nurses and other health care team members, the registered professional nurse shall be responsible for exercising that degree of judgment and knowledge reasonably expected to assure that a proper delegation has been made.

2. A registered professional nurse may not delegate the performance of a nursing task to persons who have not been adequately prepared by verifiable training and education and have not demonstrated the adequacy of their knowledge, skill and competency to perform the task being delegated.

3. A RN may not delegate non-PCA tasks to staff employed as PCA II or PCA I who are RNs from a foreign country or those enrolled in nursing school. In order to function/perform tasks that are approved under the scope of practice of a RN, staff must be licensed as a RN in New Jersey.

4. No task may be delegated which is within the scope of nursing practice and requires:
   a. The substantial knowledge and skill derived from completion of a nursing education program and the specialized skill, judgment and knowledge of a registered nurse; and
   b. An understanding of nursing principles necessary to recognize and manage complications which may result in harm to the health and safety of the patient.

WHO CAN PERFORM: RN

RESPONSIBILITY:
It is the responsibility of nursing leadership or management member, as appropriate to implement, maintain, evaluate, review and revise this policy.

APPROVED: Nurse Practice Education Council, January 10, 2003.

Beverly S. Karas-Irwin, RN
Chairperson, Nurse Practice Education Council

Linda C. Lewis, RN
Vice President, Paient Care Services

FIGURE 13-1 Sample hospital policy on delegation. (With permission from Valley Hospital.)

level of skill, and standard of education of the individual to whom you are delegating. Job descriptions will give you a broad view of what an individual is expected to do, but you must know the individual's capabilities, experience, attitude, and skills. A novice nurse will not have the competency that a nurse with 10 years of experience, a professional certification, and a clinical ladder position will have. It is also necessary to have knowledge of the individual strengths and weaknesses of each team member. A team member who just lost her mother to breast cancer may not be the best person to delegate to perform tasks for a patient with breast cancer.

The Right Direction/Communication

The right direction/communication is required of nurses as they delegate tasks to staff members. It is not enough to assign a task to a staff member; the staff member must know what is expected of them. "You will take Ms. Smith's temperature every hour starting at 8 AM, and report the temperature back to me immediately." If you tell the staff member to take the temperature every hour, they may not know when to start and may report a sudden increase in temperature to you because they have not been trained to determine when an independent nursing action is needed. Your directions must follow the 4 Cs: be clear, concise, correct, and complete. A clear communication is one that is understood by the listener. If you say, "Can you get Mrs. Jones," what are you asking? For that patient to be transported back to the unit from a test? For the staff member to assume full care for Mrs. Jones? Or to answer Mrs. Jones's bell? Tell the staff member exactly what you want done. A concise communication is one in which the right amount of communication has been given. If you are asking a PCA to take a patient's temperature, they do not need to know the physiological response to an increased temperature. It confuses the communication and wastes time. Tell the associate what they need to know. A correct communication is one that is accurate. You may have two patients named Edward Norton on your unit. It is not enough to tell the LPN to give Mr. Norton his pain medication. Which Mr. Norton are you referring to? Last, a complete communication leaves no questions on the part of the delegate. Do not assume that just because you asked a PCA to take a patient's temperature that they will know to report it to you.

Communication is a two-way activity, and it is important to create an environment where staff members feel free to say that they are not comfortable doing a task, for instance because they have not done it for a long time.

Right Supervision

The nurse remains accountable for the total care delivered to the patients on the unit. The right supervision includes "the provision of guidance, direction, oversight, evaluation and follow-up by the licensed nurse for accomplishment of a nursing task delegated to nursing assistive personnel" (NCSBN, 2005). While you will not directly perform the tasks delegated, you will be responsible for determining patient progress and outcomes of the care delivered, as well as evaluating and improving staff performance. This requires you to be able to communicate effectively to support team performance.

ACCEPTANCE OF DELEGATED ASSIGNMENT

In accepting a delegated assignment, the following decision-making algorithm is appropriate (State of New Jersey, 1999):

- Is the act consistent with your defined scope of practice?
- Is the activity authorized by a valid order and in accordance with established institutional/agency or provider protocols, policies, and procedures?
- Is the act supported by research data from nursing literature/or research from a health related field? Has a national nursing organization issued a position statement on this practice? (See Chapter 19.)
- Do you possess the knowledge and clinical competence to perform the act safely?
- Is the act to be performed within acceptable "standards of care" that would be provided under similar circumstances by reasonable, prudent nurses with similar education and clinical skills?
- Are you prepared to assume accountability for the provision of safe care?

This model will assist you if you have a question about nursing practice or the delegation of work to you.

DELEGATION FACTORS

To recap, what to delegate will depend on a number of factors (adapted from Heidenthal & Marthaler, 2005):
- Your state's nurse practice act.
- Hospital policies and procedures.

- Job descriptions.
- Staff competencies.
- Clinical situation.
- Professional standards.
- Patient needs.

What activities can usually be delegated? The following is a list of potential activities that may be delegated.

Direct Patient Care Activities

Vital signs

- Take and record blood pressure, respirations, temperature, and pulse rate.
- Obtain daily weight.
- Apply leads and connect to cardiac monitor.

Intake and output

- Measure and record intake and output.
- Collect specimens.

Activities of daily living

- Perform total or partial bed bath.
- Perform perineal care.
- Shave.
- Wash hair.
- Perform mouth care.
- Change linen and assist with making occupied bed.

Nutrition

- Feed patient.
- Calculate and record calorie count.

Skin care

- Perform back care.
- Prepare skin for procedure.
- Perform skin prep for operative procedure.

Activity and mobility

- Assist in ambulating patient.
- Perform passive and active range of motion.
- Position.
- Turn and reposition patient.
- Assist with transfers.

Respiratory support

- Set up oxygen.
- Assist patient with using an incentive spirometer.
- Assist patient with coughing and deep breathing exercises.

Procedures

- Set up patient room (suction canisters, cables for continuous cardiac monitoring, tubing for chest tubes).
- Orient patient to room environment.
- Obtain necessary supplies for sterile procedure.
- Perform postmortem care.

Indirect Patient Care Activities

Cleaning

- Clean equipment in use and stored equipment.
- Clean environment, including counter tops and desk tops.
- Clean and defrost food refrigerators.
- Clean patient care area after transfer or discharge.
- Clean patient care area after procedures are completed.
- Empty waste baskets in patient rooms and unit.
- Empty linen hampers.
- Remove meal trays.
- Clean supply carts.
- Clean and restock procedure rooms.
- Make unoccupied beds.

Errands

- Deliver meal trays.
- Obtain and deliver supplies.
- Obtain and deliver equipment.
- Obtain and deliver blood products.
- Check laboratory specimens for appropriate labeling.
- Deliver specimens to clinical laboratory.

Clerical tasks

- Place pages.
- Place and answer phone calls.
- Assemble, disassemble, and maintain patient charts.
- Transcribe physician and nursing patient care orders.
- Schedule diagnostic tests and procedures.
- Order necessary office supplies and forms.
- Sort and deliver mail.
- Keep unit log books up to date with patient admissions, transfers, and discharges.
- Maintain awareness of nursing bed assignments.

Stocking and maintenance

- Stock patient bedside supplies.
- Stock unit supplies.
- Stock utility rooms.
- Stock treatment, examination, and procedure rooms.
- Stock nourishments and kitchen supplies.
- Check electrical equipment for inspections due dates.
- Stock linen cart.

Activities That May Not Be Delegated

Nursing activities that may not be delegated include the following:

- Performing an initial patient assessment and subsequent assessments or nursing interventions that require specialized nursing knowledge, judgment, and/or skill.

- Formulating a nursing diagnosis.
- Identifying nursing care goals and developing the nursing plan of care in conjunction with the patient and/or family.
- Updating the patient's plan of care.
- Providing patient education to patient and/or family.
- Evaluating a patient's progress, or lack thereof, toward achieving desired goals and outcomes.
- Discussing patient issues with physician.
- Communicating with physicians or implementing orders from physician.
- Documenting the patient's assessment or response to therapeutic interventions in the patient's plan of care.
- Administering medications.
- Providing direct nursing care.

Adapted from American Association of Critical-Care Nurses (2004).

OBSTACLES TO DELEGATION

There are obstacles to delegation. Nurses who have worked with primary care models for much of their professional life may have difficulty in giving up aspects of nursing care. It is important to keep in mind that "effective teams focus on integrative work processes while working toward a common goal" (Anthony, Standing, & Hertz, 2000).

Barriers to delegation can arise not only on the part of the delegator, the RN, but also on the part of the delegatee, the UAP, and the situation/environment.

Characteristics that create barriers in the delegator.
- Preference for operating by oneself.
- Demand that everyone know all the details.
- "I can do it better myself" fallacy.
- Lack of experience in the job or in delegating.
- Insecurity.
- Fear of being disliked.
- Refusal to allow mistakes.
- Lack of confidence in subordinates.
- Perfectionism, leading to excess control.
- Lack of organizational skill in balancing workloads.
- Failure to delegate authority commensurate with responsibility.
- Uncertainty over tasks and inability to explain.
- Disinclination to develop subordinates.
- Failure to establish effective controls and to follow up.

Characteristics that create barriers in the delegate.

- Lack of experience.
- Lack of competence.
- Avoidance of responsibility.
- Overdependence.
- Disorganization.
- Overload of work.
- Immersion in trivia.

Characteristics that create barriers related to the situation/environment.
- One-person-show policy.
- No toleration of mistakes.
- Criticality of decisions.
- Urgency, leaving no time to explain (crisis management).
- Understaffing.

Adapted from American Association of Critical-Care Nurses (2004).

LEVELS OF CLINICAL EXPERIENCE

The use of effective delegation has been related to levels of clinical experience (Benner & Benner, 1984, cited in Carroll, 2006).

The novice nurse has limited experience with tasks and needs rules to guide actions.

The advanced beginner has enough experience to recognize patterns in work but continues to need help in setting priorities; relies on rules and protocols.

The competent nurse has been practicing 2 to 3 years; can prioritize and cope with various contingencies; requires assistance working through various situations not yet experienced.

The proficient nurse has enough experience to see the "big picture" rather than a series of individual accidents/actions; decision making is more efficient and accurate; is able to prioritize and plan even more challenging patient care.

The expert no longer relies on rules to understand a situation or to act appropriately; focuses quickly on viable solutions; is able to lead a team efficiently; can organize others' work and supervise them effectively.

So, it is important to know the nurses with whom you are working on any given day, so that you can also use their level of expertise in the planning of your delegation. The following guidelines may help RNs delegate more effectively:
- Be aware of your internal barriers to delegation.
- Never delegate a task you would not do yourself.

- Delegate to the most appropriate person, carefully considering these factors:
  - Patient acuity.
  - The activity to be performed.
  - The support person's job description.
  - Competencies of the individual who will complete the task.
- Communicate clearly. How one communicates a task can determine how successfully it will be completed. Ineffective communication is the most commonly cited reason delegated activities are not completed as expected.

(American Association of Critical-Care Nurses [AACN], 2004).

Koloroutis et al. (2007) described three scenarios that can be used as a means of determining the most appropriate method of delegation to become part of the staffing assignments of a unit. These scenarios are unit based, pairing, and partnering.

Unit-Based Scenarios

In the unit-based scenario, assistive personnel, such as the ward secretary and nursing assistant, serve the unit. The nursing assistant works off a task list usually found in the job description, and has minimal direction from, or interaction with the RNs. An example of the unit-based scenario is assigning a nursing assistant to take all the vital signs or bathe all the patients. But another nurse may ask the nursing assistant to help with picking up medications from pharmacy, while another nurse asks the NA to assist with feeding a patient.

Pairing

In a pairing scenario one RN works with an LPN and/ or an NA for the shift. However, the RN and LPN and/ or assistant are not intentionally scheduled to work the same shift each day. Delegation usually increases with pairing. In this scenario, the RN and the LPN or NA are able to discuss how care is to be prioritized and how it is to be done, and identify expected individualized outcomes for the shift

Partnering

In partnering, one RN and one LPN and/or NA are consistently scheduled to work together, making a commitment to maintain healthy interpersonal relationships, trust each other, and advance each other's knowledge

PRIORITY SETTING

Proper delegation also requires priority setting. One of the most difficult challenges facing both the nurse and the nurse manager is the prioritization of care delivered to the patients on a unit. The priorities change rapidly and the nurse manager should be aware of the unit needs at all times. To manage your priorities and to control the activity of the workplace around you, Carrick et al. (2007) suggest the three I's:

1. Identify your priorities.
2. Interact differently with others.
3. Initiate action.

To identify your priorities, list your entire job-related responsibilities on a piece of paper. Then classify the top priorities, and create a "to-do" list that you can work from during the day. Remember, this list will change as the day progresses, but keep updating it and rank your priorities as they change. This list serves as a reference for the actions of the day.

To interact differently with others, Carrick et al. (2007) recommend the following four tactics to maintain control over your time, energy, and priorities.

- Identify a time when you can handle an issue: You cannot refuse a task or patient request, but you will be able to say when you will be available to do the task. Reassuring a person that you will complete the task and giving a timeline, help to control requests and interruptions that compete for your time.
- Ask questions before taking on an assignment: Before you take on any assignment, you need to understand the scope, the intended outcome, and the deadlines.
- Ask for help when you need it: Quickly do a reality check of your time, prioritize alternatives, and then meet with the person who can help you make the right decision or complete the assignment. When asking for help, be realistic about the expectation of the other person, and be open to alternative decision making.
- Use delegation to manage your responsibilities: You cannot do it all! When delegating, be sure to explain the scope, expectations, roles, responsibilities, and authority for the task. Always be available as a resource.

To initiate action, you need to set realistic goals. To set realistic goals, be SMART: the goals need to be specific, measurable, attainable, relevant, and time bound.

As a nurse manager, you have a responsibility to control time, set appropriate priorities, and act on the priorities. In setting priorities, you will always need to keep in mind the following question: "Of all of the important things that I need to do right now, which is the most important for the patient(s)?" Is it urgent? Or just important?

SUMMARY

Delegation is one of the most challenging activities of the new manager. There is more nursing care needed than nurses to provide that care. In addition, not all care needed for a patient requires a professional nurse. Nurses must work within an interdisciplinary team and with individuals of varying capabilities and talents.

Delegation skills are developed by the new nurse over time. It involves an awareness of the total patient care needs for the patients assigned, as well as a thorough knowledge of the capabilities and competencies of staff members. Delegation is a process that results in safe and efficient patient care if it is used appropriately. It is a critical step in the delivery of nursing care.

In summary, the Four Delegation Steps identified by the National Council of State Boards of Nursing and The American Nurses Association will serve as a guideline for effective delegation: Step One – Assessment and Planning; Step Two – Communication; Step Three – Surveillance and Supervision; Step Four – Evaluation and Feedback (https://www.ncsbn.org/Delegation_joint_statement_NCSBN-ANA.pdf [pp. 7 9]).

CLINICAL CORNER

Delegation and the New Nurse

A wide range of emotions is expressed when nurses share their stories about how they learned, or if they had formal education specific to nursing delegation. Experiences vary in degree and sentiment, and very often, reactions tend to run the gamut; some are explosive "It was trial by fire!" most are questionable "I don't remember learning about that!" and all were learning experiences on what to do or what not to do in the future. Often, the responses are reflective of how the nurse was "formed." Educational background, years of experience, and formal versus extemporaneous education factor into the equation.

Clinical staff are directly impacted by these experiences. It can make or break a positive orientation/on-boarding process, develop or degrade teamwork and collaboration, and it can even be a factor if a newly hired nurse or other hospital worker decides to rethink their decision on whether to stay at the institution or even to leave the field altogether. Therefore, it is critical for faculty and staff development specialists to create solid curriculum to implement a variety of learning modalities aside from the dry, and sometimes tedious, lecture, by mixing it up with simulations, discussions, anecdotes, role-playing, and the like. The goal of the education of nurses in the art of delegation is to develop skilled, professional clinical leaders who are excellent communicators, efficient, and conscientious, and who achieve positive patient care experiences and desired outcomes.

Delegation keeps costs down, builds effective and solid teams across health care disciplines, and involves education and collaboration. It relies on an enormous team effort and mandates clear, coordinated communication skills. It is an expected nursing competency and as nurses become proficient in delegation, it allows them to make sound judgments about patients and coordinate optimal patient care (Currie, 2008).

Reflecting on my past early experiences as a new nurse "delegator," I decided to ask my current class of registered nurse (RN) to Bachelor of Science in Nursing (BSN) students the following questions:

- What do you remember about the subject of delegation?
- Were you taught this subject in nursing school?
- Did you have a degree of mastery or comfort with this skill?

Would you share your nursing delegation initiation story with me?

I share with you these stories, and of course, mine.

Personal Reflection #1 Kimberly

"I went to nursing school at a community college. I graduated in 1997 with an Associate Degree in nursing. We

Continued

CLINICAL CORNER—cont'd

Delegation and the New Nurse

were not taught how to delegate in school at all! When I started on the floor, we had a 4- to 6-week orientation. During that orientation, my preceptors showed me how to assign certain tasks to the tech. They were the ones who instructed me on what could and could not be assigned to the techs, and what had to be done by me as the nurse. They also made it clear that whatever I assigned to the tech, I was still ultimately responsible. Then one day I came in to work to find out that I was in charge. My delegation education at this level was baptism by fire. I was put in charge with no training, and part of the responsibility was to complete the assignment for the floor, as well as assign admissions as they came up. Oh, and if you screw it up, everyone will be miserable for the shift!"

Reflection #2 Deborah

"When I attended nursing school 32 years ago, we were never formally taught nursing delegation or peer delegation. We learned how to delegate from our nursing instructors. My nursing clinical rotations consisted of 8 hours of direct patient care followed by post-evaluations. Upon graduation, we knew how to function on the floor.

Today, as a preceptor for new RNs in Labor & Delivery, I think that the new graduates are not well prepared in the role of delegation. Prioritization skills are lacking and they are more focused on 'tasks' rather than the bigger picture or the 'whole picture.' I lead by example and support them in every way to make them feel comfortable and not to feel intimidated. I am currently orienting a patient care assistant (PCA) and use the same techniques as mentioned above."

Reflection #3 Michelle

"Let me share with you my operating room experience today. I needed to turn our room around quickly, but of course, safely. We had the same surgeon following himself; therefore, I needed to manage my time wisely. I helped the surgical tech open all of the instrumentation so she would not feel as if I had put it all on her. Really, I should have been seeing the patient, going over her history, obtaining the meds needed for the case, and putting some of the information in the computer. But because I myself was a tech at one time, I knew how it felt to be left on your own and open up an entire room by yourself.

After helping the tech, I went to see my patient. It took me about 15 minutes as she had a long history. When I brought my patient to the room, the tech was gone and had not communicated to me where she was going. There should always be two people in a room with a patient in case of a code, or other emergency. The tech felt it was

unfair that she did not get a break and I did. I told her that she could have said something, I would have given her more time for lunch to make up for a break; communication is key. Safety first: she was not being responsible in leaving the room and not letting me know where she was. I work hard and do lead by example."

Reflection #4 Donna

"As a new RN working nights on an orthopedic unit, I remember feeling that I had to do it all. I was afraid to ask for help from the nursing assistants because I felt intimidated by their veteran status and I was not at all confident in my new role. I didn't have a good sense of what the big picture was, how it impacted my patients, my team, and my ability to be a better nurse. I remember many times leaving late from work because I couldn't complete all my work in a timely manner. Charting was always put off until the bitter end; and when it came time to remember what needed to be charted, that became another brutal memory game."

Reflection #5 Kathleen

"As a relatively new RN, I was partnered with a licensed practical nurse (LPN) for an assignment of 10 patients. I was told I needed to hang all IV meds (intravenous medication) because they needed to be mixed and that is not in the scope of an LPN. Looking back now, I was unclear of the scope of LPN practice and the job description for what I could expect from her.

These were all my patients and my responsibility. The situations were difficult as I was unclear what I could delegate to the LPN; she was happy to keep busy with her patients and remind me she could not administer certain meds.

I found myself unprepared to delegate, not even sure what that looked or sounded like and therefore cared for the full patient load myself (at least this was my perception). Delegating to this LPN also seemed difficult to me as she was an older nurse who had been there much longer than me.

Delegation to unlicensed care providers, such as a nursing assistant and unit clerk was also something I struggled with. In this case, I had been a nursing assistant in another hospital before becoming a nurse. I think this helped me know 'what nursing assistants do' so I did not have that issue, but the nursing assistants were very experienced, and again, older than me. This was sometimes a barrier for me as a new young nurse. The nursing assistants did not always like a new and young person telling them what to do. However, I did have the opportunity to work with some amazing nursing assistants where this was not an issue and I learned plenty from them as well.

Delegation and the New Nurse

To say what I have learned since, one very important point my very experienced nurse manager taught me was to communicate with the person you are delegating to within the framework of the patient. Instead of asking the nursing assistant, 'Could you please do me a favor and take Mr. Smith to the bathroom,' we need to say, 'Our patient Mr. Smith needs to use the bathroom. Will you assist him as I am beginning a dressing change for our patient Mrs. Johnson.' She taught me that this language is more respectful and builds the staff as a team with the care of the patient in the center. The care I am requesting is to meet the patient's need, not purely my need. One other lesson learned is to be well aware of job descriptions and scope of practice for those with licenses."

Common themes come to the surface with these reflections. Often, the RN with the delegation dilemma is a new RN, with limited (if any) experience. A certain baseline level of discomfort exists and causes anxiety. Initially, the nurse views delegation as a "to-do" list of tasks that need to be completed during a certain prescribed time. Most of the delegation decisions are based on job descriptions: patient care associate, RN, other ancillary help. Rarely does a new delegator use their nursing judgment and take into consideration each person's strengths and weaknesses, who is suited to the various subtitles, etc. Delegation is a process. The nurse assesses if, when, or where assistance is needed. She/he then selects the appropriate person. The assistance is carried out under that "umbrella" supervision, and lastly, the delegation process is evaluated and feedback is shared. The nurse prioritizes the patients' needs, considers their condition, differentiates between nursing versus non-nursing tasks, and selects tasks to be delegated. The nurse then chooses the appropriate member of the team to assume the task. Nurses need to know the skill level of each team member to match the assignment appropriately (Curtis & Nicholl, 2004).

References

Currie, P. (2008). Delegation considerations for nursing practice. *Critical Care Nurse, 28*(5), 86–87.

Curtis, E., & Nicholl, H. (2004). Delegation: A key function of nursing. *Nursing Management, 11*(4), 26–31.

Donna Grotheer, MSN, RN
Hackensack Pascack UMC

EVIDENCE-BASED PRACTICE

Weydt, A. (2010). Developing delegation skills. *The Online Journal of Issues in Nursing 15*(2), manuscript 1.

Abstract

One of the most complex nursing skills is that of delegation. It requires sophisticated clinical judgment and final accountability for patient care. Effective delegation is based on one's state nurse practice act and an understanding of the concepts of responsibility, authority, and accountability. Work Complexity Assessment, a program that defines and quantifies various levels of care complexity based on the knowledge and skill required to perform the work, has demonstrated that methods of patient assignment and staff scheduling that support consistency increase what could be delegated to ancillary personnel by using the more effective assignment patterns. The author begins this article by discussing delegation and the related concepts of responsibility, accountability, and authority. Next, factors to consider in the delegation process, namely nursing judgment, interpersonal relationships, and assignment patterns, are presented. The author concludes by sharing how to develop delegation skills.

Delegation and the Related Concepts

Delegation is one of the most important tasks of a registered nurse (RN). When the RN delegates to another health care worker, the nurse must know the roles of the team members and know the patient needs. The nurse must use clinical judgment when delegating, and must know job descriptions of the team members. The RN is still responsible to be sure the tasks were carried out appropriately. The RN has the responsibility to delegate appropriately, the accountability of the tasks, and the authority to assign team members appropriate tasks.

Nursing Judgment

Delegation is based on the RN's judgment when assigning certain patients to certain health care workers.

Four guidelines for effective delegation have been identified by Koloroutis (2004, p. 136). They are:

- Delegation requires RNs to make decisions based on patient needs, complexity of the work, competency of the individual accepting the delegation, and the time that the work is done.
- Delegation requires that timely information regarding the individual patient be shared, defines specific

Continued

EVIDENCE-BASED PRACTICE—cont'd

expectations, clarifies any adaptation of the work in the context of the individual patient situation, and provides needed guidance and support by the RN.

- Ultimate accountability for process and outcomes of care, even those he or she has delegated, is retained by the RN.
- RNs make assignments and the care provider accepts responsibility, authority, and accountability for the work assigned.

Interpersonal Relationships

The RN must have proper interpersonal skills to delegate effectively to the LPN or nursing assistant. Communication is essential to transfer the tasks of delegation to the appropriate staff member. The development of a trusting relationship between the RN and the other team members is essential for the provision of safe, effective care.

The Work Complexity Assessment (WCA) defines three levels of complexity:

1. Unit-Based Scenarios

    In this setting, the health care workers are assigned tasks, for example, a nursing assistant would be assigned to do all vital signs on the unit. This allows for minimal communication with the RN. This leads to the question, "what RN is ultimately responsible for the tasks performed by the nursing assistant?"

2. Pairing

    Pairing is the second scenario in which one RN works with an LPN and nursing assistant for the shift (Koloroutis, et al., 2007). The nursing staff are paired for one shift. The next day, the nursing assistant may be paired with a different RN. Delegation increases with pairing. Prioritization of patient care should be reviewed.

3. Partnering

    In partnering, one RN and one LPN or nursing assistant are scheduled to work together. This hopefully will foster trust by working together daily (Koloroutis, et al., 2007).

Develop Delegation Skills

The development of delegation skills is learned over time. The state nurse practice acts outline the scope of practice in delegating to others. Delegation skills should be started in nursing school. This is an area where simulation in the nursing labs would be beneficial to the students.

Conclusion

The RN is the delegator of nursing tasks to licensed practical nurses (LPNs) and nursing assistants and other team members. The RN is ultimately responsible for patient care in a safe manner. The nurse practice act determines the delegation process. Responsibility, accountability, and authority all play a crucial role in safe patient delegation. The three assignment scenarios, unit based, pairing, and partnering, are used in Work Complexity Assessment. RNs must delegate effectively as an ongoing process to provide quality patient care.

Reference

Koloroutis, M., Felgen, J., Person, C., & Wessel, S. (2007). *Field guide: Relationship-based care visions, strategies, tools and exemplars for transforming practice*. Minneapolis, MN: Creative Health Care Management, Inc.

▌ NCLEX® EXAMINATION QUESTIONS

1. Which of the following is not a principle of delegation?
    A. The nursing profession determines the scope and standards of nursing practice.
    B. The registered nurse (RN) takes responsibility and accountability for the provision of nursing practice.
    C. The RN directs care and determines the appropriate use of resources when providing care.
    D. The licensed practical nurse (LPN) can delegate tasks to the nursing assistant.

2. The _____ nurse no longer relies on rules to understand a situation or to act appropriately; focuses quickly on viable solutions; is able to lead a team efficiently; can organize others' work and supervise them effectively.
    A. Novice
    B. Expert
    C. Competent
    D. Proficient

3. Barriers to delegation can arise for which of the following health care workers?
    A. Registered nurse (RN) delegator
    B. RN delegate
    C. Licensed practical nurse (LPN)
    D. All of the above

4. Some activities may not be delegated. All of the following may be delegated except:
   A. Performing an initial patient assessment
   B. Updating the patient's plan of care
   C. Providing direct nursing care
   D. Giving a registered nurse (RN) a needle and syringe, unlabeled, and telling her to administer the medication even though the RN did not see the medication prepared

5. Heidenthal and Marthaler (2005) state that what to delegate depends on all of the following factors except:
   A. Your state's nurse practice act
   B. Hospital policies and procedures
   C. What shift you are working
   D. The clinical situation

6. Who is accountable for ensuring that the registered nurse (RN) has access to documented competency information for staff to whom the RN is delegating tasks?
   A. The organization/agency
   B. The nurse leader
   C. The nurse supervisor
   D. The safety office

7. When accepting a delegated assignment, what does the nurse use per the State of New Jersey Nurse Practice Act, 1999?
   A. A nursing matrix
   B. A decision-making algorithm

C. Facility policy
D. Facility procedure

8. When delegating, the requirement of the right _____ means that you must know the competency level, job description, individual level of skill, and education of the individual to whom you are delegating.
   A. Direction/communication
   B. Person
   C. Task
   D. Circumstance

9. Many long-term care facilities assign _____ _____ as charge nurses.
   A. Registered nurses (RNs)
   B. Licensed practical nurses (LPNs)
   C. Nursing supervisors
   D. Nurse externs

10. What are the five rights of delegation per the National Council of State Boards of Nursing (1997)?
    A. Right task, right circumstance, right person, right direction/communication, right unit
    B. Right task, right circumstance, right medication, right direction/communication, right supervision
    C. Right task, right circumstance, right person, right direction/communication, right supervision
    D. Right task, right time, right person, right direction/communication, right supervision

Answers: 1. D   2. D   3. D   4. D   5. C   6. A   7. B
8. B   9. B   10. C

REFERENCES

American Nurses Association [ANA]. *Decision tree for delegation by registered nurses.* www.nursingworld.org/MainMenuCategories/ThePracticcofProfessionalNursing/NursingStandards/ANAPrinciples/PrinciplesofDelegation.pdf.aspx p. 12.

American Nurses Association [ANA]. (1992). *Position statement: Registered nurse education relating to the utilization of unlicensed assistive personnel.* http://ana.org/readroom/position/uap/uaprned.htm.

American Nurses Association [ANA] and National Council of State Boards of Nursing [NCSBN]. (2008). *Joint Statement of Delegation.* www.ncsbn.org/index.htm.

Anthony, M. K., Standing, T., & Hertz, J. E. (2000). Factors influencing outcomes after delegation to unlicensed assistive personnel. *Journal of Nursing Administration, 30*(10), 474–481.

Benner, P., & Benner, R. (1984). *From novice to expert: Excellence and power in clinical nursing practice.* Menlo Park, CA: Addison-Wesley Publishing.

Carrick, L., Carrick, L., & Yurkow, J. (2007). A nurse leader's guide to managing priorities. *American Nurse Today,* July, 40–41.

Carroll, P. (1998). Buyer beware? Using non-credentialed assistive personnel: Clinical and management perspectives. *Subacute Care Today, 1*(5), 24–28.

Carroll, P. (2006). *Nursing leadership and management: A practical guide.* Clifton Park, NY: Thomson Delmar Learning.

Heidenthal, P., & Marthaler, M. (2005). *Delegation of nursing care.* Clifton Park, NY: Thomson Delmar Learning.

Koloroutis, M. (2004). *Relationship-based care: A model for transforming practice.* Minneapolis, MN: Creative Health Care Management, Inc.

Koloroutis, M., Felgen, J., Person, C., & Wessel, S. (2007). *Field guide: Relationship-based care visions, strategies, tools and exemplars for transforming practice.* Minneapolis, MN: Creative Health Care Management, Inc.

National Council of State Boards of Nursing. (1997). *The five rights of delegation.* Chicago, IL: Author.

National Council of State Boards of Nursing [NCSBN]. (2005). *ANA and NCSBOB Joint Statement of Delegation.* Chicago, IL.

State of Kentucky. (1999). *Delegation of nursing tasks.* KRS 311A.170, 314.011, 201 KAR 20:400. www.lrc.state.ky.us/kar/201/020/400.htm.

State of New Jersey. (1999). New Jersey State Board of Nursing fact sheet: Decision making model for delegations of selected nursing tasks. *NJAC, 13*(3), 7–36. www.state.nj.us/lps/ca/nursing/ago1.htm.

Snyder, D., Medina, J., Bell, L., & Wavra, T. (eds). (2004). *American Association of Critical-Care Nurses Delegation Handbook* (2nd ed.). www.aacn.org/wd/practice/docs/aacndelegationhandbook.pdf.

14

Providing Competent Staff

OBJECTIVES

- Discuss hospital-wide and unit-based new employee orientation.
- Analyze the role of preceptor in nurse orientation.
- Compare and contrast the roles of the nurse, preceptor, and human resources in orientation.
- Analyze the progression of nursing clinical competence.

- Review the annual mandatory competencies for patient care staff.
- Compare and contrast the roles of manager and staff in performance appraisal.
- Identify the steps and progression of the staff registered nurse in the clinical ladder program.
- Discuss activities used by the nurse manager to support promotion of staff members.

OUTLINE

KEY TERMS

orientation process in which initial job training and information are provided to staff

mandatories mandatory education educational sessions and competencies that are required by accrediting agencies

competencies areas in which employees are judged to be qualified to perform

peer review the process by which practicing registered nurses systematically assess, monitor, and make judgments about the quality of nursing care provided by peers as measured against professional standards of practice

performance appraisal process in an organization by which employees are routinely evaluated according to performance standards

preceptor experienced individual who assists new employees in acquiring the necessary knowledge and skills to function effectively in a new environment

BENNER FIVE STAGES

When **new nurses enter** the workforce, it is important to realize that this is just the beginning of their professional journey. As discussed in Chapter 10, Benner (1984) posits that the nurse moves through five stages of clinical competence: novice, advanced beginner, competent, proficient, and expert. As you read this content, think of your own areas of experience in nursing. Decide where you think you fit.

Remember that you progress in professional competence as you work. Self-assessment of your current level of performance is an important function in nursing. Much of your progression will also greatly depend on the work environment. The organization provides the environment for the clinical progression of all staff, both for organizational needs and for the personal development of the nurse. Such professional work environments are evidenced in the various health care organizations that have achieved Magnet status (American Nurses Credentialing Center [ANCC], 2013).

The first experience of a novice nurse in the continuing progression toward competency occurs in the health care agency as a new employee.

STAFF COMPETENCY

The Joint Commission states that a hospital must provide the right number of competent staff to meet the needs of the patients (2014). Competent staff members are qualified and able to perform the work according to professional standards. To meet the goal of providing adequate competent staff, the hospital must carry out the following processes and activities:

- Orienting, training, and educating staff.
- Ongoing in-service and other education and training to increase staff knowledge of specific work-related issues.
- Assessing, maintaining, and improving staff competence.
- Ongoing, periodic competence assessment evaluating staff members' continuing abilities to perform throughout their association with the organization.

NEW EMPLOYEE ORIENTATION

Orientation is a process in which initial job training and information are provided to staff.

Staff orientation promotes safe and effective job performance. Some elements of orientation need to occur before staff begin to provide care, treatment, and services. Other elements of orientation can occur when staff are providing care, treatment, and services (The Joint Commission, 2014). Employees, regardless of level of competence, are required to attend orientation. Basic-to-new employee orientation is education on organization-specific functions, policies, and expectations, such as mission, vision, values, stakeholder expectations, performance improvement, basic skill evaluation, and mandatory policy review. Traditional hospital orientations can range from 3 weeks to 6 months depending on the organization and responsibilities of the nurse. The newer residency programs are ranging from 6 weeks to 1 year.

For new graduates the orientation is often expanded to allow for mentoring to the new role. The timeframe for new nurse socialization to the role, or the process of developing clinical judgment in practice, has been suggested to be as follows (Ferguson, Day, Anderson, & Rohatnsky, 2007):

- Orientation (0 to 20 days).
- Learning practice norms (orientation 4 to 6 months).
- Developing confidence (6 to 12 months).
- Consolidating relationships (12 to 18 months).
- Seeking challenges (18 to 24 months).

This does not mean that the formal orientation is 2 years, but that the length of time for a new nurse to become fully socialized to the profession and organization takes that amount of time. Once an employee accepts a new position, the orientation process is outlined. The length of orientation varies from hospital to hospital and for different groups of employees. Some hospitals differentiate between experienced staff and novice staff. Before this, a new employee will also have to complete a health physical and meet all of the medical criteria for employment, such as hepatitis B immunization and immunity status, and tuberculosis testing, etc. Some institutions require criminal background checks as well as drug screens.

Mandatory Content

The first part of orientation is usually organization specific and includes a hospital-wide orientation that may include speakers, such as the human resources representative, the infection control coordinator, the safety officer, the employee health coordinator, and the process improvement coordinator. This organization-specific orientation usually includes those educational topics that are considered mandatory by the accreditation agencies. These mandatory topics are usually reviewed on an annual basis in most health care institutions. This mandatory review allows for the determination of employee competency in knowledge in these content areas (Box 14-1).

Unit-Based Content

Next, there is unit-based or nursing-based orientation. Unit-based orientations are designed by the unit educator and nurse manager to orient the new nurse to the unit, its policies, patient needs, procedures, and protocols. For example, a nurse in a cardiac unit will receive education on electrocardiogram interpretation, cardiac drugs, cardiac arrest protocols, etc. A nurse in the labor room will receive education on fetal monitoring, neonatal resuscitation, etc. Patient care assignments will be made to match the learning of orientation. A description of the progression of orientation is shown in Figure 14-1.

PRECEPTOR MODEL

There are numerous models of nursing orientation, but most use **preceptors** to work with and evaluate the new employee during the orientation phase. New nurses are traditionally oriented to the professional role by "experienced" registered nurses who are knowledgeable in the "ways of nursing" in the organization. A preceptor can be defined as an experienced staff member who possesses excellent clinical skills and facilitates learning through caring, respect, compassion, understanding, nurturing, role modeling, and the excellent use of interpersonal

communication (Speers, Strzyzewski, & Ziolkowski, 2004). There are varied methods of choosing preceptors and pairing them with orientees. In hospitals with clinical ladders, experienced nurses are required to serve as preceptors as part of their normal responsibilities. In other institutions, preceptors are chosen based on their competencies, although in yet other institutions, nurses are chosen based on availability. This last method often results in multiple preceptors for one orientee, depending on who is available. This can result in frustration for the orientee, who may be receiving multiple messages from multiple preceptors (Hardy & Smith, 2001). Research demonstrates that proper pairing is key to the success of the preceptor program (Hardy & Smith, 2001; Horton,

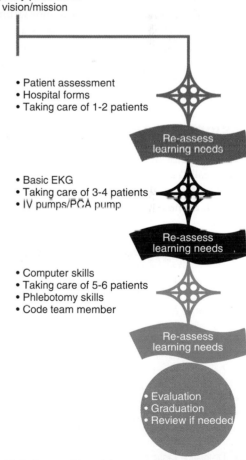

- Start orientation
- Review policy/procedures
- Hospital vision/mission

- Patient assessment
- Hospital forms
- Taking care of 1-2 patients

Re-assess learning needs

- Basic EKG
- Taking care of 3-4 patients
- IV pumps/PCA pump

Re-assess learning needs

- Computer skills
- Taking care of 5-6 patients
- Phlebotomy skills
- Code team member

Re-assess learning needs

- Evaluation
- Graduation
- Review if needed

FIGURE 14-1 A sample training roadmap. (Lee, V., & Harris, T. [2007]. Mentoring new nursing graduates. www.minoritynurse.com/features/other/080207d.html.)

BOX 14-1   New Employee Orientation: Mandatory Content

- Mission and governance
- Organizational strategic plan and objectives
- Customer contact requirements
- Code of conduct
- Fire safety
- Service excellence
- Age-specific patient content
- Infection control
- Process improvement
- Corporate compliance
- HIPAA (Health Insurance Portability and Accountability Act)
- Benefits

DiPaoli, Hertach, & Bower, 2012). Proper pairing occurs with preceptors who are selected into the role based on competencies in both clinical nursing and the ability to facilitate learning (Speers et al., 2004, Bower et al., 2012).

This model can be used to assist new employees and to reward experienced staff nurses. It provides a means for orienting and socializing the new nurse as well as providing a mechanism to recognize exceptionally competent staff nurses (Sullivan & Decker, 2013). Box 14-2 lists various functions of the preceptor.

There are also rewards for the preceptor in assisting the orientation of new nurses. The experienced nurses often feel more enthusiasm and more involved with the new staff, while the orientees express a sense of belonging to the unit (Hardy & Smith, 2001). Many preceptors use their precepting activities to support their progression up the institution's clinical ladder (Chapter 10). New graduate nurses require time to move from the role of student to expert clinician. Acting as a preceptor is an essential part of that transition (Neuman et al., 2004, Bowere et al., 2012).

Other roles involved in this orientation are discussed in Box 14-2.

RESIDENCY PROGRAMS

The Institute of Medicine report, The Future of Nursing (2006), called for the development of nurse residency programs to assist in the transition process of the new graduate, both at the new registered nurse (RN) and advanced practice registered nurse (APRN) levels. Although nurse residency programs vary in length and pay, they are usually 12-month programs designed to support baccalaureate nursing graduates as they transition into their first professional nursing role. The programs consist of a series of work and learning experiences that emphasize and develop the clinical and leadership skills necessary for the novice nurse to become a successful part of the interdisciplinary health care team. Before the development of such residency programs, new nurses often reported a lack of confidence, difficulty with work relationships, frustrations relating to the work environment, lack of time and guidance for developing organizational and priority-setting abilities, and overall high levels of stress. These factors likely contributed to the high turnover rate among new nurses, estimated at between 35% and 60% within the first year (Casey et al., 2004; Halfer and Grad, 2006). Evaluation of 12 1-year post-baccalaureate nurse residency programs found improved communication and organization skills, as well as higher perceived levels of support and reduced stress. The 12-month turnover rate among the first and second group of residents to graduate from the program was significantly lower (12% and 9%, respectively), than the average rate of 35% to 60% reported in the literature for hospitals without such a program (Krugman et al., 2006; Williams et al., 2007; Goode et al., 2009). Such 12-month residencies are highly competitive.

BOX 14-2   Preceptor Functions

- Assist new nurse to acquire knowledge and skills
- Tailor program specifically to needs
- Orient to unit
- Socialize within group
- Orient to unit functions
- Teach unfamiliar procedures
- Assist in development of skills
- Act as resource person
- Familiarize with policies and procedures
- Act as counselor
- Act as role model
- Act as time management coach
- Delegate tasks
- Assist with priority setting
- Mentor to shared governance

CONTINUED EMPLOYEE DEVELOPMENT

Accrediting agencies require that staff competence to perform job responsibilities must be assessed, demonstrated, and maintained by the human resources department in conjunction with the education department and the nurse manager (The Joint Commission, 2014). Competency in the required organizational and unit "mandatories" must be annually evaluated. The current licensure of the individual must be maintained on record. Some states require contact hours for professional license renewal. Many health care organizations provide these contact hours through their internal education or through employee benefits, which include educational advancement.

As the employee moves from novice to expert, the organization supports the individual in achieving the required competencies and additional learning required for growth. The basis for the assessment of the individual's needs and abilities is determined through the performance appraisal, peer review processes, and the educational needs assessment. These processes allow for the evaluation of the employee against stated standards. They also allow the employee to set annual goals for future development. The aggregation of these individual learning goals then becomes part of the annual education and human resource plan of the organization.

PEER REVIEW

Peer review in nursing is the process by which practicing registered nurses systematically access, monitor, and make judgments about the quality of nursing care provided by peers as measured against professional standards of practice. It is different from the standard performance appraisal in that it forms part of an annual performance appraisal process by which professional nurses judge the performance of professional peers. The peer review process stimulates professionalism through consistent accountability and promotes the self-regulation of nursing practice (ANCC, 2013).

The six principles of peer review are as follows:
1. A peer is someone of the same rank.
2. Peer review is practice focused.
3. Feedback is timely, routine, and a continuous expectation.
4. Peer review fosters a continuous learning culture of patient safety and best practice.
5. Feedback is not anonymous.
6. Feedback incorporates the nurse's developmental stage.

Peer-Review Principles

#1 A peer is someone of the same rank.
- Peer review implies that nursing care delivered by a group of nurses or an individual nurse is evaluated by individuals of the same rank or standing, according to established standards of practice.
- Peer reviewers are nurse colleagues with clinical competence similar to that of the nurse seeking peer review.
- Steps in the peer-review process are the same for all nurses and all settings.
- The key difference lies in identifying the purpose, peer group, and appropriate professionally defined standards upon which to base the review.

#2 Peer review is practice focused.
- Standards of nursing practice provide a means for measuring the quality of nursing care a client receives.

- Peer review in nursing is a process by which practicing registered nurses (RNs) systematically access, monitor, and make judgments about the quality of nursing care provided by peers, as measured against professional standards of practice.
- Peer-review activities are focused on practice decisions of professional nurses to determine the appropriateness and timeliness of those decisions.

#3 Feedback is timely, routine, and a continuous expectation
- In every health care facility in which nurses practice and for each nurse in continuous expectation.
- Individual practice and provision for peer review should be an ongoing process.
- An organized program makes peer review timely and objective.

#4 Peer review fosters a continuous learning culture of patient safety and best practice.
- The goals of every agency providing nursing care should include peer review as a culture of patient safety and best practice. It is one means of maintaining standards of nursing practice and upgrading nursing care.
- With respect to the individual, participation in the peer-review process stimulates professional growth; clinical knowledge and skills are updated.
- The purpose of peer review is to determine strengths and weaknesses of nursing care, taking into consideration local and institutional resources and constraints; to provide evidence for use as the basis of recommendations for new or altered policies and procedures to improve nursing care; and to identify areas where practice patterns indicate more knowledge is needed.
- Nurse reviewers need, or must strive to develop, a judicial temperament; the capacity and willingness to make critical decisions on the basis of evidence.

#5 Feedback is not anonymous.
- Feedback to the nurse under review is most effective when both verbal and written communication are combined.

#6 Feedback incorporates the nurse's developmental stage.
- Individuals, institutions, and the nursing profession benefit from an effective developmental stage.
- Peer-review program. With respect to the individual, participation in the peer-review process stimulates professional growth; clinical knowledge and skills are updated.

Source: Haag-Heitman, B., & George. V. (2011b). *Peer review in nursing: Principles for successful practice.* Sudbury, MA: Jones & Bartlett. www.jblearning.com.

BOX 14-3   Roles Involved in Orientation

Role of Nurse Manager
- Provide leadership in the culture of the nursing unit
- Provide supportive evaluation feedback to new nurses and experienced nurses
- Demonstrate valuing of mentoring activities
- Provide workloads that are reasonable and safe (with monitoring)
- Provide full-time employment on a single nursing unit
- Provide educational experiences
- Provide collaborative team experiences when possible

Nurse Managers' Retention Strategies
- Assist new nurses to manage stress
- Increase levels of responsibility slowly
- Maintain a level of challenge through provision of additional responsibilities
- Acknowledge continuing education needs
- Provide encouragement and support in nurses' transition
- Maintain an appropriate staff mix wherein nurses can practice safely

Human Resource Role
- Provide adequate orientation programs
- Provide ongoing support to address higher levels of learning
- Approve leaves of absence or educational study
- Support educational opportunities
- Coordinate new nurse employment on single units
- Initiate formal evaluative processes for performance appraisal
- Support a learning organization approach
- Provide resources and learning opportunities
- Acknowledge the contributions of mentors

Creative Engagement and Retention Strategies
- Support and encourage certification programs
- Facilitate service for education agreements
- Support clinical leadership
- Invest in the employee
- Provide extended learning experiences to enhance practice
- Provide adequate staff for safe patient care
- Provide oversight of new nurses by experienced nurses
- Encourage institutional commitment to mentorship
- Support "respectful workplace" initiatives

From Ferguson, L., Day, R., Anderson, C., & Rohatinsky, N. (2007). *The process for mentoring new nurses into professional practice.* Conference presentation at the National Healthcare Leadership Conference, 2007. www.healthcareleadershipconference.ca/assets/PDFs/Presentation%20PDFs/June%2012/Pier%209/The%20Process%20of%20Mentoring%20New%20Nurses%20into%20Professional%20Practice.pdf.

Peer review forms the basis of nursing accountability for current practice and the continual improvement of practice. Many institutions include peer review as the first step in the **performance appraisal** process. Roles involved in orientation are shown in Box 14-3.

PERFORMANCE APPRAISAL PROCESS

Performance appraisal originally began as a method to justify salary increases for employees. Today the performance appraisal is still used to determine rewards, but also to further assist the employee in setting performance goals for the year. Staff career progression begins with goal setting at the annual performance appraisal process.

Guidelines for Overall Performance Rating

Formal performance evaluations occur on an annual basis for most employees. These are most often done at a predetermined time, based on the human resource policies of the institution. The formal evaluation is part of the employee record and is usually a competency-based assessment of the performance of the employee during the past year. In many institutions, the competencies are related to the overall mission, vision, and goals of the organization. The evaluation forms the basis for the retention/promotion of the individual as well as the compensation adjustment. It also provides information that assists in the development of the employee's goals and objectives for the upcoming evaluation period. Box 14-4 provides guidelines for performance rating.

The nurse and the nurse manager should know the bases on which the individual is being rated. If you are the nurse being evaluated, ask for a copy of the tool being used. If the evaluation is based on the job description, make sure that both the nurse and manager have a copy. Most nursing departments develop department-wide or unit-specific goals, and all nurses, regardless of their position, are expected to contribute to these goals. Other organizations expect nurses to accomplish individual goals. It is important

BOX 14-4 Guidelines for Overall Performance Rating

University of Michigan Health System

Important Points
- There should be no surprises at evaluation time that influence an employee's overall rating.
- Overall principle is preponderance
- At applicable to level of nurse
- Developmental tool to initiate discussion in regard to level movement
- Any rating other than "meets behavioral expectations" requires rationale.

Scale	Guidelines
Behavioral expectations not met/NA	• This category is used when employees have consistently not met their job expectations over the course of the last year. • It would be expected that you would have already documented and counseled the employee on the issues that led to this overall rating.

Approaching behavioral expectations	• This category can be used for two purposes. One is to indicate performance issues that need attention, the other is to indicate performance for a new hire or someone at a new level who has not been in the position long enough to fully evaluate their performance.
	• For staff that are new to UMHHC (University of Michigan Hospitals and Health Centers) or their roles:
	  • Employment or transfer of less than 4 months (or whatever timeframe is appropriate for you to evaluate performance).
	  • Still mastering new skills and responsibilities.
	  • You expect the employee will be able to meet expectations next year.
	• For staff whose performance is less than meeting expectations:
	  • Inconsistent demonstration of framework behaviors for applicable level.
	  • Need to demonstrate growth and improvement to meet behaviors.
	  • Specific action plan should be developed to improve performance that includes measurable goals and expected outcomes.

Meets behavioral expectations	• This category is used when the employee is meeting behavioral expectations, is effective, and provides value for the organization. • Work is thorough and accurate; is accountable for own outcomes. • Contributes to the goals of the organization and the unit. • Exhibits professional demeanor. • Demonstrates commitment to meeting level expectations.

Exceeds behavioral expectations	• This category is used when the employee regularly meets expectations plus:
	  • Demonstrates excellence and exceeds expectations consistently; goes above and beyond.
	  • Continuously increases the quality and/or quantity of contribution.
	  • Demonstrates self-awareness related to performance.

to know how you are evaluating or being evaluated. Behaviors appropriate during the evaluation process are listed in Box 14-5.

As a nurse being evaluated:
- Know what you are being rated on.
- Acknowledge the peer review results.
- Before the review, carefully think about the period since your last review.
- Review the previous year's goals.
- Keep track of your performance and accomplishments along the way.
- Use examples to illustrate how you met the standard.
- Remain positive; acknowledge errors and show how you learned from them.
- Receive criticism well.
- Clarify expectations.
- Accept praise.

BOX 14-5   List of Recommended Supervisor and Staff Nurse Behaviors for Performance Appraisal

Manager Behaviors	Staff Nurse Behaviors
Records routinely scheduled observations of the nurse's performance relative to position, professional standards, and job description competencies in a variety of situations.	Uses position and professional standard expectations daily.
Validates interpretation of nurse's performance.	Documents specific patient outcomes that reflect planned nursing interventions.
Offers counsel and support as required, citing position and professional standard expectations.	Asks for clarification of expectations when there is doubt, citing position responsibilities and professional standards.
Plans a date and time collaboratively with the nurse.	
Communicates to nurse what will be needed for evaluation meeting.	Summarizes accomplishments during the evaluation period.
Confirms the interview in writing.	Prepares a list of activities that advance career to the next level.
Reviews nurse's past evaluation record.	
Completes the written evaluation.	Collaborates with the supervisor relative to date, time, and expected preparation for the evaluation interview.

Modified from Grohar-Murray, M.E., DiCroce, H. R., & Langan, J. (2011). *Leadership and management in nursing* (5th ed.). Upper Saddle River, NJ: Prentice Hall.

There are three main phases of the performance appraisal process:

1. Planning for the appraisal interview.
2. Participating in the appraisal interview.
3. Using evaluation results from both the peer review and performance appraisal.

Planning for the Interview

Preparing for the evaluation is important. In preparing, one should always list strengths and weaknesses, accomplishment of last year's goals, and future goals.

The nurse manager must also be prepared with proper documentation for this interview with specific examples of performance. There must be a correlation between the evaluation and the job description and goals of the institution.

Participating in the Appraisal Interview

This is the time for discussion specific to the employee only. The first topic of discussion is the individual's accomplishments and successes. This begins the interview on a positive note. The process should be carried out in a professional and sequential manner. If the employee is being recommended for improvement in certain areas, these specific areas must be addressed at the interview and the employee be granted a certain amount of time to improve on the lacking skills or performance. If disciplinary action is warranted because of inferior performance, the nurse manager should have means to correct the performance, such as counseling or reeducation, readily available to the employee.

Using Evaluation Results

Health care organizations have in place a method for goal attainment and outcome management. This plan may include items such as whether employee goals were met and, if not, what the plan is to assist the employee in meeting these goals in a timely manner. There may be a process improvement plan in place for evaluation of this process. Also, the employee is asked to set goals for the upcoming year along with outcome measures. These goals and outcome measures will form a portion of the next performance appraisal. The responsibilities of the supervisor and the staff nurses during the performance appraisal are listed in Box 14-6.

A sample evaluation process for a beginning nurse and a peer evaluation process is shown in Box 14-7.

The goals of the individual employees must match the goals of the unit, the department, and the institution as a whole. As the goals of all employees are set and the organizations set the strategic challenges and objectives for the next year, education and human resource plans are developed. Ongoing education, is mandated by The Joint Commission (2014) and

BOX 14-6 Supervisor and Staff Nurse Responsibilities

Supervisor Responsibilities	Staff Nurse Responsibilities
Conducts the interview.	Shares documented evidence of significant professional outcomes.
States judgments about the nurse's performance.	
Provides justification for salary.	Clarifies performance.
Encourages new goals.	States future goals.
Agrees upon future goals.	States actions to meet goals.

Modified from Grohar-Murray, M.E., DiCroce, H. R., & Langan, J. (2011). *Leadership and management in nursing* (5th ed.). Upper Saddle River, NJ: Prentice Hall.

includes in-services, training, and other activities, that should, at a minimum:

- Occur when job responsibilities or duties change;
- Increase knowledge of work-related issues;
- Be appropriate to the needs of the population(s) served and comply with law and regulation;
- Emphasize specific job-related aspects of safety and infection prevention and control;
- Incorporate methods of team training, when appropriate;
- Inform when and how to report adverse and sentinel events;
- Be offered in response to learning needs identified through performance improvement findings and other data analysis (i.e., data from staff surveys, performance evaluations, or other needs assessments);

BOX 14-7 University of Michigan Health System

Performance Evaluation Process: Self-evaluation With Peer Input

1. The nurse will select a minimum of three peers to perform a peer review.
   - Those selected must be educated in the peer review process.
   - At least one peer must be a registered nurse (RN).
   - Each nurse will be asked to evaluate the person on one or two different Framework domains, so that all five Framework domains are reviewed overall by peers. The Clinical Skills and Knowledge domain must be completed by an RN whenever possible.
2. The nurse will submit the names of their chosen peers to the manager that will be completing their performance evaluation. The nurse distributes one or two domains of the peer feedback tool to selected peers.
3. The reviewers will use the current Development Framework Peer Input tool for their appraisal. They will complete their peer tool, sign it, and return it to the nurse within 7 days.
   - Peers should circle the appropriate behavioral level. Peer reviewers would be encouraged to support their views with concrete examples on the right hand side of the page.
   - Each peer will comment on one or two different Framework domains.
4. The peer review forms are returned to the nurse, who shall review the content and summarize the information on the performance review form.

The nurse will complete the level appropriate self-evaluation portion of the staff.

5. Performance Planning and Evaluation form, with consideration of the input provided by the peer evaluation.
6. The nurse will submit their completed Staff Performance Planning and Evaluation form and their Peer Review forms to the manager. If materials are not submitted within 2 weeks of the established due date, then the managers may proceed with completing the evaluation process.

The manager will review the peer review form, peer summary, and self-evaluation and then complete the manager section of the evaluation form.

- The manager will use peer and self-evaluations as well as own knowledge of employee performance in determining ratings on the Performance Planning and Evaluation form.
- Rationale for rating other than "meets expectations," must be provided in the evaluation summary section after each domain.
- The manager will arrange an appointment with the nurse for the performance review.
7. The Peer Review forms will be returned to the nurse following the performance evaluation process, and a copy of the completed Performance Plan/Evaluation will be given to the nurse.
8. Completed evaluations are given to the administrative assistant for processing.

From University of Michigan Health System. *Performance evaluation process—Self-evaluation with peer input.* Used with permission.

- Result in documented outcomes; and
- Be documented.

Health care organizations develop myriad educational programs to further support the professional growth of employees and the mission of the organization.

As nurses progress from novice to expert, many health care facilities have a system that allows for promotion of nurses along clinical ladders. Education and benefits for progression in clinical competence form the basis for such ladders.

■ SUMMARY

Health care organizations are responsible for the level of competency of all employees. Competency assessment starts with the initial orientation for all employees and continues throughout the term of employment. Nurses progress on a continuum of competency from novice to expert during their careers according to the work of Benner (1984). This continuum forms the basis for many career development opportunities available to the nurse. These opportunities are related to job function during the peer review and performance appraisal process.

🔲 CLINICAL CORNER

Peer Review: Invigorate Your Practice

"There is only one corner of the universe you can be certain of improving, and that is your own self."
Aldous Leonard Huxley

Peer review is typically associated with the process of publishing an author's academic work that is reviewed by peers who are experts in the same field to ensure scholarly standards are met before publication. A nursing peer review process is different. This involves ongoing feedback on the individual's performance and professional development. Most often when we hear the words "peer review," they typically invoke fear in our hearts. Many express that they "feel uncomfortable" giving and receiving feedback to and from a peer, but they are okay with receiving feedback from a supervisor, who spends much less time working side by side with them. You need to ask yourself, even if you might feel uncomfortable receiving feedback from a peer, do you think your peers are not assessing and evaluating your performance? Do you think your peers have not formed opinions on the skills you excel at and the skills that you might need some mentoring in? Might your peer not have some suggestions for your continuing education that might help you grow as a professional? These are important questions to contemplate and peer review is an important topic to reflect on throughout your professional nursing career. The Institute of Medicine (2010) recognized that nursing plays a vital role in the front lines of health care and nurses should be considered full partners in health care reform. One element to assist the nursing profession in leading the changes needed to improve health care is peer review.

Nursing peer review has been recognized as a measure of accountability and a means of evaluating and improving practice (Jambunathan, 1992). The American Nurses

Association (ANA) (1988) deems that primary accountability for quality nursing care resides with the individual nurse. The nursing peer review process recognizes that in a self-regulating professional practice model, the clinical accountability for care rests solely with the clinical practicing nurse (Haag-Heitman & George, 2011b, p. 6). Peer review is a mechanism to maintain nursing standards. Each nurse is responsible for interpreting and implementing the standards of nursing practice. Nurses are stewards for patient safety and have a professional and societal responsibility to maintain competence and complete performance improvement activities. Historically, peer review has been connected with clinical nurses, single nurse specialties, or advanced practice nurses. Most recently in the 2010 edition of *Nursing's Social Policy Statement: The Essence of the Profession*, the ANA discusses the need for all levels in all areas where nurses practice to participate in peer review to regulate their own practice. Additionally, a periodic self-appraisal and peer feedback for assurance of competence and continuous professional development must be in place for all levels of nursing to achieve and maintain Magnet designation (American Nurse Credentialing Center, 2013).

What is Nursing Peer Review? Peer review is an essential component of professional practice.

The ANA defines nursing peer review as an organized effort whereby practicing professionals review the quality and appropriateness of services ordered or performed by their professional peers. Peer review in nursing is the process by which practicing registered nurses systematically assess, monitor, and make judgments about the quality of nursing care provided by peers as measured against professional standards of practice (p. 3).

Current-day peer review guiding principles include someone of the same rank; practice focused; timely, routine, and continuous feedback; a continuous learning culture of best practice; not anonymous; and feedback that incorporates the developmental stage of the nurse (Haag-Heitman & George, 2011a).

Nursing peer review is often confused with peer and annual evaluations. The annual evaluation is a managerial function and focuses on the employee's goal alignment with the organization. In addition to the annual evaluation, organizations often have clinical nurses give "peer" feedback about the nurse being evaluated to the manager. The manager summarizes it and delivers this anonymous feedback to the nurse at the time of the annual evaluation. This peer evaluation method violates current-day nursing peer-review principles. The annual evaluation is retrospective and does not allow for real-time practice assessments of the nurse's practice. A nurse manager is not a peer of a clinical nurse and the feedback is delivered anonymously. Nursing peer review should focus on role specific competencies, professional development, and outcomes. Peer review should be independent of the annual evaluation, should not be blinded from the nurse, and should be delivered by a peer of the same rank (George & Haag-Heitman, 2012).

Think of peer review as an opportunity to reflect on your practice and develop a plan on how you want to grow and develop as a professional. We tend to not reflect on our practice as often as we should. Things you should be asking yourself include the following:

- Professionally, where do I want to be 5 years from now?
- What formal education or continuing education will I need to achieve my professional goals?
- What are the external forces impacting health care and nursing?
- Is health care moving to an outpatient model of care and managing population health?
- Do I have the skills needed for an outpatient setting?
- Do I want to achieve national board certification? How will I get there?
- Who is a role model for me? Can I work with this person to improve?

All of these questions are a part of reflection on your practice, and peer review can help you move forward in your practice.

Benefits of Nursing Peer Review: Benefits of peer review are an integration of improved communication, professional autonomy, and accountability. In 2005, the American Association of Critical-Care Nurses (AACN) used evidence-based and relationship-centered principles to formulate the Six Standards of a Healthy Work Environment. Skilled communication is one of the six standards. Nurses must be as proficient in communication skills as they are in clinical skills (Barden, 2005). Blinded feedback violates the principle of skilled communication. Blinded feedback does not provide for clarification of the comment(s) or constructive pointers for behavior change to enhance growth. Through ongoing feedback by peers of equal rank, the peer review process provides the nurse with an increased awareness of professional conduct, enhances interprofessional collaboration, and allows the nurse time to reflect on their practice.

Implications: Nurses have an obligation to their organization and the professional discipline to perform nursing peer review. Nurses are the only health care providers at the front line of patient care delivery around-the-clock, and are required to be knowledgeable about many aspects, including chronic disease, medication management, evidenced-based practice, ethical decision making, evaluating trended data, and the use of complex technology, to name but a few. Working with other nurses who are clinically competent has long been cited by clinical nurses as a key feature of a satisfying and productive unit work environment (Schmalenberg et al., 2008). Healthy work environments are essential to ensure patient safety, enhance nurse's recruitment and retention, and maintain an organization's financial viability (Barden, 2005). Peer review encourages an increase in the amount of control that nurses have over their work, which promotes job satisfaction, a reduction in nursing turnover, and professionalism in nursing (Alexander, Weisman, & Chase, 1982).

The ANA and Magnet Recognition Program support the need for peer review in all levels where nursing is practiced. Typically, the attention of peer review has been a clinical focus to improve systems to reduce occurrences of negative events. This type of peer review is essential in order for nurses to deliver quality care. But just as the role of the clinical nurse has expanded, so has the role of the nurse leader. A robust peer review process must be in place for nurse leaders as well as clinical nurses. Whether the nurse is involved in direct care, an APN, nursing management, or nursing administration, peer review is needed to assist the nurse to improve their practice.

Continued

👤 CLINICAL CORNER—cont'd

Conclusion: Peer review is an essential element that defines all professional disciplines; it is not optional for a practicing professional. Other professions, such as medicine, pharmacy, and accountancy recognize the need for peer review to improve performance (Combes, 2009; Graham, 2009; Haines et al., 2010; Pan et al., 2013). Until nursing embraces the principles of peer review at all levels and implements a continual structure for peer review, nursing will not achieve significant and sustainable changes in quality and safety outcomes for patients, families, and society (George & Haag-Heitman, 2011).

Challenge yourself to think about peer review in a different light and move away from a state of uneasiness that peer review often creates. Let this Clinical Corner be the spark that will catapult you to volunteer to be a part of, or lead a team in your organization, to develop or redefine your peer review process to align with contemporary principles. Feedback is a gift. A nurse's peer is the most suitable person to give feedback to improve because that peer is working in the same role. We often see ourselves with a clear lens, but receiving feedback from another can identify opportunities for improvement. How does an individual nurse grow in their practice and in the profession without honest, direct feedback on their performance from a peer? The true value of peer review is to assist us in improving ourselves in the wonderful profession that we have chosen; nursing.

Constantly improve.

Beverly S. Karas-Irwin, DNP, RN, NP-C, HNB-BC, NEA-BC
The Valley Hospital

EVIDENCE-BASED PRACTICE

Fiedler, R., Read, E. S., Lane, K. A., Hicks, F. D., & Jeqier, B. J. (2014). Long-term outcomes of a postbaccalaureate nurse residency program: a pilot study. *Journal of Nursing Administration*, 44(7-8), 417–422.

Author Information

Author affiliations: Assistant Professor (Dr Fiedler) and Assistant Dean for Generalist Education and Professor (Dr Hicks), College of Nursing, Rush University; and Manager, Professional Nursing Practice/Educator Quality Coordinator (Dr Read), Medical Center, Rush University, Chicago, Illinois; School Health Professional (Ms Lane), Hong Kong; and Assistant Professor (Dr Jegier), The College at Brockport, New York.

Abstract

Objective

The purpose of this pilot study was to determine what influence a nurse residency program (NRP) has on long-term outcomes, including turnover rates, career satisfaction, and leadership development.

Background

Studies examining short-term outcomes of NRPs have shown positive effects. Long-term studies of NRPs have not been reported.

Methods

This descriptive study surveyed former nurse residents still employed at the facility. Data were collected by means of a demographic tool and the McCloskey/Mueller Satisfaction Scale, a job satisfaction tool.

Results

Although nursing turnover increased past the year-long residency program, it remained well below the national average. All components of satisfaction were ranked relatively high, but co-worker/peer support was most important to job satisfaction. Leadership development in the areas of certification and pursuing an advanced degree increased with longer employment, but hospital committee involvement decreased with successive cohorts.

Conclusion

Overall, the long-term outcomes of an NRP appear to have benefits to both the organization and the individual.

NCLEX® EXAMINATION QUESTIONS

1. The Joint Commission (2014) states that a hospital must provide the right number of competent staff to meet the needs of the patients. Which of the following is not a criterion that must be present to meet the goal of providing adequate competent staff?
   A. Orienting, training, and educating staff
   B. The hospital provides ongoing in-service and other education and training.
   C. Assessing, maintaining, and improving staff competence
   D. Providing full monetary compensation for conferences and nurse certifications

2. There are _____ principles of peer review.
   A. Four
   B. Five
   C. Six
   D. Seven

3. Which of the following is not necessary during a new hire orientation to a hospital?
   A. Mission
   B. Vision
   C. Performance improvement
   D. Pay scales of the entire group

4. _____ in nursing is the process by which practicing registered nurses systematically assess, monitor, and make judgments about the quality of nursing care provided by colleagues as measured against professional standards of practice.
   A. Peer review
   B. Infection control assessment
   C. Nurse supervisor evaluation
   D. Education manager

5. According to The Joint Commission (2014), accrediting agencies require that staff competence to perform job responsibilities must be assessed, demonstrated and maintained by _____.
   A. Human resources
   B. Nurse manager
   C. Education department
   D. All of the above

6. According to the Institute of Medicine's report, The Future of Nursing (2006), there was a call for the development of _____ programs to assist in the transition process of the new graduate.
   A. Residency programs
   B. Preceptor programs
   C. Clinical ladder programs
   D. Peer-review programs

7. Which of the following is an advantage for the nurse to act as preceptor to new nurses?
   A. It supports the progression in the institution's clinical ladder.
   B. Higher pay per hour is awarded to precept.
   C. Enhanced job promotion prospects
   D. The preceptor decides if the new nurse should stay on or be let go.

8. A _____ is defined as an experienced staff member who possesses excellent clinical skills and facilitates learning through caring, respect, compassion, understanding, nurturing, role-modeling, and the excellent use of interpersonal communication as per Speers, Strzyzewski, and Ziolkowski (2004).
   A. Preceptor
   B. Charge nurse
   C. Supervisor
   D. Nurse manager

9. For new graduate nurses, the orientation may:
   A. Be expanded
   B. Not be expanded
   C. Relate specifically to the age of the nurse
   D. Be given on whatever shift the nurse has been hired for

10. The part of the orientation process that includes speakers from human resources, infection control, hospital safety and security, and process improvement, is called:
    A. Hospital-wide orientation
    B. Unit-specific orientation
    C. Staff competencies
    D. Nursing orientation

Answers: 1. D   2. C   3. D   4. A   5. D   6. A   7. A   8. A   9. A   10. A

REFERENCES

Alexander, C. S., Weisman, C. S., & Chase, G. A. (1982). Determinants of staff nurses' perceptions of autonomy within different clinical outcomes. *Nursing Research*, *31*, 48–52.

American Nurses Association. (1988). *Peer review guidelines*. Kansas City, MO: Author.

American Nurses Association. (2010). *Nursing's social policy statement: The essence of the profession*. Silver Spring, MD: Author.

American Nurses Credentialing Center. (2013). *2014 Magnet application manual*. Silver Spring, MD: Author.

Barden, C. (Ed.). (2005). *AACN standards for establishing and sustaining healthy work environments*. Aliso Viejo, CA: AACN.

Combes, J. (2009). Peer perspective deepens. *Hospital Health Network*, *83*(9), 56.

George, V., & Haag-Heitman, B. (2011). Nursing peer review: The manager's role. *Journal of Nursing Management*, *19*, 254–259.

George, V., & Haag-Heitman, B. (2012). Differentiating peer review and the annual performance review. *Nurse Leader*, *10*(1), 26–28.

Graham, G. (2009). Introducing the new principles-based peer review standards. *Journal of Accountancy*, *207*(5), 39–43.

Haag-Heitman, B., & George, V. (2011a). Nursing peer review: Principles and practice. *American Nurse Today*, *6*(9), 48.

Haag-Heitman, B., & George, V. (2011b). *Nursing peer review: Strategies for successful implementation*. Burlington, MA: Jones & Bartlett.

Haines, S. T., Ammann, R. R., Beehrle-Hobbs, D., & Groppi, J. A. (2010). Protected professional practice evaluation: A continuous quality-improvement process. *American Journal of Health-System Pharmacy: AJHP: Official Journal of the American Society of Health-System Pharmacists*, *67*(22), 1933–1940.

Hardy, R., & Smith, R. (2001). Enhancing staff development with a structured preceptor program. *Journal of Nursing Care Quality*, *15*, 9–17.

Institute of Medicine. (2010). *The future of nursing: Leading change, advancing health*. www.iom.edu/Reports/2010/The-Future-of-Nursing-Leading-Change-Advancing-Health.aspx%20.

Jambunathan, J. (1992). Planning a peer review program. *Journal of Nursing Staff Development*, *8*(5), 235–239.

Pan, H., Hsu, G., Yang, T., Huang, J., Chou, C., Liang, H., & Wong, K. (2013). Peer reviewing of screening mammography in Taiwan: Its reliability and the improvement. *Chinese Medical Journal*, *126*(1), 68–71.

Schmalenberg, C., Kramer, M., Brewer, B., Burke, R., Chmielewski, L., Cox, K., & Waldo, M. (2008). Clinically competent peers and support for education: Structures and practices that work. . . article 3 in a series of 8. *Critical Care Nurse*, *28*(4), 54.

15

Group Management for Effective Outcomes

OBJECTIVES

- Discuss nurse leader responsibility regarding group management.
- Review techniques for working with groups.
- Review techniques for leading groups and meetings.
- Differentiate between functional and dysfunctional groups.
- Review the different methods used to evaluate staff performance.
- Identify the difference between supervising and evaluating the work of others.
- Review the importance of supervising and leading groups, task forces, and patient care conferences.

OUTLINE

KEY TERMS

cohesiveness degree to which the members are attracted to the group and wish to retain membership in it

committees groups that deal with specific issues involving several service areas

competing groups groups in which members compete for resources or recognition

group aggregate of individuals who interact and mutually influence each other; several individuals assembled together or who have some unifying relationship

real (command) groups groups that accomplish tasks in an organization and are recognized as legitimate organizational entities

task group several individuals who work together to accomplish specific time-limited assignments

teams real groups in which people work cooperatively with each other to achieve a goal

GROUPS AND TEAMS

Nurses work as part of a team on the unit where they are employed. This does not necessarily mean that they are all practicing team nursing, but they are part of a larger group that is responsible for the overall delivery of care on the unit. As a team member it is important to know how to work within a team, how to manage teams, and how to evaluate the performance of others.

A **group** consists of individuals who interact and influence each other. Groups exist in organizations. According to Sullivan and Decker (2009), group members include:

- Individuals from a single work group, such as a unit-based council.
- Individuals at similar job levels from more than one work group, such as a nursing retention council.
- Individuals from different job levels, such as the "night council."
- Individuals from different work groups and different job levels in the organization, such as interdisciplinary groups composing a service excellence committee.

As can be seen from this definition, there are a number of groups that function within a nursing unit. Some of these groups will be:

- Interdisciplinary teams: Sometimes called collaboratives, which are composed of the different functions caring for a patient. An example would be an ambulatory chemotherapy collaborative, in which the team composition includes the nurse, the pharmacist, the dietician, the admission clerk, and the intravenous therapist.
- Patient care team: This may be similar to the group of individuals actually providing actual care to the patient. It may be composed of all individuals responsible for care per shift or over 24 hours.
- Performance improvement team: May include individuals from various disciplines and from various levels of the organization (e.g., department head, staff nurse, environmental services member, etc.)

The nurse and nurse manager are also part of a much larger group: the patient care (or nursing) department. As a member of this larger group, it is important to support the overall goals of the patient care department and be a functional valued member of this team. The differences between groups and teams are described in Box 15-1. **Teams** are **real groups** in which individuals must work cooperatively with each other to achieve some overarching goal (Sullivan & Decker, 2009).

One of the first rules for any team, **committee**, or council is the development of the charge of the group. This is often called the bylaws or rules of the group. The development of such bylaws focuses the work of the group to the expected outcomes or committee rules stated in the bylaws.

An example of a Nursing Council Bylaws is given here.

ACTIVE LISTENING

The first rule for dealing with individuals as well as with teams is to be a good listener. As a good listener, you

---

BOX 15-1 Differences Between Groups and Teams

Groups
1. Members have a common purpose, but work independently, sometimes competitive with one another.
2. Individuals may have limited knowledge about one another.
3. Meetings serve as a forum to receive reports and coordinate activity.
4. Meetings follow an agenda with set time constraints.
5. Attendance is not essential; the group can function with absent members and substitutes.
6. The composition of the group may vary.
7. Individuals rather that the group are recognized for effectiveness.

Teams
1. Members are interdependent, collaborating for a common mission or project, never competitive with one another.
2. Trust develops from learning about one another; how to anticipate behavior.
3. Meetings serve to evaluate team effectiveness.
4. Meetings are often unstructured, allowing time for strategic planning and team development.
5. Attendance and participation of each member are essential.
6. Team members may not appoint substitutes.
7. Individual performance is secondary to team effectiveness.

Nees, T. (2010). *Seven characteristics of groups and teams.* http://leadingtoserve.com/?p=172

must listen actively. This is when the person listening is completely focused and tuned in to the individual who is speaking. The active listener is nonjudgmental and comprehends the full conversation. See Box 15-2 for guidelines on active listening.

CONDUCTING MEETINGS

Nurse managers are often asked to lead group or team meetings. Many of these may be staff meetings for the

---

BOX 15-2 Guidelines for Active Listening

1. Slow down your internal processes and seek data. Do not interrupt the speaker.
2. The more information you acquire through listening, the less interpretation you do (making up the missing pieces or motivations). The less information you have, the more interpretation you do.
3. Realize that the first words from the other person are not necessarily representative of inner thoughts and feelings. Be patient.
4. When listening, suspend your own beliefs and views and judgments, at least temporarily. Attempt to understand the perspective of the other person, particularly if it is different from yours.
5. Realize that any judgments or "labels" strongly influence the manner in which you listen to the other person.
6. Appreciate the difference between understanding other people's perspectives and agreeing with them. First strive to understand. Then you may agree or disagree.
7. Effective listening is based on an inner desire to learn about another's unique experience of the world.

Modified from Olen, D. (1992). *Communicating speaking and listening to end misunderstanding and promote friendship.* Germantown, WI: JODA Communications.

---

review of issues of importance to the unit, performance improvement teams, patient care teams, or other shared governance teams. Table 15-1 outlines some guidelines for leading group meetings (Sullivan & Decker, 2009).

These guidelines can be further adapted to delineate guidelines for leading teams (Table 15-2), such as patient care teams.

EFFECTIVE AND INEFFECTIVE TEAMS

Parker (1990) states that a team is a **group** of people with a high degree of interdependence geared toward the achievement of a goal or a **task**. Not all teams function well, and there are times when even the most qualified team has a dysfunctional day. If a team has a "bad day," it is important for the team member or leader to evaluate the reasons for the poor performance. If the reasons can be understood, it is important to alter the way the team works to increase functionality, efficiency, and patient outcomes.

An effective team is able to move the agenda forward with clear decision making, a level of understanding of the goals and actions, and the willingness of the team members to participate in the decision-making process.

The original work done by McGregor (1960) has stood the test of time and continues to show significant differences between effective and ineffective teams (Table 15-3).

Not all teams are functional! And it is very difficult for members who are working within the team to realize their level of effectiveness. If you feel the team is not working as well as it should, you may want to evaluate a team's effectiveness using a team assessment questionnaire tool.

TABLE 15-1 Guidelines for Leading Group Meetings

- Begin and end on time.
- Start with the agenda, stick to it!
- Create a warm, accepting, and nonthreatening climate.
- Arrange seating to minimize differences in power, maximize involvement, and allow visualization of all meeting activities. (A U-shape is optimal.)
- Use interesting and varied visuals and other aids.
- Clarify all terms and concepts. Avoid jargon.
- Foster cooperation in the group.
- Establish goals and key objectives.
- Keep the group focused.
- Focus the discussion on one topic at a time.
- Facilitate thoughtful problem solving based on evidence
- Allocate time for all problem-solving steps.
- Promote involvement.
- Facilitate integration of material and ideas.
- Encourage the exploration of implications of ideas.
- Facilitate the evaluation of the quality of the discussion.
- Elicit the expression of dissenting opinions.
- Summarize discussion.
- Finalize the plan of action for implementing decisions.
- Arrange for follow-up.

These guidelines can be further adapted to delineate guidelines for leading teams (see Table 15-2), such as patient care teams.

TABLE 15-2   Guidelines for Leading Teams

- Do not waste staff time.
- Create a warm, accepting, and nonthreatening climate.
- Be knowledgeable of all team members' abilities and values.
- Communicate in clear terms that are understood by all team members.
- Clarify all terms and concepts. Avoid jargon.
- Foster cooperation in the group.
- Establish goals and key objectives for the day.
- Routinely check on the performance of the group and patient outcomes to determine if changes in the plan are needed.
- Facilitate thoughtful problem solving based on evidence
- Allocate time for all changes in the delivery of care.
- Promote involvement of all members.
- Facilitate the integration of work and ideas of all team members.
- Assist other team members if needed.
- Evaluate work at the end of the shift.
- Thank all team members for the work done.
- Assist any members who need improvement.

TABLE 15-3   Attributes of Effective and Ineffective Teams

Attribute	Effective Team	Ineffective Team
Working environment	Informal, comfortable, relaxed	Indifferent, bored, tense, stiff
Discussion	Focused	Frequently unfocused
	Shared by almost everyone	Dominated by a few
Objectives	Well understood and accepted	Unclear, or many personal agendas
Listening	Respectful; encourages participation	Judgmental; much interruption and "grandstanding"
Ability to handle conflict	Comfortable with disagreement	Uncomfortable with disagreement
	Open discussion of conflicts	Disagreement usually suppressed, or one group aggressively dominates
Decision making	Usually reached by consensus	Often occurs prematurely
	Formal voting kept to a minimum	Formal voting occurs frequently
	General agreement is necessary for action; dissenters are free to voice	Simple majority is sufficient for action; minority is expected to go along with opinion
Criticism	Frequent, frank, relatively comfortable, constructive	Embarrassing and tension-producing, destructive
	Directed toward removing obstacle	Directed personally at others
Leadership	Shared; shifts from time to time	Autocratic; remains clearly with committee chairperson
Assignments	Clearly stated	Unclear
	Accepted by all despite disagreements	Resented by dissenting members
Feelings	Freely expressed, open for discussion	Hidden, considered "explosive" and inappropriate for discussion
Self-regulation	Frequent and ongoing, focused on solutions	Infrequent, or occurs outside meetings

Modified from McGregor, D. (1960). *The human side of enterprise.* New York: McGraw-Hill.

TEAM ASSESSMENT QUESTIONNAIRE

Instructions: Use the scale below to indicate how each statement applies to your team. Evaluate the statements honestly and without overthinking your answers.

3 = Usually
2 = Sometimes
1 = Rarely

_____1. Team members are passionate and unguarded in their discussion of issues.

_____2. Team members call out one another's deficiencies or unproductive behaviors.

_____3. Team members know what their peers are working on and how they contribute to the collective good of the team.

_____4. Team members quickly and genuinely apologize to one another when they say or do

_____ something inappropriate or possibly damaging to the team.

_____5. Team members willingly make sacrifices (such as budget, turf, head count) in their departments or areas of expertise for the good of the team.

_____6. Team members openly admit their weaknesses and mistakes.

_____7. Team meetings are compelling, not boring.

_____8. Team members leave meetings confident that their peers are completely committed to the decisions that were agreed on, even if they were in initial disagreement.

_____9. Morale is significantly affected by the failure to achieve team goals.

_____10. During team meetings, the most important and difficult issues are put on the table to be resolved.

_____11. Team members are deeply concerned about the prospect of letting down their peers.

_____12. Team members know about one another's personal lives and are comfortable discussing them.

_____13. Team members end discussions with clear and specific resolutions and action plans.

_____14. Team members challenge one another about their plans and approaches.

_____15. Team members are slow to seek credit for their own contributions, but quick to point out those of others.

Scoring

Combine your scores for the preceding statements as indicated below:

Dysfunction 1: Absence of Trust	Dysfunction 2: Fear of Conflict	Dysfunction 3: Lack of Commitment	Dysfunction 4: Avoidance of Accountability	Dysfunction 5: Inattention to Results
Statement 4: ___	Statement 1 : ___	Statement 3: ___	Statement 2: ___	Statement 5: ___
Statement 6: ___	Statement 7: ___	Statement 8: ___	Statement 11: ___	Statement 9: ___
Statement 12: ___	Statement 10: ___	Statement 13: ___	Statement 14: ___	Statement 15: ___
Total: ___	Total: ___	Total:	Total: ___	Total: ___

A score of 8 or 9 is a probable indication that the dysfunction is not a problem for your team.
A score of 6 or 7 indicates that the dysfunction could be a problem.
A score of 3 to 5 is probably an indication that the dysfunction needs to be addressed.
Regardless of your scores, it is important to keep in mind that every team needs constant work, because without it, even the best ones deviate toward dysfunction
(Lencioni, P. (2002) *The five dysfunctions of a team: A leadership fable.* San Francisco: Jossey-Bass.)

POWER AND CONTROL

Whenever there is a team effort, power and control usually come into play. When a person reacts to a situation at the "feeling" level, there are often blame and judgment calls. People normally would like to believe that their input and contributions are respected and used by the group. For a team to be effective, each member of the group must be able to effectively communicate, offer constructive criticism, and acknowledge the positive at every chance. (See Guidelines for Acknowledgment in Box 15-3.) A "just" culture throughout an organization will assist with such freedom in communication (see Chapter 8).

RECOGNIZE AND REWARD SUCCESS

Rewards are listed as one important principle of high-performing organizations. The Studer Group (2007, 2012) has defined nine principles of high-performing organizations. The ninth principle is to recognize and reward success. Everyone makes a difference! Start creating legends in your organization. A legend is an example of those who live the organizational values. By creating legends we establish real-life examples for others to follow. Create win-win situations for your staff. Never let great work go unnoticed! The first step in creating a legend in your organization is to reward team members for a job well done. Much of the work in creating legends

---

BOX 15-3   Guidelines for Acknowledgment

1. Acknowledgments must be specific. The specific behavior or action that is appreciated must be identified in the acknowledgment; for example, "Thank you for taking notes for me when I had to go to the dentist. You identified three key points that appeared on the test."
2. Acknowledgments must be "eye to eye."
3. Acknowledgments must be sincere, that is, from the heart. Each of us recognizes insincerity. If you do not truly appreciate a behavior or action, do not say anything. Insincerity often makes people angry or upset, thus defeating the goal.
4. Acknowledgments are more powerful when they are given in public. Most people receive pleasure from public acknowledgment and remember these occasions for a long time. For people who are shy and may prefer no public acknowledgment, this is an opportunity to work on a personal growth issue with them. Public acknowledgment is an opportunity to communicate what is valued.
5. Acknowledgments need to be timely. The less time that elapses between the event and the acknowledgment, the more powerful and effective it is and the more the acknowledgment is appreciated by the recipient.

From Yoder-Wise, P. (2011). *Leading and managing in nursing.* St. Louis: Elsevier. p. 353.

---

in your organization will be communicated through the various committees and team meetings. Such award and recognition has been documented to be related to increased nurse satisfaction (Guyton, 2012).

QUALITIES OF A TEAM PLAYER

Nurses work in a collaborative environment, yet many nurses have concerns about the lack of ability of some individuals to work as part of a team: "They just don't support us!"

Maxwell (2002) has identified 17 characteristics that make a good team player.

1. Adaptability: Inflexibility does not work in teams. Being rigid in thinking or behavior is destructive to both the individual and to the team.
2. Collaboration: Collaboration is more than cooperation. It means each person brings something to the project that adds value to the team and supports the creation of synergy.
3. Commitment: This is the passion in the face of adversity to take action and make things happen. It is the passion to do whatever it takes to accomplish the team objectives.
4. Communicate: Communication should happen early and often. Frequency of interaction with other team members, talking with them and sharing thoughts, ideas, and experiences; these are the activities that support teamwork.
5. Competence: Competence translates as someone who is capable, highly qualified, and does the job well.
6. Dependable: Team members who are dependable follow through and do what they have agreed to do, and do it well, without prodding or delay.
7. Disciplined: Discipline is doing what you really do not want to do so you can accomplish the goals you really want; includes paying attention to detail in thinking, in emotions, and in the actions you take.
8. Adding value: Helping a teammate advance or grow into a better person or team player; helping teammates advance the team; believing in your teammates before they believe in themselves, are all examples of adding value.
9. Enthusiastic: Enthusiasm focuses on becoming a highly energetic team member who has a positive attitude and believes that the team, together, can be better than anyone dreamed they could be.
10. Intentional: The team and its members have a purpose for themselves and for the team. Every action counts and is meaningful. Focusing on doing the right things in each moment and following through with these actions to their logical conclusion.
11. Awareness of the mission: Each team member has a sense of purpose and mission that drives all thoughts, ideas, and actions to do what is best for their team and their cause.
12. Prepared: Being prepared translates as being ready for every meeting and event and begins with a thorough assessment of what is needed, aligning the appropriate work with the appropriate effort, addressing the mental aspects of the right attitude, and being ready to take action.
13. Relationship oriented: The ability to be connected to other members of the team, to be in a relationship with them is the core of being relationship oriented. These relationships and the mutual respect upon which they are built create **cohesiveness** on the team.

14. Improve yourself: As a team member, you strive to continually grow and reflect, both routinely and periodically, on how well each venture or assignment went and what you could have done better. This is a process of self-reflection.

15. Selflessness: Putting others on the team ahead of yourself by being generous to team members, avoiding "playing politics," showing loyalty toward team members, and valuing interdependence among team members over the American value of being independent, are all examples of selflessness.

16. Solution focused: Do not be consumed with all of the problems associated with the endeavor. Rather, focus on finding the solutions; think about what is possible.

17. Tenacious: Being tenacious means giving your all, with determination, and refusing to stop until the goal has been accomplished.

Strong patient and nurse outcomes depend on the work of the entire team, so it is important for all staff members to understand their significance and value within the larger organizational and team structure.

INTERDISCIPLINARY TEAMS

Highly functional interdisciplinary teams are essential in today's health care system. The following are some of the different team members who work with nurses:

- Physicians;
- Dieticians;
- Case managers;
- Social workers;
- Teachers;
- Respiratory therapists;
- Physical therapists;
- Occupational therapists;
- Psychologists; and
- Pharmacists.

Having a team composed of members from varied disciplines often creates a more challenging team function in that everyone is attempting to protect their own "turf" and assume power. In the early stages of these groups, there may be some turf wars until the team forms a single identity.

Durskat and Wolf (2001) believe that three major components of smoothly functioning teams must be created:

1. Mutual trust among the members

2. A strong sense of team identity (that the team is unique and worthwhile)

3. A sense of team efficacy (that the team performs well and its members are synergistic in their manner of working together)

One area of particular concern in today's health care environment is the outcome measure of readmission. Hospitals are being penalized through penalties in reimbursement for heart failure readmission rates above the nationwide average. Interdisciplinary/interorganizational teams are being formed to oversee the development of protocols that transverse the multiple organizations that take care of the patient through the multitude of transitions of care during the chronic disease care process. Such teams need to be highly effective, organized, and outcome driven.

SUPERVISING THE WORK OF OTHERS

Nurses continuously supervise the work of others. This may include the nursing assistant, licensed practical nurse/licensed vocational nurse (LPN/LVN), other registered nurses, patient care technicians, and the unit clerk. Many conversations occur among these groups with various purposes, some of which are listed here.

- To orient, teach, and guide co-workers according to their individual learning styles and needs, consistent with their backgrounds, experience, and assignments
- To stimulate desire for self-improvement in supervisees
- To encourage supervisees to use their unique talents and develop special skills
- To model desired attitudes, skills, interests, and work habits

TYPES OF CONVERSATIONS

In the evaluation of team members, some organizations are defining team members as high-medium-low (H-M-L) performers. Essentially, high performers are people who deliver solutions. Middle performers can identify the problem, but may lack the experience or self-confidence to bring solutions. Low performers tend to blame others for the problem; they act like renters instead of owners. The Studer Group (2007) suggests that leaders rate themselves. The best leaders are always willing to perform an honest self-assessment. Are you a high, middle, or low performer? What actions will you take as a result?

Often, leaders using this exercise to rank their employees ask, "What if I have an employee who is technically excellent, but nobody wants to work with them?" To qualify as a high performer, an individual must be excellent both technically and as a team member. In fact, the Studer Group (2007) even suggests terminating the employment of those who get results, but do not role-model the organization's standards of behavior because they are so damaging to overall employee morale.

According to the Studer Group (2007), after the ranking of an employee as an H-M-L performer, an employee tracking log should be used to track the name, rating (H-M-L), initial meeting date, and follow-up date/comments. Always hold meetings with high performers first, middle performers next, and low performers last. Ordering the meetings in this way accomplishes several things. High performers, for example, can dispel fear about the meetings when other employees ask why the boss wanted to meet with them. Perhaps most importantly, leaders report that they feel energized and fortified for those difficult low-performer conversations once they have enjoyed so many positive conversations with employees they value.

H-M-L conversations are not evaluations tied to pay, so they should not take place at evaluation time. However, by repeating these meetings twice a year, conversations can complement staff evaluations so employees get the more frequent feedback they seek from managers. Leaders can help employees, especially middle performers, understand that these 15-minute meetings are opportunities for recognition, coaching, and professional development.

The objectives and outcomes are distinct for each type of conversation.

High-performer conversations: Rerecruit the best performers by giving specific positive feedback about what they do well, their accomplishments, and examples of positive attitude. Share information about where the organization is going, and ask if there is anything you can do for them to make their job better.

Middle-performer conversations: Use a support coach technique. The overall tone of the meeting must be positive. Begin by reassuring these individuals that you value their contributions and that your goal is to retain them as valuable employees. Thank them for what they do well. Then identify and discuss one specific area for development; something you would like them to improve. Complete the conversation by reaffirming their good qualities and expressing your appreciation.

Low-performer conversations: Do not start the meeting out on a positive note. Use the DESK approach:
- **D**escribe what has been observed.
- **E**valuate how you feel.
- **S**how what needs to be done.
- Ensure that employees **K**now the consequences of the continued poor performance.

Because low performers are so skilled at excuses, guilt, and indignation, these conversations can be difficult for managers. The manager needs to remain calm, objective, and clear about consequences if performance does not improve by a specified date. If the behavior has not improved, the nurse manager needs to follow through and take action. Refer to Chapter 14 for Performance Appraisal

Table 15-4 gives an example of a differentiating staff worksheet.

TABLE 15-4	**Differentiating Staff Worksheet**		
	High	**Medium**	**Low**
Definition	Comes to work on time	Good attendance	Points out problems in a negative way
	Good attitude	Loyal most of the time	Positions leadership poorly
	Problem solves	Influenced by high and low performers	Master of we/they
	You relax when you know they are scheduled	Wants to do a good job	Passive aggressive
	Good influence	Could just need more experience	Thinks they will outlast the leader
	Use for peer interviews	Helps manager be aware of problems	Says manager is the problem
	Five-pillar ownership		
	Brings solutions		
Professionalism	Adheres to unit policies concerning breaks, personal phone calls, leaving the work area, and other absences from work.	Usually adheres to unit policies concerning breaks, personal phone calls, leaving the work area, and other absences from work.	Does not communicate effectively about absences from work areas. Handles personal phone calls in a manner that interferes with work. Breaks last longer than allowed.
Teamwork	Demonstrates high commitment to making things better for the work unit and organization as a whole.	Committed to improving performance of the work unit and organization. May require coaching to fully execute.	Demonstrates little commitment to the work unit and the organization.
Knowledge and competence	Eager to change for the good of the organization. Strives for continuous professional development.	Invested in own professional development. May require some coaching to fully execute.	Shows little interest in improving own performance or the performance of the organization. Develops professional skills only when asked.
Communication	Comes to work with a positive attitude.	Usually comes to work with a positive attitude. Occasionally gets caught up in the negative attitude of others.	Comes to work with a negative attitude. Has a negative influence on the work environment.
Safety awareness	Demonstrates the behaviors of safety awareness in all aspects of work.	Demonstrates the behaviors of safety awareness in most aspects of work.	Performs work with little regard to the behaviors of safety awareness.

From The Studer Group. (2007). *The nine principles*. Retrieved November 9, 2007, from www.studergroup.com/dotCMS/knowledgeAssetDetail?inode=217849.

SUMMARY

Once you have worked on a specific unit for a period of time the culture of the hospital and the unit will become clear. Positive attitudes foster positive attitudes; negative work habits foster negative work habits. The nurse manager is charged with creating an environment conducive to high-quality patient care and staff satisfaction. The interactions within the team environment set the tone. Supervision and evaluation are part of a process of continuous improvement and staff development.

CLINICAL CORNER

Supporting a Culture of Communication at a Unit-Based Level

Maintaining a culture of communication at the unit level is of utmost importance in health care settings. It is the responsibility of every member of the unit team to support communication initiatives that may influence patient safety, continuity of care, planning of care, and positive patient outcomes. Additionally, every member of the unit team is also responsible for staying up-to-date on organizational communication.

One of the most critical times of communication at the unit level is during shift-to-shift handoff. Several methods can be implemented on units to ensure hand off is standardized and efficient, and all information is appropriately shared. On my 16-bed pediatric oncology/hematology/BMT unit, end-of-shift hand off is communicated face-to-face with the incoming nurse. To guide our patient report, we use a Kardex to communicate important information including the patient's weight, allergies, diagnosis, chemotherapy regimen, nursing orders, type of IV (intravenous) line and fluid, dressing changes, recent blood transfusions, and lab results. Often, nurses also use our electronic health record to open the patient's chart and review medications, physician notes, the nursing plan of care, and patient education. My institution also supports a culture of bedside shift reports where the outgoing and incoming nurses give hand off at the patient's bedside and do an initial safety assessment together. As my unit has moved toward this type of hand off, I have recognized the benefits that this method provides for both the nurse and the patient. Bedside hand off gives the opportunity for the plan of care to be reinforced with the patient and also allows for time to reinforce education that may have been done during the previous shift. It can give reassurance to the patient that their care will be continued because they see and hear what the nurse is discussing. In addition, it gives patients and families the opportunity to ask questions about their care. I first witnessed bedside hand off when I had a family member in the hospital. As a relative, I felt reassured witnessing the nurses discuss my grandfather's case and discuss their plans for the next shift. As the incoming nurse, I find a bedside shift report very beneficial in ensuring my patient is safe and stable. It assists me in making prioritization decisions regarding which patient to see and assess first.

The change to institute bedside reporting can be challenging at times. A journal club discussion has been one approach my unit has used to address the adjustment in hand off. The goal for the journal club was to discuss research that supports the purposes and effectiveness of bedside reporting. With nurses having a better understanding of the benefits of bedside hand off, the goal is for the hand off to be completed with every patient, every time.

An additional way to support communication at the unit level is through a team huddle at change of shift or at midshift. Team huddles at change of shift give an opportunity for each outgoing nurse to discuss important information about their patients to all of the incoming nurses. Pertinent information is shared so that all members of the team are informed about all patients. It also gives the charge nurse the opportunity to know more about every patient on the unit. A mid-shift huddle also gives the opportunity for every nurse to give an update about their patient's condition and plans for the day. Written communication among charge nurses can also be beneficial to ensure pertinent patient information is shared. Last year my unit designed a new assignment sheet to convey communication to charge nurses and administrative head nurses. This new assignment sheet involves assigning an acuity score to every patient and writing a brief note about every patient's plan. It also indicates the number of blood transfusions, the number of patients receiving chemotherapy, number of patients on isolation, and number of bone marrow infusions. We have found this new assignment sheet useful for communication between shifts as well as to our supervisors.

The communication of patient information is essential not only for nurses, but also for all members of the health care team. Daily bedside multidisciplinary rounds give the opportunity for all team members to discuss the patients' plans of care. It is essential for staff nurses to be involved in these rounds and communicate the patients' response to their treatment and plans of care. In addition to daily walking bedside rounds, my unit has implemented weekly psychosocial rounds. These rounds were developed through discussion among nurses at the Unit Based Council who recognized, through survey and feedback results, that there was a greater need to understand the patient and family's psychosocial needs. Staff nurses collaborated with our social workers to implement these rounds, with the goal of communicating more information about patients and families that would assist in planning and delivering care. Nurses have found these rounds helpful in bridging communication gaps among members of the team. To ensure nurses on off shifts can have access to what was discussed, a binder is kept in a secure place at the nurses' station with the notes from the discussion.

CLINICAL CORNER—cont'd

Supporting communication at the unit level also entails organization-wide communication regarding new or revised policies, updates from committee meetings, information from unit-based council meetings, results of quality data, and results from patient surveys. Every member of the unit team has an e-mail address supplied by the institution and is responsible for checking e-mail on a regular basis. Managers and other leaders use e-mail to communicate important information that affects nurses and patient care. Other methods used on my unit to communicate important information include bulletin boards and newsletters. Recently, many units in the hospital have designed their own newsletters to share information with staff. The newsletters are also shared with the entire patient care community through e-mail and have helped units learn more about each other. At the hospital-wide level, shared-governance-based nursing councils allow for information to be shared among units. One such council at my institution is the Staff Advisory Council. This consists of representatives from every unit-based council throughout the medical center. The purpose of this council is to "facilitate collaboration of staff nurses for the pursuit of excellence in patient care." At each monthly meeting, different units report on their yearly goals, the actions taken to meet the goals, and their outcomes. Unit representatives are responsible for communicating the information shared at this council with their own unit. Additionally, minutes from this council, as well as the other nursing councils, are available on the hospital intranet. It has become an expectation that all staff nurses are aware of information discussed at council meetings because much of the information shared affects patient care and ultimately patient outcomes.

At Hackensack University Medical Center, communication is part of the care delivery model and the professional practice model. Within both of these models, the patient is at the center and guides our nursing practice. Communication at the unit level will always be essential between staff nurses, the multidisciplinary team, and the entire health care organization to ensure all patients are treated with the best care possible and have the opportunity to achieve the best outcomes.

Gina M. Dovi, MSN, RN, CPHON
Clinical Level III Staff Nurse
Hackensack University Medical Center

EVIDENCE-BASED PRACTICE

Leonard, M., Graham, S., & Bonacum, D. (2004). The human factor: The critical importance of effective teamwork and communication in providing safe care. *Quality Safety Health Care*, 13(1), 185-190.

Susan A Nancarrow, Andrew Booth, Steven Ariss, Tony Smith, Pam Enderby & Alison Roots (2013). Ten principles of good interdisciplinary team work. *Human Resources for Health*, 11, 19. http://dx.doi.org/10.1186/1478-4491-11-19

Abstract
Background
Interdisciplinary teamwork is increasingly prevalent supported by policies and practices that bring care closer to the patient and challenge traditional professional boundaries. To date, there has been a great deal of emphasis on the processes of teamwork, and in some cases, outcomes.

Method
This study draws on two sources of knowledge to identify the attributes of a good interdisciplinary team; a published systematic review of the literature on interdisciplinary teamwork, and the perceptions of over 253 staff from 11 community rehabilitation and intermediate care teams in the United Kingdom. These data sources were merged using qualitative content analysis to arrive at a framework that identifies characteristics and proposes 10 competencies that support effective interdisciplinary teamwork.

Results
Ten characteristics underpinning effective interdisciplinary teamwork were identified
The 10 principles are:
1. Positive leadership and management attributes
2. Communication strategies and structures
3. Personal rewards training and development
4. Appropriate resources and procedures
5. Appropriate skill mix
6. Supportive team climate
7. Individual characteristics that support interdisciplinary teamwork
8. Clarity of vision
9. Quality and outcomes of care respecting
10. Understanding roles

Continued

EVIDENCE-BASED PRACTICE—cont'd

Conclusions

We propose competency statements that an effective interdisciplinary team functioning at a high level should demonstrate.

Interdisciplinary teamwork is a working method whereby multiple disciplines work together to provide care. There is no research specifically on having a systematic framework for interdisciplinary teamwork.

The main focus of this study was on inter/multidisciplinary teams: the research, interventions, and data-gathering activities that included all team members.

Characteristics of a good interdisciplinary team

These characteristics can be reformulated as competency statements that an effective interdisciplinary team functioning at a high level might be expected to demonstrate. Competencies of an interdisciplinary team:

1. Identifies a leader who establishes a clear direction and vision for the team, while listening and providing support and supervision to the team members.
2. Incorporates a set of values that clearly provides direction for the team's service provision; these values should be visible and consistently portrayed.
3. Demonstrates a team culture and interdisciplinary atmosphere of trust where contributions are valued and consensus is fostered.
4. Ensures appropriate processes and infrastructures are in place to uphold the vision of the service.

5. Provides quality patient-focused services with documented outcomes; uses feedback to improve the quality of care.
6. Uses communication strategies that promote intrateam communications, collaborative decision making, and effective team processes.
7. Provides sufficient team staffing to integrate an appropriate mix of skills, competencies, and personalities to meet the needs of patients and enhance smooth functioning.
8. Facilitates recruitment of staff who demonstrate interdisciplinary competencies, including team functioning, collaborative leadership, communication, and sufficient professional knowledge and experience.
9. Promotes role interdependence while respecting individual roles and autonomy.
10. Facilitates personal development through appropriate training, rewards, recognition, and opportunities for career development.

The study identified the need for teams to regularly invest time in the processes of team development and functioning.

The study showed evidence for a theoretical understanding and developed a framework to define the characteristics of interdisciplinary teamwork and presented the competencies for effective interdisciplinary teamwork.

NCLEX® EXAMINATION QUESTIONS

1. A(n) _____ refers to several individuals who work together to accomplish specific time-limited assignments.
   A. Task group
   B. Informal group
   C. Formal group
   D. Real group
2. One use for the electronic health information is:
   A. Education
   B. Patient care delivery
   C. Patient care management
   D. Patient care support processes
3. Regarding the different types of conversation, _____use a support coach technique; the

overall tone of the meeting must be positive. Begin by reassuring these individuals that you value their contributions and that your goal is to retain them as value.
   A. High-performer conversations
   B. Middle-performer conversations
   C. Low-performer conversations
   D. Exceptional-performer conversations
4. Durskat and Wolf (2001) believe that the major components of smoothly functioning teams must be created. They are listed as:
   A. Mutual trust among the members
   B. A strong sense of team identify
   C. A sense of team efficacy
   D. All must be present

5. _____ is the passion in the face of adversity to take action and make things happen, it is the passion to do whatever it takes to accomplish the team objectives.
   A. Commitment
   B. Communication
   C. Collaboration
   D. Adaptability

6. A _____ is an example of one who lives the organizational values.
   A. Group
   B. Supervisor
   C. Legend
   D. Team player

7. Which author/s states that a team is a group of people with a high degree of interdependence geared toward the achievement of a goal or a task?
   A. McGregor (1960)
   B. Parker (1990)
   C. Sullivan and Decker (2009)
   D. Maxwell (2002)

8. For a team to be effective, each member of the group must be able to:
   A. Effectively communicate
   B. Offer constructive criticism
   C. Acknowledge the positive
   D. Do all of the above

9. All of the factors can further be adapted to delineate guidelines for leading teams. Which of the following is not an acceptable guideline?
   A. Do not waste time
   B. Facilitate thoughtful problem solving based on evidence
   C. Create a nonthreatening environment
   D. Plan to meet after the shift to decrease interruptions

10. The first rule for any team, committee, or council is the development of the _____ of the group.
    A. Charge
    B. Team members
    C. Roles of individual team members
    D. Timeline

Answers: 1. A   2. C   4. A   5. C   6. B   7. D   8. D
9. A   10. D

REFERENCES

Durskat, V., & Wolt, S. (2001). Building the emotional intelligence of groups. *Harvard Business Review, 79*, 81–91.

Guyton, N. (2012). Nine principles of successful nursing leadership. *American Nurse Today.* August, 7(8).

Lencioni, P. (2002). *The five dysfunctions of a team: A leadership fable.* San Francisco: Jossey-Bass.

Maxwell, J. (2002). *The 17 essential qualities of a team player.* Nashville, TN: Thomas Nelson Publishers.

McGregor, D. (1960). *The human side of enterprise.* New York: McGraw-Hill.

Nees, T. (2010). *Seven characteristics of groups and teams.* http://leadingtoserve.com/?p=172.

Olen, D. (1992). *Communicating speaking and listening to end misunderstanding and promote friendship.* Germantown, WI: JODA Communications.

Parker, G. M. (1990). *Team players and teamwork.* San Francisco: Jossey-Bass.

Roussel, L. (2012). *Management and leadership for nurse administrators* (6th ed.). Burlington, MA: Jones & Bartlett.

Sullivan, E. J., & Decker, P. J. (2009). *Effective leadership and management in nursing* (6th ed.). Upper Saddle River, NJ: Pearson Prentice Hall.

The Studer Group. (2007). *The nine principles.* www.studergroup.com/dotCMS/knowledgeAsset Detail?inode=217849.

The Studer Group. (2012). *It's not rocket science: Strategies to blast your hospital into the highest patient experience stratosphere.* https://programs.gha.org/Portals/5/documents/societies/GSHHRA/2012/HANDOUT%20Rocket%20Science%20(Otten).pdf.

Yoder-Wise, P. (2011). *Leading and managing in nursing.* St. Louis: Elsevier.

16

Hospital Information Systems

OBJECTIVES

- Define electronic health records (EHRs) and electronic medical records (EMRs).
- Relate National Patient Safety Goals to the adoption of EMRs.
- Analyze the driving forces behind the implementation of electronic record keeping.
- Review the components of a hospital-wide EMR.
- Differentiate between an EMR and a hospital information system.

- Discuss obstacles to the use of EMRs.
- Analyze the role of the nurse in the implementation and use of EMRs.
- Identify the required informatics competencies of nurses.
- Discuss the future of electronic applications to enhance nursing practice.

OUTLINE

KEY TERMS

clinical information systems systems used for the collection, integration, and distribution of information to the appropriate department

computerized provider order entry (CPOE) automated systems for providers to enter patient care orders and to access decision support databases

decision support provision of assistance via a computer application for the purpose of assisting the nurse in decision making

electronic health record information relating to the past or future physical/mental health, or condition of an individual that resides in electronic systems used to capture, transmit, receive, store, or manipulate data for the primary purpose of providing health-related services

electronic medical record information relating to the medical care received by an individual; usually institution specific, residing in electronic systems that are hospital or health-system based

HEALTH CARE INFORMATICS

The Institute of Medicine Reports (2001, 2003) support the use of health care information systems to improve practices and improve patient safety. Health care informatics is seen as one method of achieving the triple aim of improving health care effectiveness, health care efficiency, and the patient experience. Informatics is regarded as a core competency of all health care professionals (Rundio & Wilson, 2013, p. 64). The keys areas of focus center on:

- National information infrastructure
- Computerized clinical data
- Clinical decision support
- Use of the Internet
- Integration of evidence-based practice

TECHNOLOGY IN HEALTH CARE

The goal of technology is to give health professionals access to the needed data and information at the time that they need it. The explosion of information technology has brought health care and nursing into a new era. The technology of health care involves much more than the **electronic medical record**, it now involves almost every aspect of our work environment. Patient beds now have alarms, scales, and sensors that detect movement. Intravenous (IV) pumps do much more than deliver the medication, they are now "smart pumps." The software they use allows an organization to create a library of medications that provides dosing guidelines by establishing concentrations, dose limits, and clinical advisories. Clinical advisories contain relevant information about a specific medication that is displayed on the smart pump screen when the drug is selected from the library. For example, a clinical alert may prompt the practitioner to use a filter with the medication they have selected for administration. Hand-held devices used by nurses in the clinical areas allow access to a great deal of clinical information. There are numerous applications that grant nurses access to view medication information, clinical lab result interpretations, and updated care protocols, allowing for the needed information to be available as the nurse is making the clinical decisions. A study of 3900 nurses in early 2012, indicated that 71% of nurses were using smartphones professionally (Dolan, 2012). This quote sums up the trend best: "But the most profound recent change is a move away from the profession's dependence on committing vast amounts of information to memory. It is not that nurses need to know less, educators say, but that the amount of essential data has exploded" (Perez-Pena, 2012). There are many applications that can assist the nurse in day-to-day practice. Some major applications are listed in Box 16-1.

BOX 16-1 Useful Apps for Nursing

Mini Nurse Lite - this free app offers information including nursing skills, IV rates, and medication dosage

Nursing best practices app – places best practices at the tip of the nurses fingertips

Informed RN Pocket Guide/Informed Emergency and Critical Care Pocket Guide – this app can provide quick answers for questions during medical emergencies.

Instant ECG – this electrocardiogram rhythms interpretation guide offers quick reference to more than 90m images of ECGs.

Critical Care ACLS Guide – useful for laying out the ACLS algorithms, as well as the rules of 9s for burns, chest x-ray interpretation and 12 lead ECG interpretation.

Epocrates Rx – basic features include drug guide, pill identifier, drug interaction checker and medical updates.

Nursing Central – smart phone app provides comprehensive disease, drug and test information. Includes Davis" Drug Guide, Taber's Medical Dictionary.

PALS Advisor – offers information on pediatric drug dosages, neonatal resuscitation and basic life support.

Heart Pro III – offers three dimensional images of the intricacies of the heart as well as typical heart rhythms to listen for in a patient.

Shift Planning – streamlined time management app that helps nurses manages tasks and schedules. Also sends auto reminders.

MediBabble Translator – translator tool for assistance with non English speaking patients.

Nurse's Pocket Guide – assessment tools and sample care plans.

Skyscape Medical Resources – features include prescription drug information, medical calculators, symptom diagnosis, medical news.

Medscape – information about drugs and diagnosis

MedCalc – Drug dosage calculator, infusion calculator. Can be individualized with specific hospital formulary concentrations.

Adapted from: Vivona, T. (2013) Useful apps for student nurses. *Nursing Times*. July 26, 2013

Evaluating Websites

In addition to these applications, there are many Internet sites that can assist nurses in all aspects of their career. There are nursing support blogs and discussion groups, but it is important to assess the veracity of a site that is accessed. Just because it is on the Internet does not mean that it is true! This poses a challenge for nurses in another area: patients have become highly educated consumers and much of the information they access is from the Internet. So both nurses and patients need to be educated on how to determine the appropriateness of the information that they find. Box 16-2 give tips for the evaluation of websites.

Although there is a wealth of data available to the nurse and patient, the transformation of this data into usable information for clinical decision making is the primary goal of all information systems in health care. The management of data is what supports decision making. Information systems provide health care staff with day-to-day information on patient flow and acuity, resource use, staffing levels, costs, budgetary balance, patient needs, patient care plans, medication usage and response, and all other documented patient-care delivery information. Nurses need to become knowledgeable on the documentation of this data into the electronic medical records, and in the means of mining and using this data to assist with improvements in care (Chapters 18, 19).

ELECTRONIC HEALTH RECORDS

A true electronic health record (EHR) is a complete record of an individual's health-related data. The U.S. Department of Health and Human Services (DHHS) is continuing to spearhead the initiative to build a national electronic health care system that would allow patients and their care givers to access their complete health records anytime and anywhere (HealthIT.gov, 2015). Over 144,000 payments totaling $7.1 billion have already been issued to professionals and hospitals by the Centers for Medicare & Medicaid Services (CMS). An estimated $22.5 billion will be paid from 2011 to 2022 to eligible providers who adopt EHR technology (Levingston, 2012).

The goal of the EHR is to have the sharing of data on a nationwide level across institutions. For example, if an individual from California entered a trauma center in New Jersey, the trauma center would be able to access the individual's record from California. Although the health care system has not reached such a level of integration, the Veterans Administration (VA) has a system that allows access to the medical record across the nation for all patients of the VA system.

The term electronic health record is loosely used to include any patient care record that is collected and stored in an electronic fashion. EHRs are real-time, patient-centered records. They make information available instantly, "whenever and wherever it is needed." And they bring together in one place everything about a patient's health. EHRs can do the following:

- Contain information about a patient's medical history, diagnoses, medications, immunization dates, allergies, radiology images, and lab and test results.
- Offer access to evidence-based tools that providers can use in making decisions about a patient's care.
- Automate and streamline providers' workflow.
- Increase the organization and accuracy of patient information.
- Support key market changes in payer requirements and consumer expectations.

One of the key features of an EHR is that it can be created, managed, and consulted by authorized providers and staff across more than one health care organization. A single EHR can bring together information from current and past doctors, emergency facilities, school and workplace clinics, pharmacies, laboratories, and medical imaging facilities (HealthIT.gov., 2015).

The IOM reports (1997, 2000, 2001) dealing with the patient safety issues facing the U.S. health care system all discussed the importance of electronic patient records in the improvement of safety, quality, and efficiency of health care in the United States. In 1991, the IOM issued a report calling for the elimination of paper-based records within 10 years. Progress has been made within a large number of acute care institutions across the country, but progress varies in other health care agencies across the transition of care. The financial costs for the implementation of such systems are high, and in this era of cost containment, many institutions do not have the financial resources to initiate such systems. The motivation is not to have a paperless system per se, but rather to make important patient information available and useable to all appropriate care givers Box 16-3 lists advantages and disadvantages of the EHR.

BOX 16-2 Tips on Evaluating Websites

The questions below will help you in evaluating web pages for use as academic sources. Be sure to look at the criteria in multiple categories before making a decision regarding the academic quality of a source.

How did you find the page?
How you located the page can give you a start on your evaluation of the site's validity as an academic resource.
- Was it found via a search conducted through a search engine? Unlike library databases, the accuracy and/or quality of information located via a search engine will vary greatly. Look carefully!
- Was it recommended by a faculty member or another reliable source? Generally, an indicator of reliability.
- Was it cited in a scholarly or credible source? Generally, an indicator of reliability.
- Was it a link from a reputable site? Generally, an indicator of reliability.

What is the site's domain?
Think of this as "decoding" the URL, or Internet address. The origination of the site can provide indications of the site's mission or purpose. The most common domains are:
- .org: An advocacy website, such as a not-for-profit organization.
- .com: A business or commercial site.
- .net: A site from a network organization or an internet service provider.
- .edu: A site affiliated with a higher education institution.
- .gov: A federal government site.
- .il.us: A state government site, this may also include public schools and community colleges.
- .uk: (United Kingdom): A site originating in another country (as indicated by the two-letter code).
- ~: The tilde usually indicates a personal page.

What is the authority of the page?
Look for information on the author of the site. On the Internet anyone can pose as an authority.
- Is the author's name visible? Does the author have an affiliation with an organization or institution?

- Does the author list their credentials? Are they relevant to the information presented?
- Is there a mailing address or telephone number included, as well as an e-mail address?

Is the information accurate and objective?
There are no standards or controls on the accuracy of information available via the Internet. It can be used by anyone as a sounding board for their thoughts and opinions.
- How accurate is the information presented? Are sources of factual information or statistics cited? Is there a bibliography included?
- Compare the page to related sources, electronic or print, for assistance in determining accuracy.
- Is the site objective? Is there a reason the site is presenting a particular point of view on a topic?
- Does the page exhibit a particular point of view or bias?
- Does the page contain advertising? This may impact the content of the information included. Look carefully to see if there is a relationship between the advertising and the content, or whether the advertising is simply providing financial support for the page.

Is the page current?
This is both an indicator of the timeliness of the information and whether or not the page is actively maintained.
- Is the information provided current?
- When was the page created?
- Are dates included for the last update or modification of the page?
- Are the links current and functional?

Does the page function well?
The ease of use of a site and its ability to help you locate information you are looking for are examples of the site's functionality.
- Is the site easy to navigate? Are options to return to the home page, tops of pages, etc., provided?
- Is the site searchable?
- Does the site include a site map or index?

www.library.illinois.edu/ugl/howdoi/webeval.html.

Researchers at the Center for IT Leadership (2010) Web Site Disclaimers studied the U.S. Department of Veterans Affairs, an early adopter of health IT and exchange, and estimated that savings from preventing adverse drug events alone totaled $4.64 billion (Byrne et al., 2010).

Although there are disadvantages to the EHR/computerized health record, the movement to health care institutions of an overall culture of safety has resulted in a strong push to implement computerized health records or hospital-wide information systems.

BOX 16-3 Advantages and Disadvantages of the Electronic Health Record

Advantages of the Electronic Health Record

- Accessible from remote sites to many people at the same time.
- Information retrieval is almost instantaneous.
- Links clinicians to protocols, expert systems, care plans, critical paths, literature databases, pharmaceutical information, and other databases of health care knowledge.
- Improved risk management and regulatory and legal compliance.
- More accurate capture of financial charges and billing efficiency.
- Increased quality outcomes, decreased mortality rates, increase safety.

Disadvantages of the Electronic Health Record

- Startup costs for hardware, software, installation, maintenance, and future upgrades are considerable.
- Learning curve for a new system of documentation is steep.
- Initial decrease in staff productivity.
- Confidentiality, privacy, and security of the information are concerns.

Adapted from Menachemi, N. & Collum, T. (2011). Benefits and drawbacks of electronic health record systems. *Risk Management and Healthcare Policy*, Pub: 4, 47–55.

Hospital information systems are large complex computer systems designed to manage information needs of a hospital. A wide range of systems is available, and most information systems are individualized to the specific health care agency or system and are not nationwide. The EHR differs from a hospital information system. A hospital information system incorporates all information used in both patient care and the management of the structures and processes that support the care delivered at a particular institution. The hospital information system is usually composed of administrative and clinical systems. The administrative information systems function to maintain and deliver the necessary information used in the daily operations of the organization. This would include financial systems, human resource systems, registration and scheduling systems, and quality data systems. The **clinical information systems** function to maintain and deliver patient-specific information and decision support systems for the delivery of safe patient care (Rousel, 2013).

The primary and secondary uses of the hospital-wide information system are as follows (adapted from Institute of Medicine [IOM], 1997):

Primary uses

- Patient care delivery.
- Patient care management.
- Patient care support processes.
- Financial and other administrative processes.

Secondary uses

- Education.
- Regulation.
- Research.
- Public health and Homeland Security.
- Policy support.

The functionality of any information system within a health care agency should address the following goals:

- Support the delivery of effective care: It has been suggested that only about 55% of Americans receive recommended medical care that is consistent with evidence-based practice guidelines (McGlynn et al., 2003; Kumar & Nash, 2011).
- Facilitate the management of chronic illness: More than half of people with chronic conditions have three or more health providers. Physicians and patients report difficulty in the coordination of care with multiple providers (Leatherman & McCarthy, 2002; Partnership for Solutions, 2002).
- Improve efficiency: Efficiency is the avoidance of waste. With the staffing and financial challenges faced by many institutions, it is imperative that processes be improved.

The core functionalities for a computerized health information system are as follows:

- Health information and data: EHRs with defined datasets, such as medical and nursing diagnoses, a medication list, allergies, demographics, clinical narratives, and laboratory test results, can ensure access to current patient data by those who need it.
- Results management: Managing all types of results (laboratory tests, radiograph results) electronically has the distinct advantage of allowing access to the results in a more efficient timeframe than with paper-based results. The automated display of results may also lead to a decrease of redundant testing (Bates & Gawande, 2003).
- Order entry: **Computerized provider order entry (CPOE)** has been shown to decrease the number of medication errors by up to 83% (Bates & Gawande, 2003).

- **Decision support:** Several studies have shown that computerized decision support improves drug dosing, drug selection, and screening for drug interactions (Abookire et al., 2000; Jao & Hier, 2010, Institute for Safe Medication Practice, 2014)
- **Electronic communication and connectivity:** Improved communication between care partners, such as pharmacy, radiology, laboratory, and nursing departments, can enhance patient safety and quality of care (Schiff et al., 2003).
- **Patient support:** A multidimensional telehealth system has demonstrated the ability to improve outcomes of patients with chronic disease (NORC [National Opinion Research Center] at University of Chicago, 2012).
- **Administrative processes:** Electronic staffing systems allow nurse managers extra time to manage care instead of creating staffing schedules.
- **Reporting and health management:** Health care agencies have manual multiple reporting.

HEALTH CARE INFORMATION MANAGEMENT SYSTEMS

There is a wide variety of hospital information systems (Figure 16-1) with which the nurse will come in contact. The most common functions are detailed here.

Patient Information Retrieval

Results of laboratory and diagnostic tests are posted to computer records in many agencies. These tests are then readily available to those who need the information.

Order Entry

Entry of physicians' orders for medications, laboratory work, diagnostic tests, and other therapies is often one of the earliest aspects of patient care that is placed on the computer. With the upgrades in technology over the past few years, some organizations are moving toward the use of hand-held computers for the creation of orders, which are then downloaded to the hospital system.

Nursing Data Entry

A computerized medication administration record (MAR) is often one of the earliest aspects of the computerized chart that is recorded. This is then followed up with computerized charting and full nursing documentation.

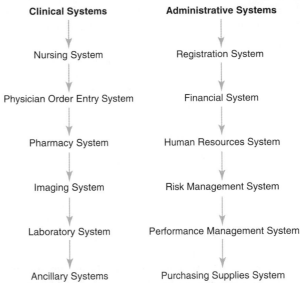

FIGURE 16-1 Health care information management system. (From Kearney Nunnery, R. [2005]. *Advancing your career: Concepts of professional nursing* [3rd ed.]. Philadelphia: F. A. Davis. Used with permission.)

Administrative Systems

Most hospitals have computerized financial and billing systems. The federal programs of Medicare and Medicaid have required that billing be done through computerized systems that can communicate with the government agency. Some of the billing systems are integrated with the patient care delivery. One such system in common use is Pyxis SupplyStation, which is integrated throughout many functions. This comprehensive system allows a facility to track cost per patient as well as the cost of inventory. Supplies and medications are stored in the system, which usually is located on each unit. Nurses enter a code and then are able to obtain the necessary supply or medication from the locked cabinet. When each supply is taken by the nurse, the machine automatically charges the patient, reorders the supply, and maintains an inventory. The Pyxis SupplyStation system is an advanced point-of-use system that automates the distribution, management, and control of medications and supplies. An automated perpetual inventory eliminates manual reorder processes. Par levels are set in the system to ensure products are ordered before a stock-out occurs.

There are numerous nurse management information systems with which the new nurse will become familiar. One such is the Automated Nurse Staffing Office System (ANSOS). Nursing management information systems provide shift reports of personnel by type needed and assigned, staffing and productivity data by unit and area, average data on the intensity of care needed, and the cost of patient care (Rousel, 2013; McKesson, 2014).

Point-of-Care Systems

Point-of-care systems may include the bedside or another point of care in the health care system. The documentation is performed wherever the patient is located. There is full accessibility of input and output patient information. One example of point-of-care systems is the smart phone. Smart phones can provide decision support systems, such as drug references, food–drug interaction indexes, and basic life support (BLS) or advanced cardiac life support (ACLS) guidelines. Some hand-held systems allow for documentation of patient care activities, which are then downloaded to the larger patient system via a docking deck. Many institutions with computerized charting have point-of-care systems located in areas near the patient so that the documentation can occur at the time of care. This allows the nurse to document in or near the patient room as soon as the information is collected. Information is also collected and recorded in other patient care devices, such as cardiac monitors, ventilators, and glucose monitors. Information from these systems can also be downloaded to the larger patient care system via an integrated EMR.

NURSING MINIMUM DATA SET

In the move toward the development of a nationwide EHR, the need arises for a standardized nursing language that can be understood across a variety of systems. The nursing minimum data set (NMDS) represents one attempt at a standardized language (Box 16-4). There are several recognized standard languages in use in nursing (Table 16-1). Many of the monitoring devices used in patient care can be integrated into the clinical information system. Most cardiac monitors, glucose monitors, and ventilators have cards installed that allow for data to flow from the device to the clinical system, thus saving documentation time. The NMDS was defined to establish uniform standards for the collection of comparable essential patient data

---

> **BOX 16-4   Elements of the Nursing Minimum Data Set (NMDS)**
>
> **Nursing Care Elements**
> 1. Nursing diagnosis
> 2. Nursing intervention
> 3. Nursing outcome
> 4. Intensity of nursing care
>
> **Patient Demographic Elements**
> 5. Personal identification*
> 6. Date of birth*
> 7. Sex*
> 8. Race and ethnicity*
> 9. Residency*
>
> **Service Elements**
> 10. Unique facility or service agency number*
> 11. Unique health record number of the patient
> 12. Unique number of the principal registered nurse provider
> 13. Episode, admission, or encounter date*
> 14. Discharge or termination date*
> 15. Disposition of patient or client*
> 16. Expected payer for most of the bill

*Elements comparable to those in the uniform minimum health data set (UMHDS).
www.nursing.umn.edu/prod/groups/nurs/@pub/@nurs/documents/asset/nurs_71413.pdf.

(Yoder-Wise, 2011, p. 203). The uniform minimum health data set (UMHDS) is a minimum set of items of information with uniform multiple data users. UMHDSs have been developed for long-term care, hospital discharge, and ambulatory care (Yoder-Wise, 2011, p. 203).

INFORMATICS COMPETENCIES FOR NURSES

As a nurse, you will need to become comfortable with the technology of the workplace. You will also need to have a working knowledge of informatics. Nursing informatics (NI) is a specialty that integrates nursing science, computer science, and information science to manage and communicate data, information, knowledge, and wisdom in nursing practice. NI supports consumers, patients, nurses, and other providers in their decision making in all roles and settings. This support is accomplished through the use

TABLE 16-1   American Nurses Association: Recognized Standardized Languages

Standardized Terminology	Problems/ Diagnoses	Interventions	Goals/ Outcomes	Reference
Complete complementary alternative medicine billing and coding reference		X		Gianinni (2005)
Home health care classification	X	X	X	Saba (1990)
International classification for nursing practice	X	X	X	International Council of Nurses (1999)
North American Nursing Diagnosis Association (NANDA) taxonomy	X			NANDA (1999)
Nursing Interventions Classification		X		McCloskey and Bulechek (2000)
Nursing management minimum data set				Huber, Delaney, & Crossley (1992)
Nursing minimum data set	X	X	X	Werley & Lang (1988)
Nursing Outcomes Classification			X	Johnson, Maas, & Moorehead (2000)
Omaha system	X	X	X	Martin & Scheet (1992)
Patient care data set	X	X	X	Ozbolt, Fruchtnight, & Hayden (1994)
Perioperative nursing data set	X	X	X	Kleinbeck (2000)
SNOMED RT	X	X	X	Spackman, Campbell, & Cote (1997)

Modified from Yoder-Wise, P.S. (2003). *Leading and managing in nursing* (3rd ed.). St. Louis: Mosby.

of information structures, information processes, and information technology (American Nurses Association [ANA], 2008). In 1992, the ANA supported nursing informatics as a specialty for registered nurses and first offered a certification examination for nursing informatics.

Nurse managers play a pivotal role in the adoption of information systems. In their leadership role, they have three levels of competency with information systems. As initial users of the information system, they need to have the following competencies:

1. Use computerized management systems to record administrative data (billing data, quality assurance data, workload data, etc.).
2. Use applications for structured data entry (classification systems, acuity level, etc.).
3. Understand client rights related to computerized information.
4. Recognize the utility of nurse involvement in the planning, design, choice, and implementation of information systems in the practice environment.
5. Incorporate a code of ethics in regard to client privacy and confidentiality.

As they become more familiar with the system, they enter a next level of competency, that of a modifier. In this role, they will have the following competencies:

1. Have an awareness of the role of nursing informatics in the context of health informatics and information systems.
2. Participate in policy and procedural development related to nursing informatics.
3. Participate in system change processes and utility analysis.
4. Participate in the evaluation of information systems in practice settings.
5. Analyze the ergonomic integrity of workstation, bedside, and portable technology apparatus in practice.
6. Participate in the design of data collection tools for practice decision making and record keeping.
7. Participate in quality management initiatives related to patient and nursing data in practice.
8. Have an awareness of the impact of implementing technology to facilitate nursing practice.
9. Evaluate security effectiveness and parameters of the system for protecting client information and ensuring confidentiality.

10. Participate in change to improve the use of informatics within nursing practice.
11. Encourage other nurses to develop comfort and competency in technology use in practice.

As they assume mastery of the competencies and progress in management, they assume a role of innovator.

1. Develop and participate in quality improvement programs using information systems.
2. Participate in patient instructional program development.

3. Participate in ergonomic design of workstations, bedside access stations, and portable apparatus equipment.
4. Maintain awareness of societal and technological trends, issues, and new developments, and apply these to nursing.
5. Demonstrate proficient awareness of legal and ethical issues related to client data, information, and confidentiality
6. Design and implement project management initiatives related to information technology for practice

SUMMARY

Information systems have become an integral part of the nursing workplace, and nurses and nurse managers need to embrace their use to assist them in making the workplace safer and more efficient. The EMR and hospital information systems are assisting the nurse to more efficiently gather the necessary patient information to make clinical decisions. As a nurse manager, you will need to role-model comfort with the use of technology for those staff members who are uncomfortable with technology. You will also need to constantly evaluate the use of technology in your practice and the efficiency of your unit.

CLINICAL CORNER

The Nurse and the Development and Implementation of the Electronic Medical Record

The electronic medical record (EMR) has, or will, become a large part of every nurse's workflow. The Institute of Medicine (IOM) has determined through the following reports: To err is human, Crossing the quality chasm, and Best care at lower cost (Institute of Medicine [IOM], 1999; 2001; & 2012) that the health care system in the United States is plagued with waste, inefficiency, medical errors, and fragmentation. It is the hope of all stakeholders that the broad adoption of a computerized medical infrastructure will support the improvement of health care in this country (Chaudry et al., 2006; Poissant et al., 2005). The introduction of information technology in health care has resulted in unexpected outcomes that affect the practice of registered nurses. Therefore it is essential that nurses have a say in how the EMR is configured and implemented in their institutions.

Once an EMR has been fully integrated into a health care system, every nurse must become proficient in its use. The EMR also presents challenges. Nurses perceive that it is time consuming and distracts them from providing individualized care. Patients interpret that the time nurses spend on the computer distances them from their Care givers. As far back as 1980 nursing theorist Virginia Henderson cautioned nurses to preserve the essence of nursing in this age of technology (Henderson, 1980). According to Benner, Hooper-Kyriakidis, and Stannard (1998) man's humanity is clearly suffering from today's technologically driven health care environment, and state that providing comfort measures, caring communication, and assisting patients and their families will not be fully actualized in a situation where there is an over-reliance on technology. Care givers also need to be aware that the roar of technology silences the subtle attempts of patients to give voice to their needs (Almerud, 2007). The sacred nurse–patient relationship is based on trust, and the conditions that are considered to be essential for the development of trust are availability and accessibility of the nurse. The EMR has the potential to interfere with this, again stressing the importance of nurse involvement in the development of the system.

As the use of the EMR becomes increasingly common in health care settings, other problems have emerged. Unintended adverse consequences (UACs) can surround the implementation and maintenance of EMRs. These range from emotional responses, new kinds of errors, changes in power structure, and overdependence on technology.

CLINICAL CORNER—cont'd

These systems cause intense emotions in users. However, many of these emotions are negative and often result in reduced efficacy of system use, particularly at the start of implementation. Changes in power structure also occur. The presence of a system that enforces specific clinical practices through mandatory data entry fields changes the power structure of organizations. Often the power of autonomy of physicians is reduced in an effort to standardize, although the power of the nursing staff, information technology specialists, and administration is increased. Another UAC, Ash et al. (2009) informs us, is that these computerized systems caused cognitive overload by emphasizing structured and complete information entry or retrieval. They go on to state that attempts to require professionals to encode data, or enter data in more structured formats, can be fruitful and are necessary for research or managerial purposes, but this does not come without a cost. Such formats are generally more time-consuming to complete and read. They noted in their studies that overly structured data entry led to a loss of cognitive focus by the clinician. When professionals are working through a case, determining a differential diagnosis, for example, the act of writing the information is integral to the cognitive processing of the case. Although this act of writing as thinking can be aided greatly by providing structure, such as the grouping of similar types of information or sequencing to guide the elucidation of a history, it is inevitably hampered by an excess of structure. Rather than helping the clinician build a cognitive pattern to understand the complexities of a case, such systems overload the user with details at odds with the cognitive model the user is trying to develop (Ash et al., 2009). One key to preventing unintended consequences is to pay attention to success factors for implementing EMRs from the start. System design is critical in preventing and managing these unintended consequences. Systems should be designed to support communication and provide the flexibility that is needed for systems to better-fit real work places (Ash et al., 2004).

The success of an EMR is directly related to its design and proper execution. Mustain et al. (2008) identified that conducting a change readiness assessment is crucial to a successful EMR implementation. They cited that factors such as leadership, culture, and professional ideals play complex roles in facilitating and hindering implementation. They identified three barriers that were continually encountered during an EMR implementation: fear, apathy, and competing priorities. The identification of these factors allowed the project's leadership team to study the current mind-set of clinicians and other team members as the project progressed. They attributed their success to this ongoing assessment.

Scott et al. (2005) determined that implementation involved several clinical components including perceptions of the system's selection, early testing, adaptation of the system to the larger organization, and adaptation of the organization to the new electronic environment. The author recommended that health care institutions use a participatory process when selecting a system. It was also discovered that different leadership roles and styles were needed at different points during the implementation. Identified during implementation were changes in clinician productivity, which required extra staffing. It was determined that software design and its complexity is what decreased clinician productivity and increased resistance to use.

Clinical content must be fine-tuned to the unique needs of nurses. Nurses need to be involved from the beginning in the design and functionality of the system they will be implementing. The key to successful implementation is that there be nurse involvement in, and great attention paid to, training and practice before implementation.

The EMR is not static. It is forever evolving. There are ongoing upgrades that involve optimizing functionality, and nurses must be an integral part of the EMR development team. Only they know how to best minimize the disruptions to care that the EMR creates. In institutions that use shared governance, nurse Informatics councils should be formed and members should provide representation from every unit. It is through their participatory involvement that the nurse at the bedside can effect change, minimize disruptions to care, and disseminate information regarding the EMR to all clinicians. The EMR is here to stay, and the nurse who is the primary care giver needs to maintain vigilance over its design and development to successfully integrate it into their work environment with as little interruption to patient care as possible.

References

Ash, J. S., Sittig, D. F., Dykstra, R., Campbell, E., & Guappone, K. (2009). The unintended consequences of computerized provider order entry: Findings from a mixed methods exploration. *International Journal of Medical Informatics, 78*(Supp 1), S69–S76.

Almerud, S. (2007). *Vigilance and invisibility: Care in technologically intensive environments* (Doctoral dissertation, Vaxjouniversitet). www.openthesis.org/document/Vigilence-Invisibility-Care-in-technology-427408.html.

Benner, P., Hooper-Kyriakidis, P., & Stannard, D. (1998). *Clinical wisdom and interventions in critical care: A thinking in action approach*. London, England: Saunders.

CLINICAL CORNER—cont'd

Chaudry, B., Wang, J., Maglione, M., Wu, S., Mojica, W., Roth, E., et al. (2006). Systematic review: Impact of health information technology on quality, efficiency, and costs of medical care. *Annals of Internal Medicine, 144,* E12–E22. web.ebsco-host.com.library.sage.edu:2048/ehost/pdfviewer/pdfviewer?vid=4&sid=41d46792-e8d1-4578-992b-a7f941537b93%40session-mgr115&hid=120.

Hendersen, V. (1980). Preserving the essence of nursing in a technological age. *Journal of Advanced Nursing, 5,* 245–260.

Institute of Medicine. (1999). *To err is human: Building a safer health system.* Washington, DC: Government Printing Office.

Institute of Medicine. (2001). *Crossing the quality chasm: A new health system for the 21st century.* Washington, DC: Government Printing Office.

Institute of Medicine. (2012). *Best care at lower cost: The path to continuously learning health care in America.* Washington, DC: Government Printing Office.

Mustain, J. M., Lowry, L. W., & Wilhort, K. W. (2008). Change readiness assessment for conversion to electronic medical records. *Journal of Nursing Administration, 38,* 379–385.

Poissant, L., Pereira, J., Tamblyn, R., & Dawasumi, Y. (2005). The impact of electronic health records on time efficiency of physicians and nurses: A systematic review. *Journal of the American Medical Informatics Association, 12,* 505–516.

Scott, J. T., Rundall, T. G., Vogt, T. M., & Hsu, J. (2005). Kaiser Permanente's experience of implementing an electronic medical record: A qualitative study. *British Medical Journal, 331,* 1313–1316.

Judy Urgo, MSN, RN
HackensackUMC

EVIDENCE-BASED PRACTICE

Westra, B., & Delaney, C.W. (2008). Informatics competencies for nursing and healthcare leaders. AMIA Annu Symp Proc. 804-808.

Abstract

Historically, educational preparation did not address informatics competencies; thus managers, administrators, or executives may not be prepared to use or lead change in the use of health information technologies. A number of resources for informatics competencies exist; however, a comprehensive list addressing the unique knowledge and skills required in the role of a manager or administrator was not found. The purpose of this study was to develop informatics competencies for nursing leaders. A synthesis of the literature and a Delphi approach using three rounds of surveys with an expert panel, resulted in identification of informatics competencies for nursing leaders that address computer skills, informatics knowledge, and informatics skills.

The goal was that all Americans have an electronic health record (EHR) by 2014. Health care leaders must be prepared to select, adopt, and implement EHRs. In the past, nursing education did not include informatics competencies. The American Organization of Nurse Executives (AONE) included it in its recent update of competencies for nursing executives. The TIGER Initiative (Technology Informatics Guiding Education) identified that all nurses in every role must be prepared to make health information technologies (HIT) a goal of the twenty-first century.

The first survey had 119 items with 38 competencies addressing computer skills, 37 addressing informatics knowledge, and 44 addressing informatics skills. Within each of the three major categories were subdivisions for easier comprehension of content areas.

Computer skills included:
- Basic software applications
- Administration applications
- Electronic communications
- Data access and decision support
- Patient documentation and monitoring
- Education
- Systems
- Research

Informatics knowledge included:
- Data
- Impact
- Ethical and legal issues
- Systems
- Education
- Research
- Usability and ergonomics

A sample of 13 nursing leaders, informaticians, and researchers was selected from the American Medical Informatics Association of Nursing Informatics Working Group, the Minnesota Organization of Nursing Leaders, and the University of Minnesota School of Nursing.

Informatics competencies for nursing leaders were developed through a review of the literature and a Delphi process that included three rounds of surveys using an expert panel of experienced nursing leaders, informaticians, and researchers. This study identifies the competencies that are unique to the role of the nursing leader.

TABLE 1

Computer Skills

Basic Software Applications
Word processing software
Spreadsheet software (e.g. Excel)
Presentation software (e.g. PowerPoint)
Internet browsers

Advanced Software Applications
Forecasting
Budgeting
Human resources
Quality assurance
Staffing/determining patient acuity
Statistical analysis
Synthesizing the whole patient picture from a multidisciplinary perspective
Planning and making decisions

Electronic Communications
Composing e-mails
Sending confidential documents
Participating in group communication

Access Data/Information
Navigating systems (e.g. file servers)
Searching information retrieval systems
Distance-learning

Patient Related Applications
Documenting patient assessments
Creating care plans
Documenting nursing interventions
Documenting outcomes of care
Monitoring trends in patient outcomes
Supporting patient education

TABLE 2

Informatics Skills

Requirements and System Selection
Develop project scope, objectives, and resources
Integrate patient care processes and nursing administrative functions in system requirements
Involve front-line staff in the development of system requirements
Involve front-line staff in the development of system selection
Specify system requirements based on the needs of the organization
Collaborate with interprofessional team in system selection process

Evaluate information systems in practice settings
Advocate for the development (or purchase) and use of integrated, cost-effective health information systems within the organization
Advocate for new applications to meet standards for interoperability

Financial
Priorities are within budget constraints and organizational priorities
Alternatives for funding information systems
Costs and benefits analysis applied for in practice, education, administration, and/or research
Financial and staffing implications of ongoing updates to information systems
Actual vs budgeted costs for implementing nursing-related information systems
Collaborate with interprofessional team around financial issues

Implementation/Management
Implementation of systems consistent with the vision, mission, strategic, and tactical plans
Use project management for implementation of IS
Manage the impact of change because of IS implementation
Front-line staff are involved in appropriate aspects of design, implementation, and testing related to their practice
Improve the use of informatics within nursing practice
Collaborate with interprofessional team to manage information systems

Ethical/Legal Concepts
Access to system information
Use of data (obtaining, storing, and disseminating text, data, images, or sounds)
Access to personal health information (PHI – HIPAA [Health Insurance Portability and Accountability Act] language)

Analysis/Evaluation
Consistency with organizational policies, external licensing, accreditation, and regulatory agency requirements
Ensure testing plans are evaluated at every phase of system implementation
Ensure that front-line staff (users) are involved in the evaluation of information systems
Collaborate with interprofessional team to evaluate information systems

Continued

EVIDENCE-BASED PRACTICE—cont'd

TABLE 3

Informatics Knowledge

Management Concepts

Management of system implementations

Avoidance of potential negative impacts

Allocating financial resources

Inclusion of nursing information within systems

Communicating a vision about the benefits

Anticipating changes in economic and business
   processes

Analysis of interprofessional workflow processes

Revising processes from workflow analysis

Decisions impacting clinical information systems (IS)
   implementation, use, and maintenance

Change management

Data Issues

Health care data standards

Importance of integrating nursing data elements in
   systems

Importance of integrating standardized nursing languages in systems

Data quality issues

Data reporting issues

Information Systems Concepts

Value of clinicians' involvement in at all appropriate
   phases

Strengths and limitations of applications related to
   software programming language or design

Strengths and limitations of applications related to
   hardware/networks

Technological trends, issues, and new developments
   as they apply to nursing

"Work arounds" and the consequences of these

Human–computer interface interactions

Ergonomics of workstation, bedside

Ergonomics of adjunct technologies

Ergonomics of portable technology

Application of IS technologies to clinical practice

Application of IS technologies to administration

Application of IS technologies to clinical research
   situations

Staff Education

Levels of informatics knowledge by roles

Methods for education

Clinical Research

Evaluating Internet resources

Methods for evaluation of IS implementation and use

Reuse of patient/administrative data for research

Application of informatics research for practice

Ethical/Legal Concepts

Patients' rights real time computerized information
   management

Principles of data integrity

Ethical principles for collection, maintenance, use, and
   dissemination of data and information

Application of HIPAA (Health Insurance Portability and
   Accountability Act) to information systems

Compliance with institutional review boards (IRBs) for
   research with data from information systems

Policies and procedures consistent with regulatory and
   accrediting requirements for IS

Intellectual property, copyright, and fair use of copyrighted material

NCLEX® EXAMINATION QUESTIONS

1. Automated systems for providers to enter patient care orders and to access decision support databases are called:
   A. Clinical information systems
   B. Decision support
   C. Computerized provider order entry (CPOE)
   D. Electronic health records

2. The core functionalities for an electronic health information system are:
   A. Health information, data, and order entry
   B. Patient census, data, and order entry
   C. Patient acuities, patient census, and incident report
   D. Incident reports and outcomes measures

3. Nursing informatics is a specialty that integrates nursing science, computer science, and information science to:
   A. Maintain and communicate data information, knowledge, and wisdom in nursing practice
   B. Manage and calculate data information, knowledge, and wisdom in nursing practice
   C. Manage and communicate data information, knowledge, and accountability in nursing practice
   D. Manage and communicate data information, knowledge, and wisdom in nursing practice

4. Nursing informatics (NI) is a specialty that integrates:
   A. Nursing science, computer science, and information science to manage and communicate data, information, knowledge, and wisdom in nursing practice.
   B. Nursing science, and information science to manage and communicate data, information, knowledge, and wisdom in nursing practice.
   C. Nursing science, computer science, and information science to manage and communicate data, information, and knowledge, in nursing practice.
   D. Computer science, and information science to manage and communicate data, information, knowledge, and wisdom in nursing practice.

5. One key feature of an electronic health record (EHR) is that it can be created, managed, and consulted by authorized providers and staff across _____ other organization(s).
   A. 1
   B. 2
   C. 3
   D. Many

6. Another use for computerized information is:
   A. Finances
   B. Billing
   C. Inventory tracking
   D. All of the above

7. Over 144,000 payments totaling _____ have already been issued to professionals and hospitals by the Centers for Medicare & Medicaid Services (CMS) to have sharing of patient data on a nationwide level.
   A. $4.1 billion
   B. $5.1 billion
   C. $6.1 billion
   D. $7.1 billion

8. A true electronic health record (EHR) is a complete record of an individual's health-related data. The _____ is continuing to spearhead the initiative to build a national electronic health care system that would allow patients and their care givers to access their complete health records anytime and anywhere (HealthIT.gov, 2015).
   A. U.S. Department of Health and Human Services (DHHS)
   B. American Nurses Association (ANA)
   C. National Institute for Occupational Safety and Health (NIOSH)
   D. Centers for Disease Control and Prevention (CDC)

9. As per Rundio and Wilson (2013, p. 64), informatics is a core competency of all health care professionals. The key areas of focus center on:
   A. National information infrastructure, computerized clinical data
   B. Clinical decision support, use of Internet
   C. Integration of evidence-based practice
   D. All of the above

10. Which of the following is not a nursing minimum data set under the service element area?
    A. Nursing outcomes
    B. Unique facility or service agency number
    C. Unique health record number of the patient
    D. The discharge or termination date

Answers: 1. C   2. A   3. D   4. A   5. D   6. D
7. D   8. A   9. D   10. A

REFERENCES

American Nurses Association. (2008). *Scope and standards of nursing informatics practice*. Washington, DC: Author. Publication.

Bates, D., & Gawande, A. (2003). Improving patient safety with information technology. *New England Journal of Medicine, 348*, 2526–2534.

Committee on Data Standards for Patient Safety. (2003). *Key capabilities of an electronic health record system: Letter report*. Washington, DC: National Academy of Sciences.

Dolan, B. (2012). *Survey: 71 percent of US nurses use smartphones*. Retrieved August 9, 2014, from http://mobihealthnews.com/17172/survey-71-percent-of-us-nurses-use-smartphones/.

Giannini, M. (2005). *The CAM and nursing coding manual*. Albany, NY: Delmar.

Goldberg, D. G., Kuzel, A. J., Feng, L. B., DeShazo, J. P., & Love, L. E. (2012). EHRs in primary care practices: Benefits, challenges and successful strategies. *The American Journal of Managed Care, 18*(2), e48–e54.

HealthIT.gov. (2015). *Fefinition of EHR*. Retrieved January 25, 2015, from http://www.healthit.gov/providers-professionals/learn-ehr-basics.

Huber, D. G., Delaney, C., & Crossley, J. (1992). A nursing management minimum data set. *Journal of Nursing Administration, 22*(7/8), 35–40.

Institute of Medicine. (1997). In Dick, R. & Steen, E. (Eds.), *The computer based record: An essential technology for health care (revised edition)*. Washington, DC: National Academies Press.

Institute of Medicine. (2000). In L. Kohn, J. Corrigan, & M. Donaldson (Eds.), *To err is human: Building a safer health system*. Washington, DC: National Academies Press.

Institute of Medicine. (2001). *Crossing the quality chasm: A new health system for the 21st century*. Washington, DC: National Academies Press.

Institute for Safe Medication Practice. (2014). *Proceedings from the ISMP Summit on the Use of Smart Infusion Pumps: GUIDELINES FOR SAFE IMPLEMENTATION AND USE*. Retrieved August 9, 2014, from http://www.ismp.org/tools/guidelines/smartpumps/.

International Council of Nurses. (1999). *International classification for nursing practice—Beta version*. Geneva, Switzerland: Author.

Jao, C., & Hier, D. (2010). Clinical decision support systems: an effective pathway to reduce medical errors and improve patient safety. In Jao, C. (Ed), *Decision Support Systems*. Rijeka, Croatia: InTech.

Kearney Nunnery, R. (2005). *Advancing your career: Concepts in professional nursing* (3rd ed.). Philadelphia: F.A. Davis.

Kumar, S., & Nash, D. (2011). *Health care myth busters: Is there a high degree of scientific certainty in modern healthcare? Scientific American*. March 25, 2011.

Leatherman, S., & McCarthy, D. (2002). *Quality of health care in the United States: A chartbook*. New York: The Commonwealth Fund.

Levingston, S. A. (2012). *Opportunities in physician electronic health records: A road map for vendors*. New York: Bloomberg Government.

McGlynn, E., Asch, S., Adams, J., et al. (2003). The quality of health care delivered to adults in the United States. *New England Journal of Medicine, 348*, 2635–2645.

Menachemi, N., & Collum, T. (2011). Benefits and drawbacks of electronic health record sys tems. *Risk Management in Health Care Policy, Vol 4*, 47–55. http://dx.doi.org/10.2147/RMHP.S12985 Published online May 11, 2011.

Mc Kesson. (2014). *ANSOS One Step Staff Scheduling*. Retrieved August 9, 2014, from http://www.mckesson.com/providers/health-systems/department-solutions/capacity-and-workforce-management/ansos-one-staff/.

North American Nursing Diagnosis Association. (1999). *Nursing diagnoses: Definitions and classification, 1999-2000*. Philadelphia: Author.

NORC at University of Chicago. *Patient Provider Telehealth Network—Using Telehealth to Improve Chronic Health Management*. Author.

Overhage, J. M., Dexter, P. R., Perkins, S. M., et al. (2002). A randomized controlled trial of clinical information shared from another institution. *Annals of Emergency Medicine, 39*, 14–23.

Partnership for Solutions, Johns Hopkins University. (2002). *Chronic conditions: Making the case for ongoing care*. Baltimore: Johns Hopkins University.

Perez-Pena, R. (January 20, 2012). A nurse need never forget. *The New York Times*, p. ED27.

Rousel, L. (2013). *Management and leadership for nurse administrators*. Boston: Jones & Bartlett.

Rundio, A., Wilson, V. (2013). *Nurse executive review and resource manual, 2nd*. Silver Spring, MD: American Nurses Credentialing Center.

Schiff, G., Klass, D., Peterson, J., Shah, G., & Bates, D. (2003). Linking laboratory and pharmacy: opportunities for reducing errors and improving care. *Archives of Internal Medicine, 163*, 893–900.

Schiff, G., & Rucker, T. (1998). Computerized prescribing: Building the electronic infrastructure for better medication usage. *JAMA, 29*, 1024–1029.

U.S. Department of Health and Human Services. (2003). *News release: HHS launches new efforts to promote paperless health care system*. Retrieved April 23, 2009, from http://www.hhs.gov/news/press/2003pres/20030701.html.

University of Illinois. (2014). *Tips and tricks for evaluating web sites*. Retrieved August 9, 2014, from http://www.library.illiois.edu/ugl/howdoi/webeval.html.

Vivona, T. (2013). Useful apps for student nurses. *Nursing Times,* July 26, 2013.

Werley, H. H., & Lang, N. M. (1988). The consensually derived nursing minimum data set elements and definitions. In H. H. Werley, & N. M. Lang (Eds.), *Identification of the nursing minimum data set* (pp. 402–411). New York: Springer.

Yoder-Wise, P. (2003, 2011). *Leading and managing in nursing* (3rd ed.). St. Louis: Mosby.

Ethical and Legal Issues in Patient Care

KEY TERMS

advance directive document that allows the competent patient to make choices regarding health care before it is needed

autonomy provides for the privilege of self-determination in deciding what happens to one's body in health care

beneficence duty to do good to others; to maintain a balance between benefits and harm; to provide all patients, including the terminally ill, with caring attention; and to treat every patient with respect and courtesy; requires that care providers contribute to the health and welfare of the patient and not merely attempt to avoid harm to the patient or client

bioethics ethics specific to health care

corporate liability responsibility of an organization for its own wrongful conduct

durable power of attorney for heath care decisions document that permits an individual to give a surrogate or proxy the authority to make decisions for that person in the event that they become incompetent

ethics science that deals with the principles of right and wrong and of good and bad, and governs our relationships with others. It is based on personal beliefs and values

informed consent consent for treatment given by a patient after three requirements are met: the patient has the capacity to consent, consent is voluntary, and the patient receives information regarding treatment in a manner that is understandable

Institutional Review Board (IRB) a group that has been formally designated to approve, monitor, and review biomedical and behavioral research involving humans with the alleged aim to protect the rights and welfare of the subjects. This group performs critical oversight functions for research conducted on human subjects that are scientific, ethical, and regulatory. Research review panels that determine the legal and ethical protection of subjects participating in medical research

justice principle of fairness in which an individual receives what is due, owed, or legitimately claimed; the treating of all parties equally, regardless of economic or social background, and learning the state's and organization's laws for reporting abuse; requires that individuals be given what they deserve or can legitimately claim

living will advance directive that indicates what an individual dictates regarding treatment or lifesaving measures in the future

morality behavior in accordance with custom or tradition that usually reflects personal or religious beliefs

nonmaleficence principle of doing no harm: observing safety rules and precautions and keeping skills up-to-date. Prohibits deliberate harm and demands weighing risks with the benefits of treatment (Grohar-Murray & Langan, 2011)

Omnibus Budget Reconciliation Act (OBRA) of 1987 one provision of this act provides patients with the right to be free from any physical or chemical restraint imposed for the purpose of discipline or convenience and not required to treat medical symptoms

Patient Self-Determination Act federal law requiring every heath care facility receiving Medicare or Medicaid to provide written information to adult patients concerning their right to make health care decisions

personal liability responsibility and accountability of individuals for their own actions or inactions

policies and procedures written standardized protocol that is authorized by the health care organization

restraint direct application of physical force to a patient, with or without the patient's permission, to restrict freedom of movement; the physical force may be human, via mechanical devices, or a combination thereof

risk management clinical and administrative activities that organizations undertake to identify, evaluate, and reduce the risk of injury to patients, staff, and visitors and the risk of loss to the organization itself

tort private or civil wrong or injury, including action of bad faith breach of contract, for which the court will provide a remedy in the form of an action for damages

ETHICAL DECISION MAKING

Today's nurses are in the public eye in the discussion of many different ethical issues and dilemmas, such as technology that maintains life for severely premature infants, technology that advances the life of severely brain-damaged patients, stem cell research, the issues of what constitutes brain death, transplant and donor programs, and end-of-life decisions. Concern for ethics has also moved beyond the clinical arenas to the business of health care, with the potential for Medicare fraud, suspect business decision making, and the protection of patient information. Ethical decision making will have an impact on your clinical professional role, your leadership role, and your research role. Professions are defined in part by the ethics that define their practice. One of the hallmarks of a profession is the existence of a code of ethics that governs the practice of the members of the profession. Nursing and nurses have long been recognized for their commitment to high ethical standards.

Ethical decision making is required when there is an ethical dilemma. Ethical dilemmas occur when there is a conflict between two or more ethical principles.

Common Ethical Principles and Their Rules

1. Beneficence: Duty to do good and to protect the patient's welfare. An example is carefully adhering to infection-control principles for all patients.
2. Nonmaleficence: Principle of doing no harm. Nurses who maintain their skills are practicing the principle of "doing no harm."
3. Justice: Principle of fairness in which an individual receives what is owed. All patients receiving the same level of culturally competent care is an example.
4. Autonomy: Respect for individual liberty and the person's right to self-determination. Informed consent is an example of adherence to the principle of autonomy.
5. Fidelity: Duty to keep one's word. Senior leaders adhering to all contracts is an example of leadership fidelity.
6. Respect for others: Right of people to make their own decisions, such as not telling a patient what he "should do" but allowing him to make his own decision.
7. Veracity: Obligation to tell the truth. As a professional, this would be a requirement to admit mistakes promptly or to not lie to a patient about bad news.

(List adapted from Little, 2003, p. 469.)

Such a conflict comes into place with the conflict between (a) the principle of autonomy (the duty to respect the patient's choice) and the duty to do only what the patient wants and (b) the principle of beneficence (the duty to protect the patient's welfare) and the duty to do only what the patient needs. An example would be the conflict that arises when a patient refuses dialysis that will prolong their life. Another example would be the situation where the family does not want their frail elderly mother given the news that her grandson has been hospitalized with a life-threatening injury. The conflict here is between veracity and self-respect. The decision of what to do is guided by beneficence. Often there is no correct decision. There are many questions that arise in clinical care, such as the following (Schroeder, 1995):

• When do we refrain from using technology?
• When do we stop using technology, once it is started?
• Who is entitled to technology? Those who can pay? Those who are uninsured? Everyone, no matter what?

In addition to the clinical situations that cause ethical conflicts, nurses and health care personnel bring their own values and beliefs into the dilemma. There are times where the beliefs of the health care personnel themselves are the dilemma. An individual with a strong religious belief in the sanctity of life may have ethical conflicts about DNR (do-not-resuscitate) orders or abortions. Cultural values and traditions may also be at the center of ethical dilemmas. Nurses and patients may believe that talking about death invites death to the door. It is important to be aware of your beliefs and to not let them interfere with the legal and professional requirements of your position. If you have beliefs that will prevent you from performing some of the requirements of your position, it is necessary to inform your supervisor, so that the patient needs can always be met.

TRADITIONAL ETHICAL THEORIES

The study of ethics has resulted in different theories that are used to guide decision making. Box 17-1 provides traditional ethical theories.

As a nurse, you will be guided by both ethical theories and your own personal values and beliefs and professional expectations (American Nurses Association [ANA], 2015; International Council of Nurses [ICN], 2009). The fundamental values of nursing are expressed in the Code of Ethics for Nurses. They are the values, such as respect for patient autonomy, acting in the patient's best interest, and maintaining professional competence, that all nurses commit to uphold when they enter the profession.

> **BOX 17-1 Traditional Ethical Theories**
>
> Utilitarianism:
> - Decisions based on what will provide the greatest good for the greatest number of people.
> - For example, the decision to force people with pulmonary tuberculosis into treatment is ethical, according to this theory, because it protects the greater population from infection.
>
> Teleology (or consequentialist theory):
> - The value of a situation is determined by its consequences.
> - Thus the outcome, not the action itself, is what counts; sometimes referred to as the "all's well that ends well" ethical approach.
>
> Deontology (or formalism):
> - An act is good only if it springs from good will.
> - This ethical theory does not allow for actions based on the concept of "the end justifies the means" (Little, 2003).

Kelly-Heidenthal, P. (2004). *Essentials of nursing leadership and management.* Clifton Park, NY: Thomson Delmar Learning.

AMERICAN NURSES ASSOCIATION'S CODE OF ETHICS FOR NURSES

Nurses must always act as patient advocates. The Nightingale Pledge in 1893 was viewed as the first code of ethics for nurses. The American Nurses Association approved the most recent Code of Ethics for Nurses in 2015.

Revised Code of Ethics for Nurses

1. The nurse practices with compassion and respect for the inherent dignity, worth, and unique attributes of every person.
2. The nurse's primary commitment is to the patient, whether an individual, family, group, community or population.
3. The nurse promotes, advocates for, and protects the rights, health, and safety of the patient.
4. The nurse has the authority, accountability, and responsibility for nursing practice; makes decisions; and takes action consistent with the obligation to promote health and to provide optimal care.
5. The nurse owes the same duties to self as to others, including the responsibility to promote health and safety, preserve wholeness of character and integrity, maintain competence, and continue personal and professional growth.
6. The nurse, through individual and collective effort, establishes, maintains, and improves the ethical environment of the work setting and conditions of employment that are conducive to safe, quality health care.
7. The nurse in all roles and settings, advances the profession through research and scholarly inquiry, professional standards development, and the generation of both nursing and health policy.
8. The nurse collaborates with other health professionals and the public to protect human rights, promote health diplomacy, and reduce health disparities.
9. The profession of nursing, collectively through its professional organizations, must articulate nursing values, maintain the integrity of the profession, and integrate principles of social justice into nursing and health policy (ANA, 2015).

INTERNATIONAL COUNCIL OF NURSES' INTERNATIONAL CODE OF ETHICS FOR NURSES

The International Council of Nurses' (ICN) International Code of Ethics for Nurses, most recently revised in 2006, is a guide for action based on social values and needs. The code has served as the standard for nurses worldwide since it was first adopted in 1953. The code is regularly reviewed and revised in response to the realities of nursing and health care in a changing society. The code makes it clear that inherent in nursing is respect for human rights, including the right to life, to dignity, and to be treated with respect. The ICN International Code of Ethics for Nurses guides nurses in everyday choices and supports their refusal to participate in activities that conflict with caring and healing.

International Council of Nurses' International Code of Ethics for Nurses

1. Nurses and people

   The nurse's primary professional responsibility is to people requiring nursing care. In providing care, the nurse promotes an environment in which the human rights, values, customs, and spiritual beliefs of the individual, family, and community are respected. The nurse ensures that the individual receives sufficient information on which to base consent for care and related treatment. The nurse holds in confidence personal information and uses judgment in sharing this information. The nurse shares with society the responsibility for initiating and supporting action to meet the health and social needs of the public, in particular those of vulnerable populations. The nurse also shares responsibility to sustain and protect the natural environment from depletion, pollution, degradation, and destruction.

2. Nurses and practice

The nurse carries personal responsibility and accountability for nursing, practice, and maintaining competence by continual learning. The nurse maintains a standard of personal health such that the ability to provide care is not compromised. The nurse uses judgment regarding individual competence when accepting and delegating responsibility.

The nurse at all times maintains standards of personal conduct that reflect well on the profession and enhance public confidence. The nurse, in providing care, ensures that uses of technology and scientific advances are compatible with the safety, dignity, and rights of people.

3. Nurses and the profession

The nurse assumes the major role in determining and implementing acceptable standards of clinical nursing practice, management, research, and education. The nurse is active in developing a core of research-based professional knowledge.

The nurse, acting through the professional organization, participates in creating and maintaining equitable social and economic working conditions in nursing.

4. Nurses and coworkers

The nurse sustains a cooperative relationship with coworkers in nursing and other fields. The nurse takes appropriate action to safeguard individuals when their care is endangered by a co-worker or any other person (ICN, 2006; copyright © 2006).

One mark of a profession is the establishment of determination of ethical behavior for its members. In addition to the American Nurses Association (ANA) and ICN codes, specialty nursing organizations and hospitals have developed codes of ethical behavior.

To assist you in dealing with the complex ethical issues that exist, hospitals have formed ethics committees. These committees are interdisciplinary and include representatives from clinical nursing, administration, medicine, social work, pharmacy, legal, and clergy. The work of ethics committees lies in three areas (Agich & Younger, 1991; Dalgo & Anderson, 1995):

- Education (seminars and workshops for committee members).
- Policy and guideline recommendations (specific hospital policies).

- Case review (analyzes patient cases and provides clear options).

As a nurse, you have the right to call on the ethics committee for a referral. Cases are often referred to the ethics committee for discussion. Issues commonly addressed by ethics committees are end-of-life issues, organ donation, and futility-of-care issues.

A systematic approach to the identification and meaning of ethical issues has been suggested by the University of Washington School of Medicine. The recommended "work-up" includes review of medical indications, patient preferences, quality of life, and contextual issues. This work-up describes "what is." Then the decision making moves to the next phase and involves questions such as:

- What is the issue?
- Where is the conflict?
- What is this case about? Is it similar to other cases encountered? What is known about them?
- Is there a precedent? Is there a paradigm case (e.g. Karen Ann Quinlan, Nancy Cruzan, Terri Schiavo, Jahi McMath)?
- Who is involved and what roles do they play?

(Rundio & Wilson, 2013, p. 143.)

END-OF-LIFE ISSUES

End-of-life issues frequently revolve around the issue of advance directives. An **advance directive** is an end-of-life decision made by a patient in advance of the actual need. Many individuals confuse an advance directive with a do-not-resuscitate (DNR) order, but they are not the same.

The Patient Self-Determination Act of 1990 requires that all individuals receiving medical care must be given written information about their rights under state law to make decisions about their care, including the right to accept medical or surgical treatment. This information needs to include information about their rights to formulate advance directives.

An advance directive instructs health care personnel on the patient's desires for care in certain circumstances. An advance directive, sometimes called a "**living will**," is a set of instructions documenting a person's wishes regarding medical care intended to sustain life. It is used if a patient becomes terminally ill, incapacitated, or unable to communicate or make decisions. Everyone has the right to accept or refuse medical care. A living will protects the patient's rights and removes the burden for making decisions from family, friends, and physicians. The ethical dilemma exists if the patient's family refuses to allow the advance directive to be used or if a health care professional refuses to implement the directives.

ORGAN DONATION

Although organ donation is a personal choice, there may be times when an ethical dilemma may ensue with carrying out this wish. For example, if a person has decided to be an organ donor and has made this clear on their driver's license, at the time of death, the family may strongly disagree with this decision. Some other ethical questions surrounding organ donation include:

- Do people have the right to petition for organs across the internet?
- If someone purchases an organ, is the health care system under any obligation to perform the transplant?
- Is it acceptable to purchase organs?
- Should healthier transplant candidates be given preference for organs?

(Adapted from Rundio & Wilson, 2013, p. 147.)

Some states have mandated that a request be made for organ or tissue donation at the time of a patient's death. In hospitals where organ transplantations are done, there is usually a full-time organ donation coordinator. Nurses may be called on to request organ donations if the facility where they are employed charges nurses with this responsibility. Again, the nurse should be very direct in making these requests so there are no miscommunications, saying, for example, "Have you considered organ donation for your loved one?"

Written consent and hospital policies and procedures must be strictly followed. There is no cost to the donor family. The usual funeral expenses still apply.

Facts: Did You Know?

As of January 2015 more than 122,344 people in the United States were on the waiting list for a lifesaving organ transplant.

- A name is added to the national transplant waiting list every 12 minutes.
- Seven percent of people on the waiting list, more than 6500 each year, die before they are able to receive a transplant.
- On average, 18 people die every day from the lack of available organs for transplant.
- One deceased donor can save up to eight lives through organ donation and can save and enhance more than 100 lives through the lifesaving and healing gift of tissue donation.

- Organ recipients are selected based primarily on medical need, location, and compatibility.
- To date, 597,166 transplants have occurred in the United States since 1988.
- Organs that can be donated after death are heart, liver, kidneys, lungs, pancreas, and small intestines. Tissues include corneas, skin, veins, heart valves, tendons, ligaments, and bones.
- The cornea is the most commonly transplanted tissue. More than 40,000 corneal transplants take place each year in the United States.
- A healthy person can become a "living donor" by donating a kidney, or a part of the liver, lung, intestine, blood, or bone marrow.
- More than 6000 living donations occur each year. One in four donors is not biologically related to the recipient.
- The buying and selling of human organs is not allowed for transplants in America, but it is allowed for research purposes.
- In most countries, it is illegal to buy and sell human organs for transplants, but international black markets for organs are growing in response to the increased demand around the world.

(The American Transplant Foundation, 2014. www.americantransplantfoundation.org/about-transplant/facts-and-myths/.)

Organ Procurement Organizations

Organ procurement organizations (OPOs) are a unique component of health care. By federal law, they are the only organizations that can recover organs from deceased donors for transplantation. There are 58 federally designated organ procurement organizations throughout the United States and its territories. Organ procurement organizations are generally structured to include clinical services, hospital development, donor family services, and public education.

The federal conditions of participation for organ donation, adopted in 1998, require hospitals to refer all deaths to OPOs for evaluation and to work collaboratively with the OPO on an approach for consent (New Jersey Sharing Network, 2014a).

Religious Views

The following are the views of various religious groups on organ donation and transplantation (American Council on Transplantation, 2007).

African Methodist Episcopal (AME) and African Methodist Episcopal Zion (AME Zion)

Organ and tissue donation is viewed as an act of neighborly love and charity by these denominations. These groups encourage all members to support donation as a way of helping others.

Amish

The Amish will consent to transplantation if they know that it is for the health and welfare of the recipient. They would be reluctant to donate their organs if the outcome was known to be questionable; however, nothing in the Amish understanding of the Bible forbids them from using modern medical services.

Baptists

Organ and tissue donation is advocated as an act of charity. In 1988, the Southern Baptist Convention passed a resolution supporting donation as a way to alleviate suffering and to have compassion for the needs of others.

Buddhists

Buddhists believe that organ and tissue donation is a matter of individual conscience.

Catholics

Catholics view organ donation as an act of charity, fraternal love, and self-sacrifice. Transplants are ethically and morally acceptable to the Vatican.

The Church of Christ Scientist

The Church of Christ Scientist takes no specific position on transplants or organ donation as distinct from other medical or surgical procedures. Church members usually rely on spiritual rather than medical means of healing. They are free to choose the form of medical treatment they desire, including organ transplantation. The decision of organ donation is left to the individual.

Hindu

Hindus are not prohibited by religious law from donating; it is considered an individual decision.

Jehovah's Witnesses

Jehovah's Witnesses do not encourage organ donation, but believe it is a matter for individual conscience according to the Watch Tower Bible and Tract Society, the legal corporation for the religion. The group does not oppose donating or receiving organs; however, all organs and tissue must be completely drained of blood before transplantation.

Judaism

Judaism teaches that saving a human life takes precedence over maintaining the sanctity of the human body.

Latter-Day Saints (Mormons)

According to church leaders, Latter-Day Saints (Mormons) are not prohibited by religious law from donating their organs or receiving transplants. The decision is a personal one.

Mennonites

Mennonites have no prohibition against organ donation and transplantation. Church officials state such decisions are individual ones.

Muslims

The Muslim Religious Council initially rejected organ donation by followers of Islam in 1983, but it has since reversed its position provided that donors consent in writing in advance. The organs and tissues of Muslim donors must be transplanted immediately and not be stored in organ banks.

Protestants

Protestantism encourages and endorses organ donation. Protestants respect the individual's conscience and a person's right to make decisions regarding their own body.

Quakers

Quakers do not oppose organ donation and transplantation. The decision is an individual one.

Seventh-Day Adventists

Seventh-Day Adventist officials have stated organ donation and transplantation to be acceptable practices for members. The decision is an individual one.

FUTILITY OF CARE

Ethical dilemmas often arise in patient care situations where there are concerns about the futility of care. The ethical conflict arises when the principle of beneficence ("do not harm") is called into question. Will further treatment benefit the patient? This is a time when a consultation with the ethics committee may be appropriate.

Some hospitals are offering a more humane approach to the DNR request. Families often misinterpret the DNR order as an order to do nothing. The intent of the order is to "allow a natural death" (AND). It is also important to understand that a decision not to receive "aggressive medical treatment" is not the same as withholding all medical care. A patient can still receive antibiotics, nutrition, pain medication, and other interventions when the goal of treatment becomes comfort rather than cure. This is called palliative care, and its primary focus is helping the patient remain as comfortable as possible.

Physician Orders for Life-Sustaining Treatment (POLST) is a form that gives seriously ill patients more control over their end-of-life care, including medical treatment, extraordinary measures (such as a ventilator or feeding tube), and CPR. The National POLST Paradigm is an approach to end-of-life planning based on conversations between patients, loved ones, and health care professionals designed to ensure that seriously ill or frail patients can choose the treatments they want, or do not want, and that their wishes are documented and honored. Unlike other documents, such as an advance directive, a completed POLST form is an actual medical order that becomes a part of the individual's medical record. It also is valid in all health care settings (Figure 17-1).

ORGANIZATIONAL ETHICS

A hospital's behavior toward its patients and its business practices has a significant impact on the patient's experience of, and response to, care. Thus, access, treatment, respect, and conduct affect patient rights. Access to hospital care is a major ethical issue in health care. Does a hospital have the right to refuse to care for a patient who does not have adequate insurance?

As a manager, you will be responsible for setting the ethical tone on your unit and guaranteeing that all patient and employee rights are respected. You will also have to practice ethically in all leadership and managerial actions. This will mean protecting the rights of your staff and providing a professional work environment. Staff members need to be able to work in an environment where they are free to report issues of concern. Hospitals have created departments of corporate compliance to oversee the reporting, documentation, and continued improvement of areas of organizational ethical concern.

Senior leaders of the organization are responsible for the safe stewardship of the organization in both business practices and all areas of clinical care.

Hospitals are legally and ethically obligated to uphold the following patient rights to:
- Participate in treatment decisions;
- Provide informed consent to treatment;
- Receive considerate and respectful care;
- Review records;
- Be informed of hospital policies; and
- Expect reasonable and appropriate continuity of care after hospitalization.

The Patient Care Partnership of the American Hospital Association replaced what was originally named the Patients' Bill of Rights (Box 17-2). The partnership informs patients about what they should expect during their hospital stay with regard to their rights and responsibilities.

RESEARCH

As a nurse, you will participate in clinical research during your career. The ethical requirements of research should be well understood and be part of your work. Hospitals and other workplaces participating in research involving human subjects have **Institutional Review Boards** (IRBs) that set guidelines for the research and approve all research studies that occur in the institution. Although the regulations for IRBs are federal law (U.S. Code of Federal Regulations, Department of Health and Human Services [DHHS] Title 45, Part 46, entitled *Protection of Human Subjects*, as well as the U.S. Food and Drug Administration [FDA] Title 21, Part 50 and Title 21, Part 56), they have arisen in light of ethical violations of the rights of patients.

The IRB's primary concerns are to determine that:
- The rights and welfare of the human subjects are protected adequately;
- The risks to subjects are outweighed by the potential benefits of the research;
- The selection of subjects is equitable; and
- Informed consent will be obtained and documented.

LEGAL ISSUES

State Board of Nursing

As a nurse you are well aware that you are held accountable for all of your actions both as an individual nurse

continued on page 15

Combined Advance Directive for Health Care
(Combined Proxy and Instruction Directive)

I understand that as a competent adult, I have the right to make decisions about my health care. There may come a time when I am unable, due to physical or mental incapacity, to make my own health care decisions. In these circumstances, those caring for me will need direction concerning my care and will turn to someone who knows my values and health care wishes. I understand that those responsible for my care will seek to make health care decisions in my best interests, based upon what they know of my wishes. In order to provide the guidance and authority needed to make decisions on my behalf:

I, _____, hereby declare and make known my instructions and wishes for my future health care. This advance directive for health care shall take effect in the event I become unable to make my own health care decisions, as determined by the physician who has primary responsibility for my care, and any necessary confirming determinations. I direct that this document become part of my permanent medical records.

In completing Part One of this directive, you will designate an individual you trust to act as your legally recognized health care representative to make health care decisions for you in the event you are unable to make decisions for yourself.

In completing Part Two of this directive, you will provide instructions concerning your health care preferences and wishes to your health care representative and others who will be entrusted with responsibility for your care, such as your physician, family members and friends.

Part One: Designation of a Health Care Representative

A) Choosing a Health Care Representative:

I hereby designate:

name _____

address _____

city _____ state _____

telephone _____

as my health care representative to make any and all health care decisions for me, including decisions to accept or to refuse any treatment, service or procedure used to diagnose or treat my physical or mental condition, and decisions to provide, withhold, or withdraw life-sustaining measures. I direct my representative to make decisions on my behalf in accordance with my wishes as stated in this document, or as otherwise known to him or her. In the event my wishes are not clear, or a situation arises I did not anticipate, my health care representative is authorized to make decisions in my best interests, based upon what is known of my wishes.

FIGURE 17-1 Combined advance directive for health care. (From NJ Commission on Legal and Ethical Problems in the Delivery of Health Care (NJ Bioethics Commission), March 1991.)

I have discussed the terms of this designation with my health care representative and he or she has willingly agreed to accept the responsibility for acting on my behalf.

_____

B) Alternate Representatives: If the person I have designated above is unable, unwilling, or unavailable to act as my health care representative, I hereby designate the following person(s) to act as my health care representative, in order of priority stated:

1. name_____   2. name_____
address_____   address_____
city_____ state_____   city_____ state_____
telephone _____   telephone _____

Part Two: Instruction Directive

In Part Two, you are asked to provide instructions concerning your future health care. This will require making important and perhaps difficult choices. Before completing your directive, you should discuss these matters with your health care representative, doctor, and family members or others who may become responsible for your care.

In **Sections C and D,** you may state the circumstances in which various forms of medical treatment, including life-sustaining measures, should be provided, withheld, or discontinued. If the options and choices below do not fully express your wishes, you should use **Section E,** and/or attach a statement to this document that would provide those responsible for your care with additional information you think would help them in making decisions about your medical treatment. **Please familiarize yourself with all sections of Part Two before completing your directive.**

C) General Instructions. To inform those responsible for my care of my specific wishes, I make the following statement of personal views regarding my health care.

Initial ONE of the following two statements with which you agree:

1. _____ I direct that all medically appropriate measures be provided to sustain my life regardless of my physical or mental condition.

2. _____ There are circumstances in which I would not want my life to be prolonged by further medical treatment. In these circumstances, life-sustaining measures should not be initiated and if they have been, they should be discontinued. I recognize that is likely to hasten my death. In the following, I specify the circumstances in which I would choose to forgo life-sustaining measures.

If you have initialed statement 2, on the following page please initial each of the statements (a, b, c) with which you agree:

FIGURE 17-1, cont'd

Continued

a. _____ I realize that there may come a time when I am diagnosed as having an incurable and irreversible illness, disease, or condition. If this occurs, and my attending physician and at least one additional physician who has personally examined me determine that my condition is **terminal,** I direct that life-sustaining measures that would serve only to artificially prolong my dying be withheld or discontinued. I also direct that I be given all medically appropriate care necessary to make me comfortable and relieve pain.

In the space provided, write in the bracketed phrase with which you agree:

To me, terminal condition means that my physicians have determined that:

_____

[I will die within a few days] [I will die within a few weeks]
[I have a life expectancy of approximately _____ or less (enter 6 months or 1 year)]
b. _____ If there should come a time when I become **permanently unconscious,** and it is determined by my attending physician and at least one additional physician with appropriate expertise who has personally examined me, that I have totally and irreversibly lost consciousness and my capacity for interaction with other people and my surroundings, I direct that life-sustaining measures be withheld or discontinued. I understand that I will not experience pain or discomfort in this condition, and I direct that I be given all medically appropriate care necessary to provide for my personal hygiene and dignity.

c. _____ I realize that there may come a time when I am diagnosed as having an **incurable and irreversible** illness, disease, or condition that may not be terminal. My condition may cause me to experience severe and progressive physical or mental deterioration and/or a permanent loss of capacities and faculties I value highly. If, in the course of my medical care, the burdens of continued life with treatment become greater than the benefits I experience, I direct that life-sustaining measures be withheld or discontinued. I also direct that I be given all medically appropriate care necessary to make me comfortable and to relieve pain.

(Paragraph **c.** covers a wide range of possible situations in which you may have experienced partial or complete loss of certain mental or physical capacities you value highly. If you wish, in the space provided below you may specify in more detail the conditions in which you would choose to forgo life-sustaining measures. You might include a description of the faculties or capacities, which, if irretrievably lost would lead you to accept death rather than continue living. You may want to express any special concerns you have about particular medical conditions or treatments, or any other considerations, that would provide further guidance to those who may become responsible for your care. If necessary, you may attach a separate statement to this document or use **Section E** to provide additional instructions.)

Examples of conditions that I find unacceptable are:

_____
_____
_____
_____

FIGURE 17-1, cont'd

D) Specific Instructions: Artificially Provided Fluids and Nutrition; Cardiopulmonary Resuscitation (CPR). On page 3 you provided general instructions regarding life-sustaining measures. Here you are asked to give specific instructions regarding two types of life-sustaining measures—artificially provided fluids and nutrition and CPR.

In the space provided, write in the bracketed phrase with which you agree:

1. In the circumstances I initialed on page 3, I also direct that artificially provided fluids and nutrition, such as feeding tube or intravenous infusion,

_____

[be withheld or withdrawn and that I be allowed to die]
[be provided to the extent medically appropriate]

2. In the circumstances I initialed on page 3, if I should suffer a cardiac arrest, I also direct that cardiopulmonary resuscitation (CPR)

_____

[not be provided and that I be allowed to die]
[be provided to preserve my life, unless medically inappropriate or futile]

3. If neither of the above statements adequately expresses your wishes concerning artificially provided fluids and nutrition or CPR, please explain your wishes below.

_____

_____

_____

E) Additional Instructions: You should provide any additional information about your health care preferences that is important to you and that may help those concerned with your care to implement your wishes. You may wish to direct your health care representative, family members, or your health care providers to consult with others, or you may wish to direct that your care be provided by a particular physician, hospital, nursing home, or at home. If you are or believe you may become pregnant, you may wish to state specific instructions. If you need more space than is provided here you may attach an additional statement to this directive.

_____

_____

_____

F) Brain Death: The state of New Jersey recognizes the irreversible cessation of all functions of the entire brain, including the brain stem (also known as whole brain death), as a legal standard for the declaration of death. However, individuals who cannot accept this standard because of their personal religious beliefs may request that it not be applied in determining their death.

FIGURE 17-1, cont'd

Continued

Initial the following statement only if it applies to you:

_____To declare my death on the basis of the whole brain death standard would violate my personal religious beliefs. I therefore wish my death to be declared solely on the basis of the traditional criteria of irreversible cessation of cardiopulmonary (heartbeat and breathing) function.

G) After Death-Anatomical Gifts: It is now possible to transplant human organs and tissue in order to save and improve the lives of others. Organs, tissues, and other body parts are also used for therapy, medical research, and education. This section allows you to indicate your desire to make an anatomical gift and if so, to provide instructions for any limitations or special uses.

Initial the statements that express your wishes:

1. _____ **I wish** to make the following anatomical gift to take effect upon my death:

A. _____ any needed organs or body parts.
B. _____ only the following organs or parts

_____

for the purposes of transplantation, therapy, medical research or education, or

C. _____ my body for anatomical study, if needed.
D. _____ special limitations, if any;

_____

If you wish to provide additional instructions, such as indicating your preference that your organs be given to a specific person or institution, or be used for a specific purpose, please do so in the space provided below.

_____
_____
_____

2. _____ **I do not wish** to make an anatomical gift upon my death.

Part Three: Signature and Witnesses

H) Copies: The original or a copy of this document has been given to the following people (Note: If you have chosen to designate a health care representative, it is important that you provide him or her with a copy of your directive):

1. name _____   2. name _____

address _____   address _____

city _____ state _____   city _____ state _____

telephone _____   telephone _____

FIGURE 17-1, cont'd

I) Signature: By writing this advance directive, I inform those who may become entrusted with my health care of my wishes and intend to ease the burdens of decision making that this responsibility may impose. I have discussed the terms of this designation with my health care representative and he or she has willingly agreed to accept the responsibility for acting on my behalf in accordance with this directive. I understand the purpose and effect of this document and sign it knowingly, voluntarily, and after careful deliberation.

Signed this _____ **day of** _____, 20 _____ .

signature _____

address _____

city _____ state _____

J) Witnesses: I declare that the person who signed this document, or asked another to sign this document on his or her behalf, did so in my presence, that he or she is personally known to me, and that he or she appears to be of sound mind and free of duress or undue influence. I am 18 years of age or older, and am not designated by this or any other document as the person's health care representative.

1. witness _____

address _____

city _____ state _____

signature _____

date _____

2. witness _____

address _____

city _____ state _____

signature _____

date _____

New Jersey Commission on Legal and Ethical
Problems in the Delivery of Health Care
(The New Jersey Bioethics Commission)
March 1991

FIGURE 17-1, cont'd

BOX 17-2   Patient Bill of Rights

The Patient Care Partnership: Understanding Expectations, Rights, and Responsibilities

The American Hospital Association's Patient Care Partnership states that the patient has the following rights:

High-quality hospital care

Patients have the right to be provided with the care needed, with skill, compassion, and respect.

A clean and safe environment

There are hospital **policies and procedures** in place to ensure that patients have an environment free from errors, abuse, and neglect.

Involvement in your care

Patients are entitled to be made aware of the benefits and risks of treatments, whether treatments are experimental or part of a research study, what can be expected from treatment and any long-term effects it might have on quality of life, what should be done after discharge, and the financial consequences of uncovered services or out-of-network providers. Patients should inform health care providers of any past illnesses, surgeries, hospital admissions, allergies, and all medications and dietary supplements taken. Patients should also inform health care providers of any health care goals and values or spiritual beliefs that are important to the well-being of the patient. It should be made clear who the power of attorney is, if the patient has a living will, or advance directives in place.

Protection of your privacy

Patients' privacy must be protected at all times once in the health care system. Patients will receive a Notice of Privacy Practices that describes the specific hospital privacy plan and means of accomplishing this.

Help when leaving the hospital

The hospital personnel will identify sources of follow-up care such as home care or ordering equipment needed for home.

Help with your billing claims

The hospital billing department will file health care claims and assist the patient with any questions regarding the bill and patient coverage.

Adapted from American Hospital Association.(2015). *Patient bill of rights.* www.aha.org/content/00-10/pcp_english_030730.pdf.

and as the nurse managing the care of others. It is important, therefore, to have an understanding of legal issues and their impact on the profession. The first contact that you will have will be the state licensing authority and the laws of that authority. The first thing you will do after graduation is pass the NCLEX examination.

Upon passing this milestone, you will receive your license to practice professional nursing. This license is given by the individual state where you are practicing and the license is governed by the statutory regulations of that particular state.

State boards of nursing in each state define those actions and duties of a nurse that are allowable by the profession guided by the state's practice act and common law. Nurse practice acts affect all areas of nursing practice. Nurse practice acts set educational standards, examination requirements, and licensing requirements and regulate the nursing profession in each particular state. State boards of nursing exist to foster public protection, to ensure consumer protection from fraud and abuse, and to respond to changes in the health care practice environment. The National Council of State Boards of Nursing (NCSBN) serves as a central clearinghouse, ensuring that individual state actions are enforced in all states in which an individual nurse may hold licensure.

Because each state has its own practice act and regulations, all nurses need to know the provisions of the practice act of the state in which they are licensed. This is especially important in the areas of diagnosis and treatment that differ from state to state. The addresses and web addresses of the various state boards are listed in Chapter 21.

If you are a nurse licensed in one state while practicing telenursing or giving telephone triage in another state, it is imperative you know the nursing regulations of the state in which your care is being delivered. With the advent of multistate licensures, nurses licensed in one state may legally practice in some other states without obtaining additional licensure. The state in which you practice is the state under whose regulations you are accountable. Not all states have multistate licenses, so again it is imperative that you know about the practice requirements of your state.

Disciplinary Action by the State Board of Nursing

As a nurse manager, you are also responsible for the monitoring of the practice of employees under your supervision and ensuring that they remain current with their licensure. A list of all individuals who hold nursing licenses, registered nurses, and licensed practical nurses, is maintained by the vice president of nursing. The nurse must show the original state license to the vice president of nursing or his or her designee when the new nursing license has been issued. Many state boards of nursing now have online licensee directories that give you the status of an individual's license.

The nurse and the nurse leader are responsible for protecting the license of nurses in the organization. Disciplinary actions by the state board of nursing will occur if a complaint about a nurse's action triggers an investigation. Potential situations that may trigger an investigation include the following:

- Impaired nursing practice (see Chapter 9).
- Negligence.
- Incompetence.
- Abuse.
- Fraud.
- Practicing beyond the scope of the license.

Corporate Liability

Corporate liability is the responsibility of an organization for its own wrongful conduct. The health care facility must maintain an environment conducive to quality patient care. Corporate liability includes (1) the duty to hire, supervise, and maintain qualified, competent, and adequate staff; (2) the duty to provide, inspect, repair, and maintain reasonably adequate equipment; and (3) the duty to maintain safety in the physical environment (Sullivan & Decker, 2009).

Malpractice

In the delivery of patient care, there is always a potential for malpractice and negligence. Malpractice refers to "any misconduct or lack of skill in carrying out professional responsibilities" (Sullivan & Decker, 2009). It is also defined as failure of a professional person to act as other prudent professionals with the same knowledge and education would act under similar circumstances.

This is one of the reasons nurses need to maintain personal malpractice insurance. The employing organization maintains blanket malpractice coverage for all employees, but it is highly recommended that individuals purchase their own personal nursing liability insurance. Most commonly, nurses are subject to legal liability arising from malpractice and negligence. Nursing negligence malpractice occurs when the nurse's actions do not meet the standard of care, when the nurse's actions are unreasonable, or when the nurse fails to act and causes harm. Harm related to nursing clinical practice commonly arises from negligent acts and omissions (unintentional torts) and a variety of intentional acts

(intentional torts) such as invasion of privacy, assault and battery, or false imprisonment (Aiken, 2004). See Box 17-1 for reasons that nurses should have personal malpractice insurance.

Tort Law

A tort is a "private or civil wrong or injury, including action of bad faith breach of contract, for which the court will provide a remedy in the form of an action for damages" (*Black's Law Dictionary*, 1996, cited in Martin & Cain, 2003).

A tort can be any of the following (Carroll, 2006, p. 279):
1. Denial of person's legal rights.
2. Failure to comply with public duty.
3. Failure to perform private duty that harms another person.

A tort can be unintentional, such as malpractice or neglect, or intentional, such as assault and battery or invasion of privacy (Fiesta, 1999). For malpractice to exist, the following elements must be present (Carroll, 2006, p. 280):
1. A duty exists: This is automatic when a patient is in a health care facility.
2. A breach of duty occurs: The nurse did something that should not have been done or did not do something that should have been done.
3. Causation: The nurse's action directly led to a patient injury.
4. Injury: Harm comes to the patient.
5. Damages: Compensate the patient for injury.

Negligence

Negligence refers to the failure of an individual to perform an act (omission) or to perform an act (commission) that a "reasonable, prudent person would not perform in a similar set of circumstances" (Sullivan & Decker, 2009). Negligence is also defined as the failure to exercise the proper degree of care required by the circumstance.

Common negligence allegations in nursing include the following:
- Medication errors.
- Patient falls.
- Use of restraints.
- Equipment injuries.
- Failure to take appropriate nursing action.
- Failure to follow hospital procedure.
- Failure to supervise treatment.

An institution's policies and procedures describe the performance expected of nurses. Deviation from this expected performance can result in a liability for negligence or malpractice. A nurse failing to adhere to institutional policy runs the risk of the employer denying the nurse defense in a lawsuit.

Charting

Most malpractice/negligence lawsuits take place years after the actual event. When a nurse is named in a lawsuit, it is likely that the memory of the event will have greatly diminished. The documentation in the patient care record may be the most reliable source of information. Therefore, a nurse's charting ability serves a double purpose of reminding of the care delivered to that particular patient. Documentation on an electronic medical record has become standardized in many facilities. Such electronic documentation is usually standard driven, making it easier for the nurse to document appropriately. But if the nurse needs to document in a nonelectronic record it is important to remember the rules of nursing documentation (Box 17-3).

Review Table 17-1 to determine FLAT charting (factual, legible, accurate, timely).

Standard of Care

Box 17-3 shows a standard of care for pain management. This standard of care would form the basis for the expectation of care delivered to all patients within an institution. Deviation from this care can be defined as malpractice. As stated earlier, the clinical problems that most commonly lead to malpractice/negligence lawsuits are restraints, medication errors, patient falls, privacy violations, and other adverse events. Therefore, it is important for the nurse and nurse manager to practice according to established policy and procedure.

Incident Reports

The filing of an incident report forms the basis of organization-wide reporting from a risk management perspective. The purpose of an incident report is to provide a factual account of an incident or an adverse event to ensure that all facts surrounding the incident are reported. The incident reporting system provides the risk manager with an opportunity to investigate all serious situations. Aggregated data from incident reports are used by management to improve health care processes within the organization and for the early identification of emerging problems. Refer to your agency for the process for incident reporting. In general, incident report forms should be completed by the following:

1. Staff member involved in the occurrence.
2. Staff member who discovered the incident.
3. Staff member to whom the incident was reported.

Incident reports should be completed as soon after the occurrence as possible. Accurately record all details of the incident and objectively describe the description of the incident and actions taken in response to it. It is important not to provide subjective information stating what should or could have been done to avoid the incident. If a document includes this information, the nurse can be asked in court why he or she did not take those actions to avoid the incident. The report also needs to include patient assessment and monitoring after the incident (Carroll, 2006).

Nurses can also be mentioned as parties in medical malpractice. In such situations, a nurse's liability is determined by the state's nurse practice act and the institution's policies and procedures. Above and beyond personal liability for personal clinical practice, nurses also have accountability and liability for their acts of delegation and supervision. As a primary care coordinator, the nurse manages the environment of care delivery. Ensuring staff competence and reporting incompetent practice are key. The nurse manager can also be held accountable for the negligence of contract employees (agency nurses) even though they are not employees of a particular institution. This is why it is important that the nurse managers are aware of skills, competencies, and knowledge of all staff working with them. Nurse managers also need to be aware of legal issues in the area of human resources. They will need to be aware of hiring standards, performance review standards, management of employees with problems, compliance with union contract, and terminations.

Health Care Information

Invasion of privacy and confidentiality is a tort violation. The Health Insurance Portability and Accountability Act (HIPAA) was enacted in 1996 to give people control over their personal information. It also made organizations that create or receive personal information accountable for protecting it. Information disclosed by patients is confidential and should be available only to authorized

---

BOX 17-3 Memorial Sloan-Kettering Cancer Center

III The Standard of Care For the Patient with Pain

Nursing Diagnosis:

Pain, Acute and/or Chronic related to:

- Disease
- Treatment
- Procedure
- Other, specify

General Outcomes:

1. Patient will report adequate pain relief.
2. Patient will have minimal side effects from analgesic regimen.
3. Patient will be satisfied with his/her pain management.

Outcome Criteria:

The Patient will:

1. be assessed for pain at least every 12 hours and prn in the inpatient setting and at each outpatient visit.
2. report pain intensity (e.g., using 0-10 scale or categorical).
3. report satisfaction of relief of pain.
4. experience minimal side effects from analgesic regimen.

The Patient/Family/Caregiver will:

5. describe the pain management plan including rationale, drug, route, dose, frequency, and potential side effects and whom to notify for questions or problems.
6. notify the physician or nurse if pain is not adequately controlled or if questions, problems, or concerns about pain management arise in either the inpatient, outpatient or home setting.
7. participate with the interdisciplinary team to determine the most effective and cost-efficient pain management program.
8. describe their responsibilities in pain management.

Assessment:

Pain assessment is the cornerstone of all effective pain management. A thorough assessment leads clinicians to the etiology of the pain itself and to other new diagnoses that may be treatable. The choice of a specific treatment depends upon a full assessment and the identification of specific pain syndromes. The assessment assists the clinician in more fully understanding the patient's pain problem and how the pain affects daily life. Also, repetitive assessments are necessary for the evaluation of the current pain treatment plan.

1. Assess and document pain intensity and satisfaction with relief regularly, at least every twelve hours for inpatients and with each clinic visit for outpatients.
2. Assess and document pain systematically including location(s), intensity, quality, onset, duration, precipitating and relieving factors (including use of analgesics and proper analgesic history), occurrence of breakthrough pain, satisfaction with relief and presence and severity of side effects (especially constipation).
3. Consider impact of pain on sleep, mood, appetite, activity, usual functioning in self-care and job, and role in family and community.
4. Assess and document the patient's knowledge of his/her pain along with attitudes and values regarding pain and its meaning.
5. Assess and document the presence of factors which impact on patient suffering: anxiety, depression, anger, attitude towards disease, attitude towards treatment.
6. Assess for the presence of social, practical, and financial supports that impact on the plan for pain management.
7. Review current disease state and extent of disease, results of recent imaging studies, current therapy, future therapy, and coexisting conditions.

Interventions:

1. Collaborate with multidisciplinary team and advocate for pain control options most appropriate for the patient, family, caregiver, and setting.
2. Administer prescribed analgesics and deliver interventions in a timely, logical, and coordinated manner.
3. Review with patient how to describe the severity of his/her pain (e.g., 0-10 scale or categorical scale), satisfaction with relief, and presence and severity of side effects.
4. Monitor ongoing effectiveness of analgesic regimen and other interventions. Document medication administration and effectiveness of analgesic regimen in accordance with policy.
5. Consult with MD/NP/PA or Advanced Practice Nurse of Primary Service about:
   - appropriate modifications in analgesic regimen.
   - treatment of analgesic-related side effects (*refer to following nursing diagnosis related to side effects of analgesics*).
6. Ensure that conversions from opioid to opioid and route to route are accurate.
7. Alter environment to provide comfort (e.g., decrease lighting and noise, provide privacy, limit visitors as patient wishes.)
8. Facilitate use of nonpharmacologic interventions (e.g., relaxation, focused breathing, distraction) when appropriate.
9. Provide patient/family/caregiver with information about medication, dose, route, frequency, and potential side effects. (Refer to specific nursing diagnosis related to individual side effects as appropriate).
10. Explore patient/family/caregiver concerns about the use of opioids.

Continued

BOX 17-3 Memorial Sloan-Kettering Cancer Center—cont'd

11. Provide information to allay fears and correct misconceptions (specifically in relation to addiction, tolerance, physical dependence).
12. Review with patient, family and caregiver their responsibility in pain management:
    - Understanding the nature of the pain, treatment, and expected response to treatment.
    - Understanding the rationale, drug, dose, frequency, and side effects of prescribed analgesics.
    - Obtaining medications, renewing prescriptions, and monitoring medication supply.
    - Reporting to MD/NP/PA or RN any new or unrelieved pain, change in pain location, quality or intensity, and side effects from analgesic regimen.
13. Consult with Advanced Practice Pain Management Nurses as needed.
14. Discuss with MD/NP/PA regarding consult with Anesthesiology Pain Management Group or Neurology Pain Service.
15. Include pain management in discharge plan. Identify need for home assessment and intervention. Communicate plan to ambulatory office practice nurse.
16. Document plan, interventions and outcomes.

Aspects of the pain management are specific to certain patient populations. To provide as comprehensive a standard as possible without redundancy, population-specific concerns will be covered at the end of the nursing diagnosis section. There information will be found related to the following groups: patients with acute pain, chronic pain, and chronic pain with acute pain episodes; pediatric and geriatric patients; patients with altered communication and those with a history of substance abuse.

Nursing Diagnosis:

Lack of knowledge, patient/family/caregiver related to aspects of pain management which may include but are not limited to:
- pain/etiology of pain
- understanding of principles and methods of pain management
- analgesics (nonopioid, opioid, and adjuvant analgesics)
- equipment/devices used to provide analgesics
- potential side effects of analgesics
- potential for physical dependence/tolerance/addiction
- nonpharmacologic interventions
- expected participation in the analgesic regimen.

Lack of knowledge is based on nursing assessment that the patient/family/caregiver lacks the information necessary to enable them to be active, informed participants in the plan of care. Knowledge deficit encompasses all dimensions of learning: cognitive, psychomotor, and affective. In relation to pain management, patients, their families, and caregivers need information about pain and the medications and the regimens ordered. For those who need special equipment to deliver their pain medication, it is important to provide opportunities to practice with that equipment. They also need information and reassurance to allay fears and concerns about opioid use, specifically, addiction, tolerance, and physical dependence.

A knowledge deficit does not apply if the individual is unable to understand the information or change behavior because of cognitive or physical impairments that may be related to medications such as opioids or other organic causes. To apply the concept of knowledge deficit, the nurse must assess and recognize the patient's, families' and caregivers' basic knowledge about the cause of pain and its treatment and plan to **provide the right information, in the right way, at the right time.**

Outcome Criteria:

In addition to the general outcomes listed in Pain, Acute and/or Chronic..., the patient/family/caregiver will:
1. Notify the MD/NP/PA or RN of any new or unrelieved pain, change in pain location, quality or intensity, and side effects from analgesic regimen.
2. Identify cause of pain.
3. State the rationale of prescribed analgesic regimen.
4. Identify the medications, doses, route, frequency, and potential side effects of prescribed analgesics.
5. Use equipment related to pain management appropriately.
6. Comply with the analgesic regimen.
7. Use nonpharmacologic methods as appropriate.
8. Express an understanding of the differences between physical dependence, tolerance, and addiction.

Assessment:

Assess and document patient, family and caregiver's knowledge regarding:
1. nature of pain, treatment, and expected response to treatment.
2. how to report pain intensity and relief.
3. specific prescribed analgesic regimen (drug, dose, route, frequency, and potential side effects [specifically constipation]).
4. physical dependence, tolerance, addiction, and other concerns related to the use of opioids.
5. use of special equipment (if applicable).
6. the role and responsibility of patient, family, and caregiver in pain management.
7. availability of resources at MSKCC and in the community.

BOX 17-3   Memorial Sloan-Kettering Cancer Center—cont'd

Interventions:

1. Assist patient, family and caregivers in understanding the pain and its causes.
2. Teach the patient, family, and caregivers methods of reporting pain intensity and relief.
3. Explain specific prescribed analgesic regimen (drug, dose, route, frequency, and potential side effects), concepts of physical dependence, tolerance, and addiction, and clarify any other misconceptions related to the use of opioids.
4. Provide information (print, audio, video) about:
   - analgesics and adjuvants, their action, dose, route, frequency, and potential side effects.
   - use of special equipment (if applicable).
   - various nonpharmacologic interventions (if appropriate).
5. Review with patient, family, and caregivers information regarding route of administration:
   - **Neural blockade and neurolytic procedures:**
     purpose of prognostic block (to predict the efficacy of a permanent ablating procedure); reinforce teaching initiated by Anesthesia Pain Management (APMG)
   - **Epidural catheter:**
     rationale for using the epidural route
     basic concepts about the use of opioids and/or local anesthetics
     possible side effects and their treatment
     setting realistic goals/expectations concerning pain relief
     progression from epidural analgesia to oral medications (if applicable)
   - **IV, Subcutaneous or Epidural Patient-Controlled Analgesia (PCA)**
     goals for PCA therapy
     prescribed programmed analgesic regimen
     how to give a PRN "rescue" dose for anticipated or breakthrough pain
     reasons for notifying the nurse (e.g., increased pain, sleepiness, hallucinations, nausea, vomiting, itching, urinary retention)
   - **Discharge instructions for patients going home with IV, subcutaneous, or epidural PCA:**
     home health care (hi-tech) agency follow-up
     operation of PCA pump, e.g., changing batteries, start/stop
     dressing change procedures
     assessment of epidural catheter site, IV access site, or subcutaneous needle insertion site
     universal precautions when handling and disposing of needles
     method of needle disposal
     delivery of supplies
     follow-up appointments
     emergency phone numbers
   - **Additional information specific for patients being discharge with a subcutaneous needle for intermittent or continuous infusions:**
     changing subcutaneous needle every 5 days or more often if redness or other discoloration, tenderness, swelling, bleeding, or drainage occurs
     use of proper technique when inserting subcutaneous needle
6. Provide instructions and allow opportunity to practice using equipment (pumps, etc.) needed for the prescribed analgesic regimen.
7. Allow time for patient/family/caregiver to express concerns, ask questions, discuss analgesic regimen, and demonstrate skills.
8. Provide patient/family/caregiver with name and phone numbers of resources at MSKCC and in the community who will assist you with pain management.
9. Review with patient and family their responsibility in pain management:
   - Understanding the nature of pain, treatment, and expected response to treatment.
   - Understanding the rationale, drug, dose, frequency and potential side effects of prescribed analgesics.
   - Obtaining medications, renewing prescriptions, and monitoring medication supply.
   - Reporting to MD/NP/PA or RN any new or unrelieved pain, change in pain location, quality, intensity or side effects from analgesic regimen.
10. Document plan, interventions, and outcomes.

NOTE: This is taken from a more comprehensive document, "Care of the Patient in Pain: Standard of Oncology Nursing Practice" by the Pain Standard Committee.

personnel. Nurses must obtain permission to release information to family members and close friends, as well as to others. This makes it difficult when nurses attempt to release information over the telephone. The nurse must identify the caller as an appropriate receiver of such information. Also, photographs, research information, or videos of the patient may not be used without specific signed releases. Computerized information also needs to be protected. Nurses charting on a hallway computer must not leave information visible on the computer screen

TABLE 17-1 **FLAT Charting**
1. Factual—What you see, not what you think happened
2. Legible—No erasures; corrections should be made with a single line drawn through the error and initialed
3. Accurate and complete—For example, color of tracheostomy secretions
4. Timely—Completed as soon after the occurrence as possible

From Kelly-Heidenthal, P., & Marthaler, M. T. (2005). *Delegation of nursing care* (p. 145). Clifton Park, NY: Thomson Delmar Learning.

to individuals in the hallway. Of particular concern is the increasing use of social media. Many employer policies do not address nurses' use of social media to discuss workplace issues on personal devices. A nurse may face serious consequences for inappropriate use of social media. Instances of inappropriate use of social and electronic media may be reported to the Board of Nursing. Depending on the laws of jurisdiction, the Board of Nursing may investigate reports of inappropriate disclosures on social media sites on the grounds of unprofessional conduct, unethical conduct, mismanagement of patient records, and breach of confidentiality. (*A Nurse's Guide to Social Media.* www.ncsbn.org/NCSBN_SocialMedia.pdf). Some tips in dealing with social media follow in Box 17-4

INFORMED CONSENT

Nurses will often be called on to witness patient consent. There are three elements of informed consent (Nathanson, 1996, cited in Rowland & Rowland, 1997, p. 188):

1. Information and knowledge:

   For any patient to make a valid decision regarding a treatment, they must have adequate information to consider. Health care providers are responsible for informing patients of the diagnosis, prognosis, available alternatives to treatment recommended, risks and benefits of treatment options, and the risks of not accepting treatment. This information must be presented to a patient in understandable terms. Both The Joint Commission (2014) and the American Hospital Association require that hospitals meet a patient's communication needs.

2. Competence:

   Adults over 18 years of age in most states are legally competent and capable of giving valid consent for medical treatment. The patient must be of sound mind and free from any legal or mental impediments from making a binding decision regarding health care. Therefore, a patient who has a legal guardian or is a minor may not be legally competent to give consent. Each state has different rules about age of competence; it is therefore necessary to be mindful of the states' legalities.

3. Voluntariness:

   For a patient's consent to be voluntary, the patient must freely elect to undergo the treatment without any sort of physical or psychological coercion. If the person is intimidated, threatened, or coerced by health care personnel, there could be a lack of valid consent.

Regarding the physician's responsibility in the communications process, the physician providing or performing the treatment and/or procedure (not a delegated representative) should disclose and discuss the following with the patient:

- The patient's diagnosis, if known.
- The nature and purpose of a proposed treatment or procedure.
- The risks and benefits of a proposed treatment or procedure.
- Alternatives (regardless of their cost or the extent to which the treatment options are covered by health insurance).
- The risks and benefits of the alternative treatment or procedure.
- The risks and benefits of not receiving or undergoing a treatment or procedure.

In turn, the patient should have an opportunity to ask questions to elicit a better understanding of the treatment or procedure, so that they can make an informed decision to proceed or to refuse a particular course of medical intervention (American Medical Association, 2008).

The consent for treatment is given by a patient after three requirements are met: the individual has the capacity to consent, consent is voluntary, and the individual receives information regarding treatment in a manner that is understandable to him or her (Sullivan & Decker, 2009).

Individual capacity to consent is determined by age and competence. The legal age is determined by state laws. Competency is determined when an individual has the ability to make choices and understands the consequences of their choices. When individuals make

BOX 17-4   How to Avoid Disclosing Confidential Patient Information

With awareness and caution, nurses can avoid inadvertently disclosing confidential or private information about patients. The following guidelines are intended to minimize the risks of using social media.

- Nurses must recognize that they have an ethical and legal obligation to maintain patient privacy and confidentiality at all times.
- Nurses are strictly prohibited from transmitting by way of any electronic media any patient-related image. In addition, nurses are restricted from transmitting any information that may be reasonably anticipated to violate patient rights to confidentiality or privacy, or otherwise degrade or embarrass the patient.
- Nurses must not share, post, or otherwise disseminate any information or images about a patient or information gained in the nurse/patient relationship with anyone unless there is a patient-care-related need to disclose the information or other legal obligation to do so.
- Nurses must not identify patients by name, or post or publish information that may lead to the identification of a patient. Limiting access to postings through privacy settings is not sufficient to ensure privacy.
- Nurses must not refer to patients in a disparaging manner, even if the patient is not identified.
- Nurses must not take photos or videos of patients on personal devices, including cell phones. Nurses should follow employer policies for taking photographs or videos of patients for treatment or other legitimate purposes using employer provided devices.
- Nurses must maintain professional boundaries in the use of electronic media. Similar to in-person relationships, the nurse has an obligation to establish, communicate, and enforce professional boundaries with patients in the online environment. Use caution when having online social contact with patients or former patients. Online contact with patients or former patients blurs the distinction between a professional and personal relationship. The fact that a patient may initiate contact with the nurse does not permit the nurse to engage in a personal relationship with the patient.
- Nurses must consult employer policies or an appropriate leader within the organization for guidance regarding work-related postings.
- Nurses must promptly report any identified breach of confidentiality or privacy.
- Nurses must be aware of and comply with employer policies regarding use of employer-owned computers, cameras, and other electronic devices, and use of personal devices in the workplace.
- Nurses must not make disparaging remarks about employers or co-workers. Do not make threatening, harassing, profane, obscene, sexually explicit, racially derogatory, homophobic, or other offensive comments.
- Nurses must not post content or otherwise speak on behalf of the employer unless authorized to do so, and must follow all applicable policies of the employer.

(*A nurse's guide to social media.* www.ncsbn.org/NCSBN_SocialMedia.pdf.)

choices without force, fraud, deceit, or duress, they are acting voluntarily. And the information must contain all of the following (Sullivan & Decker, 2009):

1. An explanation of the treatment to be performed and the expected results
2. A description of the anticipated risks and discomforts
3. A list of potential benefits
4. A disclosure of possible alternatives
5. An offer to answer the patient's questions
6. A statement that the patient may withdraw his or her consent at any time

Nurses are often asked to witness a patient's informed consent. In signing the document, the nurse is witnessing the patient's signature, not validating the patient's complete understanding. A nurse has a right to refuse to sign if they think that any of the above information is not met.

Patient Restraints

Basic human rights are not forfeited on entry into a health care facility. A competent patient has the right to refuse **restraints** unless he or she is at risk of harming others. Improper use of restraints may constitute assault or false imprisonment. If a patient has to be restrained, the patient has a right to the least restrictive restraint use at all times. Injuries resulting from improper use of restraints often are a cause of legal complaints.

The Omnibus Budget Reconciliation Act (OBRA) of 1987 gives patients the right to be free from any physical or chemical restraint imposed for the purpose of discipline or convenience and not required to treat medical symptoms.

Restraint use must meet the following requirements:
1. There is a physician's order for specific duration and circumstances for use.
2. PRN (pro re nata) orders are not permitted.
3. There is continuous assessment and reassessment of patient as per hospital policy.
4. Informed consent for use must be given (if the patient unable to give consent, proxy consent is necessary).

Patient Self-Determination Act

The Patient Self-Determination Act provides legislative support to the expression of a patient's consent to or refusal of medical treatment, even when the patient is no longer able to verbalize them. Patients who can verbalize refusal of care are allowed to sign out "against medical advice" (AMA). Health care organizations have policies and procedures surrounding patients signing out AMA. In this situation the nurse documents in detail the events leading to the refusal of care and documents patient awareness of the consequences of refusal. Patients who are unable to verbalize consent or refusal can do so with the following documents:
1. Advance medical directive
2. Durable power of attorney
3. Health care proxy
4. Living will
5. POLST

Advance Medical Directive

Advance medical directives are written instructions expressing an individual's health care wishes in the event of incapacitation. A sample is shown in Figure 17-1.

Durable Power of Attorney

These are legal instructions enabling an individual to act on another's behalf. In health care, it is often part of an advance medical directive. Figure 17-2 is an example of such instructions.

Health Care Proxy

Documents delegate the authority to make health care decisions to another when the patient has become incapacitated.

Living will and POLST documents were discussed earlier in this chapter.

Nurse's Responsibility in Advance Directives

Most health care organizations have policies for the documentation of patient self-determination documents. Nurses are required to ask patients and families if there are advance directives on initial assessment. These documents are then placed in the chart for future reference if necessary. State statutes regarding advance directives vary from state to state, so it is important to know state practice.

Good Samaritan Laws

Although nurses are legally covered for professional actions within the workplace, there are often concerns about professional actions in times of emergency outside of the health care institution. Good Samaritan laws have been enacted to encourage professionals to render help in an emergency or accident situation. The Hawaii Good Samaritan Act reads: "Any person who in good faith renders emergency care, without remuneration or expectation of remuneration, at the scene of an accident or emergency to the victim of the accident or emergency shall not be liable for any civil damages resulting from the person's acts or omission, except for such damages as may result from the person's gross negligence or wanton acts or omissions" (U.S. Legal Definitions, 2008).

Durable Power of Attorney for Health Care Decisions
■ *Take a copy of this with you whenever you go to the hospital or on a trip* ■

It is important to choose someone to make healthcare decisions for you when you cannot make or communicate decisions for yourself. Tell the person you choose what healthcare treatments you want. The person you choose will be your agent. He or she will have the right to make decisions for your healthcare. If you DO NOT choose someone to make decisions for you, write NONE on the line for the agent's name.

I, _____ , SS# _____ (optional), appoint the person named in this document to be my agent to make my healthcare decisions.

This document is a Durable Power of Attorney for Healthcare Decisions, My agent's power shall not end if I become incapacitated or if there is uncertainty that I am dead. This document revokes any prior Durable Power of Attorney for Healthcare Decisions. My agent may not appoint anyone else to make decisions for me. My agent and my care-givers are protected from any claims based on following this Durable Power of Attorney for Healthcare. My agent shall not be responsible for any costs associated with my care. I give my agent full power to make all decisions for me about my healthcare, including the power to direct the withholding or withdrawal of life-prolonging treatment, including artificially supplied nutrition and hydration/tube feeding. My agent is authorized to:

- Consent, refuse or withdraw consent to any care, procedure, treatment, or service to diagnose, treat or maintain a physical or mental condition, including artificial nutrition and hydration;
- Permit, refuse, or withdraw permission to participate in federally regulated research related to my condition or disorder
- Make all necessary arrangements for any hospital, psychiatric treatment facility, hospice, nursing home, or other health-care organization; and, employ or discharge healthcare personnel (any person who is authorized or permitted by the laws of the state to provide healthcare services) as he or she shall deem necessary for my physical, mental, or emotional well-being;
- Request, receive, review and authorize sending any information regarding my physical or mental health, or my personal affairs, including medical and hospital records; and execute any releases that may be required to obtain such information;
- Move me into or out of any state or institution;
- Take legal action, if needed;
- Make decisions about autopsy, tissue and organ donation, and the disposition of my body in conformity with state law; and
- Become my guardian if one is needed.

In exercising this power, I expect my agent to be guided by my directions as we discussed them prior to this appointment and/or to be guided by my Healthcare Directive (*see reverse side*).
If you DO NOT want the person (agent) you name to be able to do one or other of the above things, draw a line through the statement and put your initials at the end of the line.

Agent's name _____ Phone _____ Email _____

Address

*If you do **not** want to name an alternate, write "none."*

Alternate Agent's name _____ Phone _____ Email _____

Address _____

Execution and Effective Date of Appointment
My agent's authority is effective immediately for the limited purpose of having full access to my medical records and to confer with my healthcare providers and me about my condition. My agent's authority to make all healthcare and related decisions for me is effective when and only when I cannot make my own healthcare decisions.

SIGN HERE for the *Durable Power of Attorney* and /or *Healthcare Directive* forms. Many states require notarization. It is recommended for the residents of all states. Please ask two persons who are not related to you or financially connected to your estate to witness your signature.

Signature _____ Date _____

Witness _____ Date _____ Witness _____ Date _____

Notarization:

On this _____ day of _____ , in the year of _____ , personally appeared before me the person signing, known by me to be the person who completes this document and acknowledged it as his/ her free act and deed.

IN WITNESS WHEROF, I have set my hand and affixed my official seal in the Court of _____ ,

State of _____ , on the date written above.

Notary Public _____

Commission expires _____

FIGURE 17-2 Sample durable power of attorney. Reprinted with permission from the center for Practical Bioethics.

Continued

Healthcare Treatment Directive

■ *If you only want to name a Durable Power of Attorney for Healthcare Decisions, draw a large X through this page.*■

I, _____ , SS# _____ , want everyone who cares for me to know what
healthcare I want.   (optional)

I always expect to be given care and treatment for pain or discomfort even if such care may affect how I sleep, eat, or breathe.

I would consent to, and want my agent to consider my participation in federally regulated research related to my disorder or condition.

I want my doctor to try treatments/interventions on a time-limited basis when the goal is to restore my health or help me experience a life in a way consistent with my values and wishes. I want such treatments/interventions withdrawn when they cannot achieve this goal or become too burdensome to me.

I want my dying to be as natural as possible. Therefore, I direct that no treatment (including food or water by tube) be given just to keep my body functioning when I have

- • a condition that will cause me to die soon, or

- • a condition so bad (including substantial brain damage or brain disease) that I have no reasonable hope of achieving a quality of life that is acceptable to me.

An acceptable quality of life to me is one that includes the following capacities and values. (Describe here the things that are most important to you when you are making decisions to choose or refuse life-sustaining treatments.)

_____

_____

_____

_____

Examples:	• recognize family or friends	• make decisions	• communicate
	• feed myself	• take care of myself	• be responsive to my environment

If you do not agree with one or other of the above statements, draw a line through the statement and put your initials at the end of the end of the line.

In facing the end of my life, I expect my agent (if I have one) and my caregivers to honor my wishes, values, and directives. For further clarification, please refer to my *Caring Conversations* Workbook, which is located at _____ .

**Be sure to sign the reverse side of this page even if you do not wish
to appoint a Durable Power of Attorney for Healthcare Decisions**

Talk about this form and your ideas about your healthcare with the person you have chosen to make decisions for you, your doctors, family, friends, and clergy. Give each of them a completed copy.

You may cancel or change this form at any time. You should review it often. Each time you review it, put your initials and the date here. _____

This document is provided as a service by the Center for Practical Bioethics.
For more information, call the Center for Practical Bioethics at 816-221-1100
Email – *bioethic@practicalbioethics.org* • Website – *www.practicalbioethics.org*

FIGURE 17-2, cont'd

SUMMARY

As a nurse, you will be confronted with ethical and legal dilemmas throughout your career. The nature of these dilemmas will change as science and technology advance. It is important, however, to recognize that as a nurse and nurse leader, you are responsible for the following:

- Creating an ethically and legally principled environment.
- Upholding standards of conduct established by the profession.
- Being committed to bringing about any changes needed.
- Being dedicated to ethical and legal principles.

- Role-modeling the ethical, legal, and professional behavior of those working under your supervision; this governs:
  - Interactions with people requiring nursing care;
  - Responsibility for maintaining competence in nursing practice;
  - Responsibility for meeting the health needs of the public;
  - Maintaining cooperative relationships with members of the interdisciplinary health care team; and
  - Determining and implementing desirable standards of nursing practice and education (ICN International Code of Ethics for Nurses, cited in Little, 2003; Carroll, 2006).

CLINICAL CORNER

Nursing Role in Physician Orders for Life-Sustaining Treatment Discussion and Documentation

A daughter leaves her elderly mother sitting in a chair watching television when she goes to get her a glass of water to take her evening medications. She returns to find her mother slumped over in the chair. The daughter immediately calls 911 and holds her dying mother's hand waiting for help to arrive. The emergency medical technician (EMT) squad arrives and finds her mother to be pulseless and not breathing. They begin cardiopulmonary resuscitation (CPR), attach the automated external defibrillator (AED), and prepare to intubate. The daughter asks them to stop and informs them that her mother has an advance directive and her wishes are to not be resuscitated. The EMT requests a copy of her mother's POLST (Physician Orders for Lift-Sustaining Treatment). The daughter responds that she is not familiar with a POLST and that her mother does not have one. The EMT informs the daughter that in the absence of a POLST they must continue with the resuscitation efforts. Her mother is intubated and transferred to the hospital, where the efforts to revive her mother are not successful. The daughter is left knowing that her mother's wishes for end-of-life care had not been honored.

The POLST translates the client's end-of-life care wishes into a provider-ordered plan of medical care. Once completed, the POLST, unless amended, functions as standing provider orders to be followed regardless of the setting in which care is being provided. The POLST, as a component of advanced care planning, ensures that the wishes of the client concerning end-of-life care are honored.

Families are frequently unaware of their loved ones' wishes for end-of-life care. It is often difficult for clients and family members to think about dying as a loved one approaches the end of life. Many times the client is ready and interested, but the family is unwilling to engage in these important discussions. As difficult as these issues are to address, advanced care planning alleviates the need for care givers to make these decisions once the client no longer has the capacity to do so for themself. It ensures that the client's wishes are being followed in situations where family members are in disagreement regarding end-of-life care. The nurse can assist in facilitating these often-difficult conversations between the client and family. During these discussions the nurse educates the client and family on the purpose of the POLST, and how it relates to other advanced care-planning documents, such as a living will and advance directive, in ensuring that end-of-life care wishes are followed. At the conclusion of these discussions, if the client wishes to initiate a POLST, the nurse advocates on their behalf by relaying the client's request to discuss completing a POLST to their physician or advanced practice nurse, following whatever steps are necessary to aid in its completion.

The physician or advanced practice nurse discusses the various treatment options and their implications, and how they can best be tailored to meet the client's end-of-life care plan. A POLST is completed and signed by the provider and the client or designated health care representative. The POLST serves as the set of medical orders for

Continued

CLINICAL CORNER—cont'd

providing end-of-life care to the client and is considered to be valid provider orders across all settings.

When a client with a POLST presents for care to the emergency room (ER), the nurse informs the ER provider and other members of the health care team of its existence. The POLST is incorporated into the client's medical record and stands as client medical orders until the provider incorporates the POLST into the treatment plan for the client. This holds true even if the POLST is signed by a physician or advanced practice nurse not associated with the institution. It is preferred to have the original signed POLST as part of the medical record, but a photocopy of the document will be honored until the original can be produced. The original POLST is returned to the client upon discharge from the ER.

For the client admitted to the hospital, the nurse will enquire during the admission interview about the existence of a POLST. If it is determined that the client has a POLST, the nurse will obtain the POLST from the client and incorporate it into the hospital record. The nurse then communicates its existence to the attending physician or advanced practice nurse, as well as other members of the health care team. The POLST is followed as valid medical orders until the practitioner has incorporated the wishes expressed by the client in the POLST into the hospital plan of care. This holds true even if the POLST is signed by a physician or advanced practice nurse not associated with the institution. Although the provider orders should reflect the wishes expressed by the client in the POLST, they should be written in a manner that adheres to the institution's specific policies and procedures. Any decision by a provider to deviate from the orders set out in the POLST should be documented in the medical record. Any ethical concerns the nurse might have regarding the POLST orders should be directed to the appropriate institutional body for handling such matters, such as a hospital ethics committee. The POLST should be reviewed before discharge. If a change in the client's health status warrants it, the POLST can be amended and signed by the practitioner and the client or designated representative. At discharge the original copy of the POLST is returned to the client. If the client is being transported by emergency medical personnel to their home or to another institution, the nurse will inform the medical team of the existence of the POLST and ensure it is readily accessible to them in the transfer documents.

In the community setting, the nurse should advise the client to prominently display the POLST in a place in the home that can be readily seen by responding emergency personnel, such as on the refrigerator or on the wall above the bed. Clients in the community should be told to carry the POLST with them at all times when they leave their home. In situations that warrant it, the nurse should first administer the level of care as ordered by the POLST and then contact the physician or advanced practice nurse for further orders.

Una M. Doddy, RN, DNPc, MPH, MBA
Clinical Instructor of Nursing
Ramapo College of NJ

EVIDENCE-BASED PRACTICE

Abstract

Nursing turnover is a problem not only in the United States, but world-wide.

There is a direct correlation between a facility's ethical climate and the nurses' commitment. This study was to determine the correlation between nurses' perception of ethical climate and organizational commitment in teaching hospitals in the southeastern region of Iran. It was a descriptive study. The sample size was 275 nurses working in four teaching hospitals in the southeastern region of Iran. The Ethical Climate Questionnaire and the Organizational Commitment Questionnaire were used. The study found a positive correlation among professionalism, caring, rules, independence climate, and organizational commitment.

The nursing shortage exists in other countries, not just in the United States. This article is focused on the nursing shortage in Iran.

The importance of the study

There is no published research, before this study, to evaluate the correlation between ethical climate and nurses' organizational commitment.

Review of the literature

The authors reviewed a study by Tsai and Huang (2008) on Taiwanese nurses, a study by Filipova (2007), a study by Cullen et al. (2003), and a study by Shafer (2009).

EVIDENCE-BASED PRACTICE—cont'd

Organizational commitment

This is when an employee is positive about the institution where they work, accepting the values of the workplace and would like to remain an employee at the facility.

Ethical climate

Victor and Cullen state there are five distinct types of organizational ethical climate: caring, professionalism, rules, independence, and instrumental (Victor & Cullen, 1987).

Caring. A caring climate may be based on the utilitarianism ethical criterion in which the most important concern is what is best for others and people look out for each other's interests, while the primary goal is to offer the greatest good for the greatest number of people.

Professionalism. This dimension is related to the deontology ethical criterion. In this climate, the first consideration is whether a decision violates law and codes. People are expected to strictly follow legal or professional standards, and the law or ethical code of the profession is the major consideration. People are expected to comply with legal and professional standards over and above all other considerations.

Rules. The rules climate is related to the deontology ethical criterion. Based on this climate, it is very important to follow the organization's rules and procedures strictly, and everyone is expected to do so. People in facilities with this climate follow organization policies to the letter.

Independence. The independence dimension is associated with the deontology ethical criterion. In this climate people are expected to follow their own personal and moral beliefs. Each person decides for themselves what is right or wrong; in other words, people are guided by their own personal ethics.

Instrumental. This dimension is associated with the egoistic criterion, and its primary goal is to provide personal benefits. In this climate, people protect their own interests above all else and are mostly out for themselves.

Method

This was a descriptive analytical study done in 2011. The sample size was 88 people. It was then upgraded to include 185 people, then up to 300 people. The questionnaires were done.

Results

Some 275 nurses from city hospitals in the southeastern region of Iran participated in the study. It was found that the climate has a direct and significant correlation only with affective commitment. In addition a caring climate has a direct and significant correlation with affective and normative commitments. The same was also found to apply to a climate of independence. An instrumental climate has no significant correlation with affective commitment.

Discussion

The study found that there was a correlation between ethical climate and organizational commitment. Ethical climate causes employees to have a positive correlation with job satisfaction.

Conclusion

The results of this study showed a positive and significant correlation between hospital climate and organizational commitment of nurses.

References

Borhani, F., Jalali, T., Abbaszadeh, A., & Haghdoost, A. (2014). Nurses' Perception of Ethical Climate And Organizational Commitment. *Nursing Ethics*, *21*(3), 278–288.

Cullen, J. B., Parboteeah, K. P., & Victor, B. (2003). The effect of ethical climate on organizational commitment: A two study analysis. *Journal of Business Ethics*, *46*, 127–141.

Filipova, A. (2007). *Perceived organizational support and ethical work climates as predictors of turnover intention of licensed nurses in skilled nursing facilities*. Kalamazoo, MI. PhD Thesis, Western Michigan University.

Shafer, W. E. (2009). Ethical climate, organizational-professional conflict and organizational commitment: A study of Chinese auditors. *Accounting, Auditing & Accountability Journal*, *22*(7), 1087–1110.

Tsai, M. T., & Huang, C. C. (2008). The relationship among ethical climate types, facets of job satisfaction, and the three components of organizational commitment: A study of nurses in Taiwan. *Journal of Business Ethics*, *80*, 565–581.

Victor, B., & Cullen, J. B. (1987). A theory and measure of ethical climate in organizations. *Research in Corporate Social Performance & Policy*, *9*, 51–71.

NCLEX® EXAMINATION QUESTIONS

1. You are the nursing supervisor and there is a patient that will be going to the operating room for a kidney transplantation. It is the ultimate responsibility of _____to check and ensure that the organ donor and recipient are correct.
   A. Surgeon
   B. Anesthesiologist
   C. Registered nurse and surgeon
   D. Surgeon and anesthesiologist

2. Another name is added to the organ donation list every _____minutes
   A. 5
   B. 6
   C. 7
   D. 12

3. Issues that are commonly addressed by ethics committees are:
   A. End-of-life issues, organ donation, futility-of-care issues
   B. End-of-life issues, organ donation, change in the durable power of attorney
   C. Organ donation, futility-of-care issues, pediatric patient issues
   D. Organ donation, do not resuscitate order, Jehovah's Witness issues

4. The American Nurses Association approved the revised code of ethics in 2015. There are _____ codes.
   A. 9
   B. 10
   C. 12
   D. 20

5. What is the document that permits an individual to give a surrogate or proxy the authority to make decisions for that person in the event that they become incompetent?
   A. Living will
   B. Durable power of attorney for health care decisions
   C. Advance directive
   D. Informed consent

6. Duty to do good to others; to maintain a balance between benefits and harm; to provide all patients, including terminally ill, with caring attention; and to treat every patient with respect and courtesy. What is the requirement that care providers contribute to the health and welfare of the patient and not merely attempt to avoid harm to the patient or client?
   A. Beneficence
   B. Nonmaleficence
   C. Personal liability
   D. Corporate liability

7. Which of the following sets educational standards, examination requirements, and licensing requirements and regulates the nursing profession in each particular state?
   A. The National League for Nursing (NLN)
   B. Nurse practice acts
   C. State board of nursing
   D. The National Council of State Boards of Nursing

8. Hospitals are legally and ethically obligated to uphold patient rights, which include the right to:
   A. Review records; family can also review records
   B. Participate in treatment decisions and to provide consent to treatment
   C. Be informed of hospital bylaws and hospital attorneys' names and telephone numbers
   D. Expect reasonable care after hospitalization

9. The Organ Procurement and Transplantation Network (OPTN) is a(n)_____network.
   A. State
   B. Local
   C. National
   D. International

10. The difference between **bioethics** and **ethics** is:
   A. Bioethics is specific to health care; ethics deals with the principles of right and wrong.
   B. Bioethics is specific to health care; ethics deals with the principles of right and wrong, good and bad.
   C. Bioethics is specific to health care; ethics deals with the principles of right and wrong, good and bad with no issues of beliefs and values.
   D. Bioethics is specific to health care, ethics is the science that deals with the principles of right and wrong and of good and bad, and governs our relationships with others. It is based on personal beliefs and values.

Answers: 1. C   2. D   3. A   4. A   5. B   6. A   7. B   8. B   9. C   10. D

REFERENCES

Agich, G. J., & Younger, S. J. (1991). For experts only? Access to hospital ethics committees. *Hastings Center Report*, *21*(5), 17–25.

American Council on Transplantation. (2007). *Religious concerns about transplantation*. www.sharenj.org/religiou.html.

American Hospital Association. (2015). *Patient bill of rights*. www.aha.org/content/00-10/pcp_english_030730.pdf.

American Nurses Association. (2015). *Code of ethics for nurses with interpretive statements*. Silver Spring, MD: American Nurses Publishing. www.nursingworld.org/ethics/chcode.htm.

American Transplant Foundation Transplant Facts and Myths. (2014). www.americantransplantfoundation.org/about-transplant/facts-and-myths/.

Carroll, P. (2006). *Nursing leadership and management: A practical guide*. Clifton Park, NY: Delmar Thomson Learning.

Dalgo, J. T., & Anderson, F. (1995). Notes from the field: Developing a hospital ethics committee. *Nursing Management*, *26*(9), 104–106.

DeLaune, S. C., & Ladner, P. K. (2002). *Fundamentals of Nursing*. Clifton Park, NJ: Delmar Thomson Learning.

Grohar-Murray, M. E., & Langan, N. (2011). *Leadership and management in nursing* (3rd ed.). Upper Saddle River, NJ: Prentice Hall.

International Council of Nurses [ICN]. (2006). *The ICN code of ethics*. Geneva: Switzerland.

International Council of Nurses [ICN]. (2009). www.icn.ch/icncode.pdf, www.icn.ch/ethics.htm.

Kelly-Heidenthal, P. (2004). *Essentials of nursing leadership and management*. Clifton Park, NY: Thomson Delmar Learning, 295.

Little, C. (2003). Ethical dimensions of patient care. In P. Kelly-Heidenthal (Ed.), *Nursing leadership and management* (pp. 266–279). Clifton Park, NY: Thomson Delmar Learning.

Memorial Sloan Kettering. (2015). Standard of care pain management. http://prc.coh.org/html/standard%20of%20care-Memorial%20Sloan.asp.

Nathanson, M. (1996). *Home Health Care Law Manual*. Gaithersberg, MD: Aspen Publishers.

National Council of State Boards of Nursing. (2014). *A nurse's guide to social media*. www.ncsbn.org/NCSBN_SocialMedia.pdf.

New Jersey Sharing Network. Health care professionals. (2014a). www.sharenj.org/.

New Jersey Sharing Network. Fast Facts. (2014b). http://www.sharenj.org/fastfacts.htm.

NJ Hospital Association. (2014). *POLST*. www.njha.com/media/201361/POLSTWhite.pdf.

Rowland, H., & Rowland, B. (1997). *Nursing administration handbook* (4th ed.). Gaithersberg, MD: An Aspen Publication, Aspen Publishers, Inc.

Rundio, A., & Wilson, V. (2013). *Nurse executive review and resource manual*. Silver Spring, MD: ANCC.

Schroeder, S. (1995). Cost containment in US healthcare. *Academic Medicine*, *70*, 861–866.

Stecher, J. (2008). Allow natural death vs. do not resuscitate. *American Journal of Nursing*, *108*, 11.

Sullivan, E., & Decker, P. (2009). *Effective leadership and management in nursing*. Upper Saddle River, NJ: Prentice Hall.

The Joint Commission. (2014). *Comprehensive accreditation manual*. Oakbrook Terrace, IL: Author.

Tomey, A. M. (2004). *Guide to nursing management and leadership* (7th ed.). St. Louis: Mosby, 75.

US Legal Definitions. (2008). *Good Samaritan laws & legal definition*. Retrieved from http://definitions.uslegal.com/g/good-samaritans/.

WEBSITES

www.nursingworld.org
www.jointcommission.org/
www.optn.org/
www.organdonor.gov/
www.ncsbn.org

SECTION 4

New Knowledge, Innovations, and Improvements

SECTION OUTLINE

Magnet-recognized institutions conscientiously integrate evidence-based practice and research into clinical and operational processes. There are established evolving programs related to evidence-based practices, and research that supports and improves practice. Such work environments continually support the advancement of patient care and the clinical inquiry of the nurses supporting high-quality patient care.

Innovations in patient care, nursing, and the practice environment are the hallmark of organizations receiving Magnet recognition. Establishing new ways of achieving the triple aim of the Institute of Medicine (IOM) high-quality patient-centered, effective and efficient care is the outcome of transformational leadership, empowering structures and processes, and exemplary professional practice in nursing.

This section will deal with the outcomes of practice environments that support quality care. It will deal with the responsibility of the nurse in the continuing improvements in practice, the use of evidence in delivery of care, and the nursing role in research.

18

Improving Organizational Performance

OBJECTIVES

- Identify the key focus of performance improvement.
- Discuss trends in quality improvement.
- List three drivers of quality.
- Outline two models of performance improvement.
- Identify three clinical outcome measures.
- Identify major patient safety goals.
- Describe four nursing outcomes specific to desired specialty.
- Relate a clinical activity to a performance model.

OUTLINE

KEY TERMS

lean management performance improvement model dealing with minimization of waste in processes.

National Patient Safety Goals set of nationwide goals set by The Joint Commission, to focus performance in areas of patient safety.

outcome measurable result related to a strategic objective.

retrospective review analysis of past events, usually through a chart audit.

risk management organized program to prevent the incidence of preventable accidents, injuries, and errors.

root-cause analysis retrospective review of the event, to evaluate potential causes of the problem or sources of variation in the process.

sentinel event unexpected occurrence involving death or serious physical or psychological injury.

Six Sigma performance improvement model based on the idea of minimal defects and concerns.

IMPROVING ORGANIZATIONAL PERFORMANCE

The year 1998 was pivotal in the quest for improvement in health care. In that year, the Institute of Medicine (IOM) issued a report, To Err Is Human: Building a Safer Health System, detailing the problem of medical errors in health care. The Advisory Commission on Consumer Protection and Quality also released a report calling for a national commitment to improve quality, concluding that "there is no guarantee that any individual will receive high quality care for any particular health problem … the health care industry is plagued … with errors in health care" (Advisory Commission on Consumer Protection and Quality, 1998). It was found that these quality concerns occur typically because of ways in which care is organized. Health care organizations were challenged to ensure that services were safe, effective, patient-centered, timely, efficient, and equitable.

Performance improvement (PI) has been shown to be a powerful tool to help health care organizations become safer and more efficient and patient-centered. Total quality management (TQM), which is also referred to as PI or quality improvement (QI), has been used in industry since the 1950s, and has been related to improvements in productivity and quality.

HISTORICAL PERSPECTIVES

In the 1950s, the Joint Commission on Accreditation of Healthcare Organizations was formed, and the evaluation of care delivered in health care institutions began. During the 1960s, the American Nurses Association began to develop standards of nursing practice, which became the basis for early quality assurance (QA) programs. In the 1970s, the U.S. Congress established Professional Standards Review Organizations (PSROs) to review the quality and cost of care delivered to Medicare and Medicaid recipients. QA required audits of care. These audits measured basic compliance, emphasizing what was done "wrong," but did little to advance a philosophy of learning from performance.

Health care costs became a major issue in the 1980s, and society began to question the efficiency and effectiveness of health care (Phelps, 1997). Health care administrators turned to industry for lessons learned in managing efficiency. Industry had adopted quality management techniques in the 1950s. An early proponent was W. Edwards Deming, who worked with the Japanese automotive industry after World War II. His 14-point management philosophy is the underpinning of TQM. The 14 points follow:

1. Create constancy of purpose toward improvement of product and service, with the aim to become competitive and to stay in business, and to provide jobs.
2. Adopt the new philosophy. We are in a new economic age. Western management must awaken to the challenge, must learn their responsibilities, and take on leadership for change.
3. Cease dependence on inspection to achieve quality. Eliminate the need for inspection on a mass basis by building quality into the product in the first place.
4. End the practice of awarding business on the basis of price tag. Instead, minimize total cost. Move toward a single supplier for any one item, on a long-term relationship of loyalty and trust.
5. Improve constantly and forever the system of production and service, to improve quality and productivity, and thus constantly decrease costs.
6. Institute training on the job.
7. Institute leadership. The aim of supervision should be to help people and machines and gadgets to do a better job. Supervision of management is in need of an overhaul, as well as supervision of production workers.
8. Drive out fear, so that everyone may work effectively for the company.
9. Break down barriers between departments. People in research, design, sales, and production must work as a team, to foresee problems of production and in use that may be encountered with the product or service.
10. Eliminate slogans, exhortations, and targets for the workforce asking for zero defects and new levels of productivity. Such exhortations only create adversarial relationships, as the bulk of the causes of low quality and low productivity belong to the system and thus lie beyond the power of the work force.
11. a. Eliminate work standards (quotas) on the factory floor. Substitute leadership.
    b. Eliminate management by objective. Eliminate management by numbers, numerical goals. Substitute leadership.
12. a. Remove barriers that rob hourly paid workers of their right to pride in workmanship. The responsibility of supervisors must be changed from sheer numbers to quality.
    b. Remove barriers that rob people in management and engineering of their right to pride in workmanship. This means, abolishment of the annual or merit rating and management by objective.
13. Institute a vigorous program of education and self-improvement.

14. Put everybody in the company to work to accomplish the transformation. The transformation is everybody's job (Deming, 2000a).

Deming believed that an industry consists of multiple processes and decisions, which are interrelated, and developed a "system of profound knowledge" (Deming, 2000b):

- All work consists of multiple processes.
- Differences in work are the result of the system of work, not individual worker performance.
- New work designs are based on our understanding of how work processes relate to one another.
- An understanding of what motivates people.

His model for improvement was the PDCA (Plan–Do–Check–Act) cycle, which remains in widespread use today. Juran (1989) elaborated on Deming's work in TQM. He believed that quality "did not happen by accident," but was the result of a quality trilogy: planning, control, and improvement. In 1960, Crosby defined quality as the extent to which processes were in conformance with the requirements of the customer. He was known for believing that things should be done "right the first time" and for the philosophy of "zero defects" (Nielsen et al., 2004). Although these three proponents of quality improvement focused on work processes, Donabedian (1992) contributed the idea of outcome as part of the overall quality structure. Outcomes involve the results achieved, and they reflect the effectiveness of the process components. This outcomes focus allows institutions to measure themselves against the standards and the competition. A compendium of past and present quality terms is presented in Table 18-1.

KEY FOCUS OF PERFORMANCE IMPROVEMENT

This focus on outcomes has moved health care from a compliance model toward one of "best practice." Although accrediting bodies and federal regulators set minimum standards of compliance, many hospitals are now moving toward a model of "best in class." Examples of organizations that recognize such "best practice" are the American Nurses Association and its Magnet Award for Nursing, and the Malcolm Baldrige National Quality Award for performance excellence. Hospitals winning the Magnet Award can be accessed at: www.nursecredentialing.org/findamagnethospital. aspx. The hospitals that have been recognized by

TABLE 18-1 Past, Present, and Evolving Quality Terms

Past Quality Terms	Present Quality Terms	Evolving Quality Terms
Quality control	Total quality management	Quality management
Quality assurance	Continuous quality improvement	Quality improvement
		Performance improvement
		Performance excellence
		Outcomes performance
		Value added performance

Adapted from Yoder-Wise, P. (2003). *Leading and managing in nursing* (p. 175). St. Louis: Mosby.

receiving the Malcolm Baldrige National Quality Award can be accessed at: http://patapsco.nist.gov/Award_Recipients/index.cfm.

The key focus of PI includes:

- Meeting and exceeding the needs of the customer/stakeholder.
- Building organizational learning into each work process.
- Continually evaluating and improving work processes.
- Assessing all customer requirements and needs.
- Being data driven.
- Continually looking at current performance.
- Constantly striving to "do it better."

It is vital to remember that all PI must be "data driven" and not based on anecdote.

DRIVERS OF QUALITY

The key focus of the quality movement is meeting the needs of the customer. In organizations striving for "best practice," this may mean exceeding the needs of the customer. According to the IOM (1998) the key Domains of Quality are effectiveness, efficiency, equity, patient-centeredness, safety, and timeliness. The Institute for Healthcare Improvement's triple aim focuses on improving the patient experience of care (including quality and satisfaction); improving the health of populations; and reducing the per capita cost of health care (2015).

Obviously, the key customers of health care are the patient and family; they are at the center of all drivers of quality. Other customers of the hospital include the physicians and the community. North Mississippi Health System defines patients and families as their key customers. They identify their key stakeholders as the members of the community, the active and referring physicians, local employers, and third party payers. The key requirements of these customers and stakeholders are listed in Table 18-2.

What is important is that each set of customers have specific requirements that need to be met by the health care organization. The degree to which these key requirements are met forms a base for the patient satisfaction measures of the institution. Other customers include regulators, partners, and payers.

Quality outcomes also are a key requirement of the patient and the community. How do hospitals measure quality outcomes? There are a variety of means.

OUTCOME MEASURES

The key to PI is the "result" of all actions taken to improve patient care. Although it is important to "do

what we say we do," it is more important to "do it well." So just how well do we deliver patient care?

Patient care units have an abundance of data available to them. One common outcome used by patient care units is patient satisfaction. A majority of health care organizations across the United States measure patient satisfaction. Two of the common vendor satisfaction measures are Press Ganey and Gallup. These data can be segmented to list the performance of specific units/shifts. The key requirements of the patient/family at North Mississippi Health System are listed in Figure 18-1. They were identified as provision of quality care, being nice, no waiting, and low cost. The key requirements of other stakeholders are also listed.

Patient satisfaction surveys are customized to include information on the key requirements of the patients of an institution. With the use of nationwide surveys, hospitals can compare their performance with that of other local hospitals, of similar hospitals, and of best-in-class performers. Figure 18-2 provides an example of a patient satisfaction data set. This graph shows that from 2009 to 2011 in six of the health

TABLE 18-2   Key Customer and Stakeholder Groups and Requirements

Group	Requirements	Outcome Measure *
Customer group: Patients (including families)	Provide me with quality care	Various outcome measures, mortality rates, time on ventilator post-coronary artery bypass grafting (CABG), guidelines for stroke management, inpatient core measures, etc.
	Be nice to me	Patient satisfaction measures
	Don't keep me waiting	Emergency services wait time
	And be low cost	Labor costs, cost of care
Stakeholder groups: Community (health and wellness)	Provide me with community health programs	Proactive community prevention and wellness results, outpatient diabetes management outcomes
	And teach me more about nutrition and obesity	NMHS (Nursing, Midwifery and Health Systems) health plan cholesterol levels
Active and referring medical staff	Provide high-quality care to my patients	Quality of care outcomes
	Collaborate with me	Physician satisfaction
	Make it easy for me to practice/refer	Physician satisfaction
Local employers and 3rd party payers	Provide me with easy access to quality and cost-effective health care/plan solutions	Community health assessment indicator, not-for-profit health care ratings,

*For specific measures, see application section 7.
From North Mississippi Health System. (2012). Baldrige Application.
http://patapsco.nist.gov/Award_Recipients/PDF_Files/2012_North_MS_Application_Summary.pdf.

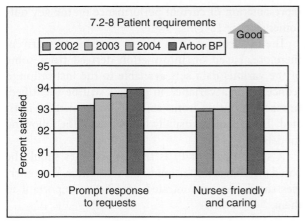

FIGURE 18-1 North Mississippi Health System. (2012). Baldrige Application figure 7.2-7 http://patapsco.nist.gov/Award_Recipients/PDF_Files/2012_North_MS_Application_Summary.pdf page 45 our nurses validate that PEOPLE who provide a caring culture is a distinctive CC (core competency). Our nurses consistently score above the national and state TOP BOX comparisons.

facilities of the North Mississippi Health System, patients felt that "nurses always communicated well" at a rate above the top box state mean and national top box national mean.

Other data sets available to the nurse include the National Database of Nursing Quality Indicators (NDNQI), a program of the American Nurses Association National Center for Nursing Quality. The database collects and evaluates unit-specific and nurse-sensitive data from hospitals in the United States and internationally. Participating facilities receive unit-level comparative data reports to use for QI purposes. Nursing-sensitive indicators reflect the structure, process, and outcomes of nursing care (Box 18-1) (American Nurses Association, 2013).

Nurses will need to know outcomes that directly affect their unit. Common outcomes for all units are infection rates, patient satisfaction, and performance on The Joint Commission (TJC)'s Core Measures. The core measures are specific to the unit, so it is important to know which measure or indicator reflects your

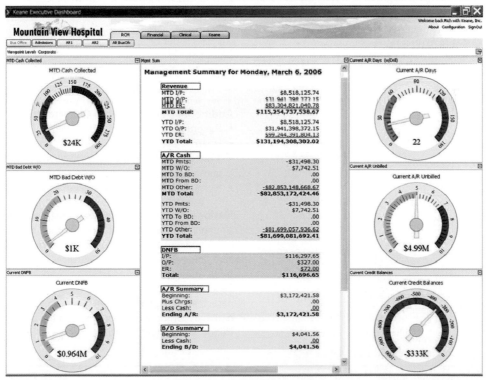

FIGURE 18-2 Scorecard. Clinical Dashboard Metrics. www.dashboardzone.com/hospital-dashboard-clinical-dashboard-metrics.

unit and your level of performance. The initial core measures include heart failure, acute myocardial infarction, pneumonia, surgical infection, and pregnancy. Others measures are pain management and children's asthma care. Participating hospitals collect data related to their performance on the specific measures, and these measures are then reported to TJC. This data set allows for nationwide comparison on performance. TJC's Core Measures are available at: www.jointcommission.org/PerformanceMeasurement/PerformanceMeasurement/default.htm.

There are also a wide variety of other outcomes that are used by hospitals, and they include financial measures (e.g., cash on hand, market share, and length of stay), human resource measures (e.g., employee satisfaction and productivity), and ethical measures (e.g., community service and financial audits). Hospitals determine the outcomes to be used as part of the strategic planning process. Reporting of the identified outcomes often occurs via a scorecard, which gives a visual representation of current performance on the key outcomes (Figure 18-2).

The first rule of PI is that it must be data driven; therefore, based on information derived from some of the various data sets available to the institution, a "concern" or a variance in process will be identified. In reaction to this "concern," a PI project will be initiated. These projects usually follow one of the following models.

A second rule of PI is that PI activities should be based on what is important to the customers. Your energies should be concentrated on what is important to them.

MODELS OF QUALITY

FOCUS Method
F: Focus on an opportunity for improvement.
O: Organize a team involved with the process.
C: Clarify the current process.

BOX 18-1 Menu of Indicators Currently Being Collected

The menu of indicators currently being collected:
- Nursing hours per patient day (NHPPD) NQF
  - Registered nurses (RN) hours per patient day
  - Licensed practical/vocational nurses (LPN/LVN) hours per patient day
  - Unlicensed assistive personnel (UAP) hours per patient day
- Nursing turnover
- Nosocomial infections NQF
- Patient falls NQF
- Patient falls with injury NQF
  - Injury level
- Pressure ulcer rate
  - Community-acquired
  - Hospital-acquired
  - Unit-acquired
- Pediatric pain assessment, intervention, reassessment (AIR) cycle
- Pediatric peripheral intravenous infiltration
- Psychiatric physical/sexual assault
- RN education/certification
- RN survey
  - Job satisfaction scales
  - Practice environment scale (PES) NQF

- Restraints NQF
- Staff mix NQF
  - RN
  - LPN/LVNs
  - UAP
  - Percent agency staff

Additional Data Elements Collected
- Patient population; adult or pediatric.
- Hospital category, e.g., teaching, nonteaching, etc.
- Type of unit (critical care, step-down, medical, surgical, combined med-surgical, rehabilitation, & psychiatric).
- Number of staffed beds designated by the hospital

National Comparison Groups and Reports
National comparison data for the indicators are grouped based on patient (adult/pediatric) and unit type: critical care, step-down, medical, surgical, combined med-surgical, rehabilitation, psychiatric, and staffed bed size. Teaching and Magnet status is identified as it relates to participating hospitals. The quarterly reports provide the national comparison along with unit performance data trended over eight quarters.

American Nurses Association. (2013). Nursing sensitive indicators.
www.nursingworld.org/MainMenuCategories/ThePracticeofProfessionalNursing/PatientSafetyQuality/Research-Measurement/The-National-Database/Nursing-Sensitive-Indic August 16, 2014. ators_1.

U: Understand the causes of variation in the process.

S: Based on evidence, Select the improvement.

Plan–Do–Study–Act (PDSA) Cycle

This model is based on Deming's PDCA model that was discussed earlier.

Plan: Plan a change, with activity aimed at improvement.

Do: Carry it out.

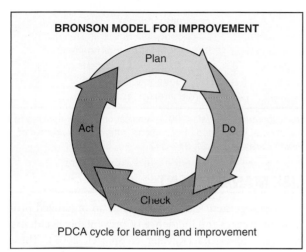

BRONSON MODEL FOR IMPROVEMENT

Plan

Act

Do

Check

PDCA cycle for learning and improvement

FIGURE 18-3 PDCA model. Bronson Methodist Hospital. (2007). Baldrige application. http://baldrige.nist.gov/PDF_files/Bronson_Methodist_Hospital_Application_Summary.pdf.

Check/Study: Study the results: what happened? What did you learn? Did the change work?

Act: Adopt the change; rework the change.

Many organizations combine these models into a PDCA-FOCUS model (Figure 18-3).

As organizations have matured in the PI journey, a new process, Six Sigma, is being used in conjunction with PDSA. The objective of Six Sigma quality is to reduce process variation to no more than 3.4 "defects" per 1 million. DMAIC (define, measure, analyze, improve and control) is the acronym used in Six Sigma. It is a data-driven quality strategy for improving processes (Box 18-2).

EVIDENCE-BASED PRACTICE

This model describes the integration of research evidence with clinical experience to improve outcomes. The process for evidence-based practice includes (Sackett et al, 2000) the following:

- Formulation of a question from current clinical concerns.
- Access of relevant research.
- Analysis of the evidence using established criteria.
- Plan change in practice.
- Implement change in practice.
- Evaluate results.

BOX 18-2 Six Sigma: DMAIC

Define the customer, their critical to quality (CTQ) issues, and the core business process involved.
- Define who the customers are, their requirements for products and services, and their expectations.
- Define project boundaries; the stop and start of the process.
- Define the process to be improved by mapping the process flow.

Measure the performance of the core business process involved.
- Develop a data collection plan for the process.
- Collect data from many sources to determine types of defects and metrics.
- Compare to customer survey results to determine shortfall.

Analyze the data collected and process map to determine root causes of defects, and opportunities for improvement.

- Identify gaps between current performance and goal performance.
- Prioritize opportunities to improve.
- Identify sources of variation.

Improve the target process by designing creative solutions to fix and prevent problems.
- Create innovative solutions using technology and discipline.
- Develop and deploy implementation plan.

Control the improvements to keep the process on the new course.
- Prevent reverting back to the "old way."
- Require the development, documentation, and implementation of an ongoing monitoring plan.
- Institutionalize the improvements through the modification of systems and structures (staffing, training, incentives).

Six Sigma is a registered trademark and service mark of Motorola, Inc.

As a nurse, you will be asked to participate in process improvement teams. These teams are usually formed in reaction to a "concern" or variance in a process. These teams are usually interdisciplinary in nature and form the "O" of the PDCA-FOCUS model. You will receive team-based education as you join the team. You will also receive "just in time" training on the multiple data collection methods used by improvement teams. These include Pareto analysis, surveys, audits, cost-benefit analysis, decision matrix, and fishbone diagram. Some teams will have a certified Six Sigma member who is responsible for data interpretation. As you mature in improvement, you will receive education specific to the institution's model.

LEAN CULTURE

The underlying principle of "lean" is that all processes contain waste. Womack and Jones (2003) define **lean** as a "way to do more and more with less and less—less human effort, less equipment, less time, and less space—while coming closer to providing customers with what they want" (p. 15).

One of the challenges of implementing lean in health care is that it requires people to identify waste in the work in which they are so invested (Table 18-3). All workers want to feel their work is valuable, perhaps most especially health care workers. Recognizing that much about their daily tasks is wasteful and does not add value can be difficult for health care professionals. A nurse who is hunting for supplies is doing it to serve the needs of patients. Nurses may not see this as wasted time and may not stop to wonder why those supplies aren't where they need them every time they need them. But if the supplies were always readily available, the time nurses spend hunting for them would instead be devoted to something more appropriate to their skills and expertise (Miller, 2005, p. 8).

TABLE 18-3   Value and Waste Examples in Health Care

Lean thinking	Health care
Value adding time	Diagnostic and care time
	Diagnostic time (collecting and analyzing clinical information)
	Active care time (clinical interventions)
	Passive care time (under observation, no interventions)
Nonvalue adding time (waste)	Diagnostic and care time
	Superfluous time (not needed diagnostics, observations or interventions)
	Administrative time

From Joosten, T., et al., (2009). Application of lean thinking to health care: Issues and observations. *International Journal of Health Care Quality, 21,* 341–347.

RISK MANAGEMENT

Risk management can be defined as an organized program to prevent the incidence of preventable accidents, injuries, and errors (Kavaler & Spiegel, 2003). These errors, accidents, and injuries incur unintended cost to the institution, and the risk management department is charged with defining the situations that place the health care institution at risk.

The **National Patient Safety Goals** further emphasize the importance of the risk management function (Box 18-3). These goals were formed based on the Institute of Medicine (IOM) 1998 report. This is a nationwide initiative with an overall goal of making specific improvements in patient safety of hospitals across the nation. The goals highlight problem areas and focus on system-wide solutions.

BOX 18-3   National Patient Safety Goals (2013)

1. Improve the Accuracy of Patient Identification.
Use at least two patient identifiers when providing care, treatment, or services.

Rationale:
Wrong-patient errors occur in virtually all stages of diagnosis and treatment. The intent for this goal is two-fold: first, to reliably identify the individual as the person for whom the service or treatment is intended; second, to match the service or treatment to that individual. Acceptable identifiers may be the individual's name, an assigned identification number, telephone number, or other person-specific identifier.

2. Improve the Effectiveness of Communication Among Caregivers.
Report critical results of tests and diagnostic procedures on a timely basis.

Rationale:
Critical results of tests and diagnostic procedures fall significantly outside the normal range and may indicate a life-threatening situation. The objective is to provide the responsible licensed caregiver these results within an established time frame so that the patient can be promptly treated.

BOX 18-3 National Patient Safety Goals (2013)—cont'd

3. Improve the Safety of Using Medications

Label all medications, medication containers, and other solutions on and off the sterile field in perioperative and other procedural settings. Note: Medication containers include syringes, medicine cups, and basins.

Rationale:

Medications or other solutions in unlabeled containers are unidentifiable. Errors, sometimes tragic, have resulted from medications and other solutions removed from their original containers and placed into unlabeled containers. This unsafe practice neglects basic principles of safe medication management, yet it is routine in many organizations. The labeling of all medications, medication containers, and other solutions is a risk-reduction activity consistent with safe medication management. This practice addresses a recognized risk point in the administration of medications in perioperative and other procedural settings.

4. Reduce the Risk of Health Care–Associated Infections.

Comply with either the current Centers for Disease Control and Prevention (CDC) hand hygiene guidelines, or the current World Health Organization (WHO) hand hygiene guidelines.

Rationale:

According to the CDC, each year millions of people acquire an infection when receiving care, treatment, and services in a health care organization. Consequently, health care–associated infections (HAIs) are a patient safety issue affecting all types of health care organizations. One of the most important ways to address HAIs is by improving the hand hygiene of health care staff. Compliance with the WHO or CDC hand hygiene guidelines will reduce the transmission of infectious agents by staff to patients, thereby decreasing the incidence of HAIs.

5. The Hospital Identifies Safety Risks Inherent in its Patient Population.

Identify patients at risk for suicide.

Rationale:

Suicide of a patient when in a staffed, round-the-clock care setting is a frequently reported type of sentinel event. Identification of individuals at risk for suicide while under the care of or following discharge from a health care organization is an important step in protecting these at-risk individuals.

6. Introduction to the Universal Protocol for Preventing Wrong Site, Wrong Procedure, and Wrong Person Surgery

The Universal Protocol applies to all surgical and nonsurgical invasive procedures. Evidence indicates that procedures that place the patient at the most risk include those that involve general anesthesia or deep sedation, although other procedures may also affect patient safety. Hospitals can enhance safety by correctly identifying the patient, the appropriate procedure, and the correct site of the procedure.

The Universal Protocol is based on the following principles:
- Wrong-person, wrong-site, and wrong-procedure surgery can and must be prevented.
- A robust approach using multiple, complementary strategies is necessary to achieve the goal of always conducting the correct procedure on the correct person, at the correct site.
- Active involvement and use of effective methods to improve communication among all members of the procedure team are important for success.
- To the extent possible, the patient, and as needed, the family are involved in the process.
- Consistent implementation of a standardized protocol is most effective in achieving safety.

Universal protocol requires the following:
1. Conduct a pre-procedure verification process.
2. Mark the procedure site.
3. A time-out is performed before the procedure.

2013 Joint Commission National Patient Safety Goals.
www.spectrumhealth.com/shr_providers/education/SHR_Ed/2013_Joint Commission.pdf August 16, 2014; or www.jointcommission.org/assets/1/6/2014_HAP_NPSG_E.pdf

Many health care institutions have integrated the risk management and PI activities. This relates to the process management nature of the risk management function. For example, Goal 2 (improve staff communication) integrates activities of both a risk management department and PI. Lessons are being learned from the aviation and race car industries in the area of handoffs, and processes are being designed to further enhance patient safety and reduce adverse events. The risk management department also investigates all identified accidents, injuries, errors, and adverse events. TJC requires all health care institutions to report sentinel events. A sentinel event is:
- An unexpected occurrence involving death or serious physical or psychological injury, or the risk thereof.

BOX 18-4   Patient Handoffs

Patient handoffs occur thousands of times a day in hospitals. Patients are transferred from unit to unit, brought to surgery, from surgery to the post-anesthetic care unit (PACU), and from PACU transferred to a unit. Many handoffs go off without a hitch, but devastating mistakes can happen during any of them.

"If you transfer a patient to the intensive care unit (ICU) after surgery and the ventilator isn't ready, you're really riding on the edge" of patient safety, says Allan Goldman, head of the pediatric intensive care unit at Great Ormond Street Hospital and a chief architect of the hospital's collaboration with Ferrari.

A 2005 study in *The Wall Street Journal* found that nearly 70% of all preventable hospital mishaps occurred because of communication problems, and that many of these breakdowns occur during patient handoffs.

In 2003, the surgeons at London's Great Ormond Street Hospital noted the efficiency of the pit stops of the Ferrari race car team, and concluded that patient handovers were haphazard in comparison. The physicians traveled to Italy to meet with individuals at Ferrari headquarters and began to incorporate some of the lessons learned in their own processes. For instance, in a Formula One race, the "lollipop man" (with the paddle) ushers the car in and signals the driver when it is safe to go; it is not always clear in the hospital who is in charge.

Back in London, the physicians also sought the advice of two jumbo jet pilots and wrote a seven-page protocol for patient handoffs. After numerous improvements and changes, "information handover omissions" fell 49%, and the number of technical errors fell 42%.

From Naik, G. (2006, November). Hospital races to learn lessons of Ferrari crew. *The Wall Street Journal.*

Serious injury specifically includes loss of limb or function. The phrase "or the risk thereof" includes any process variation for which a recurrence would carry a significant chance of a serious adverse outcome.

- Such events are called "sentinel" because they signal the need for immediate investigation and response.
- The terms "sentinel event" and "medical error" are not synonymous; not all sentinel events occur because of an error, and not all errors result in sentinel events.

When a sentinel event is identified, a root-cause analysis is performed by a team that includes those directly involved in the process. This **root-cause analysis** is a **retrospective review** of the event, to evaluate potential causes of the problem or sources of variation in the process. In a root-cause analysis of the "hand off" procedure in the discussion of hand offs (Box 18-4), it was found that there was no systemized process for the hand off and that multiple failures of communication occurred because of this lack of process. This process was then changed and evaluated, and the outcomes were positive.

The major outcome of PI is the creation of a learning organization (Baldrige, 2014, p. 2). This means that learning:

- Is a regular part of daily work.
- Is practiced at personal, unit, and organizational levels.
- Results in solving problems at their source ("root cause").
- Is focused on building and sharing knowledge throughout the organization.
- Is driven by opportunities to affect significant, meaningful change.

This is the outcome of institution-wide PI.

SUMMARY

Nurses and organization administrators should continually learn from their performance. Health care organizations have a long history of collecting information on performance, but in the past 10 years, the emphasis on performance has changed as the health care environment has become more competitive. TJC requires organizations to collect information on the Core Measures and to determine how the individual hospital is performing. Nurses should know the levels of performance based on actual data. These results may be shown in dashboard form to allow the reader to make a quick determination of performance to target based on color. The use of data for PI is one means of continually learning about one's performance and making improvements based on reviews of performance. As a new nurse, it will be important to realize that as nurses in clinical practice, the review of data provides the opportunity to improve our practice to better meet the needs of the patient.

CLINICAL CORNER

Health care is evolving and more challenging with advanced technology, electronic documentation, regulatory requirements, and increased public reporting of quality information, transparency, and hospital penalties for poor outcomes.

Nurses are faced with increasing demands to participate in a variety of quality performance activities within a hospital setting. A hospital's culture determines the magnitude of initiatives for quality improvement and the role of a nurse. New graduates are faced with challenges in learning to be a patient advocate, a team player, and communicator to ensure the voice of the patient is heard. Since nurses are the essential care givers in the hospital, they can profoundly influence the quality of care provided, in addition to patient outcomes. Subsequently, the pursuit of providing high-quality care is dependent on the commitment and critical thinking of a nurse.

Nurses are a safety net to prevent real time medication errors by following the seven rights to medication administration; prevent falls by ensuring an accurate risk assessment is completed, and the environment is evaluated for safety; and assessing the integrity of the patient's skin to prevent and/or identify pressure ulcers, which can ultimately lead to an infection, complications, and impact patient outcomes. Hand off communication is critical in the health care arena between all direct care providers, the patient, and family to ensure that safe, evidence-based care is delivered to every patient. Health care is challenging and as a nurse we took an oath to be a "patient advocate." Florence Nightingale once said, "For the sick it is important to have the best."

Florence Nightingale: Examination for Inquiry on Scutari (20 Feb 1855). In Great Britain Parliament, Report upon the State of the Hospitals of the British Army in Crimea and Scutari, House of Commons Papers (1855), Vol. 33 of Sess 1854-55, 343. Science quotes on:| Best (42) | Importance (106) | Sick (6)

Terri Szucs, MSN, RN, CPHQ
Director of Quality, St. Joseph's Regional Medical Center
Paterson, NJ

EVIDENCE-BASED PRACTICE

Hostetter, M., Klein, S. (2011). Using Patient-Reported Outcomes to Improve Health Care Quality. *Quality Matters*, December/January

Quality Matters offers reports on emerging models and trends in health care quality improvement and interviews with leaders in the field.

This report addresses patient-reported outcomes measures (PROMs). It discusses that PROMs are a critical component of assessing whether clinicians are improving the health of patients. PROMs evaluate whether or not the services provided improved patients' health and sense of well-being. An example is patients are asked to assess their general health, ability to complete various activities, mood, level of fatigue, and pain.

The ultimate measure of health system performance is whether or not it helps people recover from an acute illness, live well with a chronic condition, and face the end of life with dignity. The only way to obtain this information is to ask the patients.

The future is patient-reported measures to evaluate performance and effectiveness of treatments. The Department of Health and Human Services Office of the National Coordinator for Health and Human Services Office of the National Coordinator for Health Information Technology plans to incorporate PROMs into standards.

In the United States PROMs are in the early stages of development for use in clinical practice. PROMs used at Dartmouth-Hitchcock Medical Center's Spine Center have been collecting data since 1997, using a survey with questions about health and well-being.

PROMs are used at the University of Pittsburgh Medical Center (UPMC). The tool has been useful to help clinicians identify patients with depression, and older adults with mobility limitations.

Obstacles to PROMs are that its use is not widespread in the United States, time spent is not billable, and providers may not see the value of implementation of them.

To have PROMs more widely used, the computer-generated surveys must be easy for the patient to understand.

Future PROM development is expected to build on the National Institutes of Health's Patient Reported Outcomes Measurement Information System. This is a program begun in 2004 that allows clinicians, researchers, and patients together to define and validate PROMs

Continued

for care of patients with human immunodeficiency virus (HIV), cancer, and disabilities. The different domains looked at were pain, fatigue, depression, and social or physical functioning.

Dewalt is testing the Patient Reported Outcomes Measurement Information System (PROMIS) measures among four groups of pediatric patients: sickle cell disease, nephrotic syndrome, asthma, and cancer. They are looking at "the kid's point of view."

Patient-reported outcome measures will be essential to the work of the Patient-Centered Outcomes Research Institute (PCORI) (wwww.pcori.org/), according to Sherine Gabriel, M.S., M.Sc., professor of medicine and epidemiology at the Mayo Clinic and chair of PCORI's methodology committee.

The U.K.'s National Joint Registry (www.njrcentre.org.uk/njrcentre/default.aspx) offers one model for the use of PROMs in comparative effectiveness research. Since 2002, the joint registry has collected data on all hip, knee, and ankle replacements that take place in England and Wales. Revision rates and mortality data are collected for 8 years. One example of an outcome data is that there was a voluntary recall of hip replacements by the manufacturer.

Experts feel that outcomes data at the organizational, regional, and national levels is one of the most promising ways to make use of PROMs.

NCLEX® EXAMINATION QUESTIONS

1. The National Patient Safety Goals:
   A. Form the basis of all process improvement activities
   B. Are a nationwide initiative
   C. Are mandated by the Institute of Medicine (IOM)
   D. Will improve patient safety
2. One model of quality is FOCUS PDCA (Plan-Do-Check-Act). The U stands for:
   A. Understand the causes of variance in the process
   B. Underlying causes for assessment
   C. Unlikely reason for a variance
   D. Understand the end result of the process improvement
3. Nurses need to know the outcomes that directly affect their unit. Common outcomes for all units are:
   A. Infection rates
   B. Patient satisfaction
   C. Performance on The Joint Commission Core Measures
   D. All of the above are correct
4. Two of the common vendor satisfaction measures are:
   A. Press Ganey and Gallup
   B. Press Ganey and The Joint Commission
   C. Gallup and Occupational Safety and Health Administration (OSHA)
   D. Gallup and National Institute of Occupational Safety and Health (NIOSH)
5. Organizations that recognize "best practice" are:
   A. American Nurses Association
   B. American Nurses Credentialing Center Magnet Status
   C. Malcolm Baldrige National Quality Award
   D. Press-Ganey Questionnaire
6. Which of the following is not one of W. Edwards Deming's 14-point management philosophy?
   A. Institute training on the job
   B. Cease dependence on inspection to achieve quality
   C. Adopt the new philosophy
   D. Begin the practice of awarding business on the basis of price tag
7. A goal of organizational learning is to make learning:
   A. The end product of all data collection
   B. Part of all activities within the organization
   C. Required of all employees in clinical positions
   D. Match the goals of The Joint Commission (TJC)
8. "Lean" refers to:
   A. The attempt to make do with the smallest amount possible
   B. A type of financial arrangement in which dollars are saved
   C. Getting rid of waste in all work processes
   D. The streamlining of all patient processes for cost saving

9. A root-cause analysis:
   A. Focuses on risk management
   B. Is a Six Sigma model
   C. Determines process variation
   D. Is a prospective review

10. Six Sigma is a model of quality focusing on:
    A. Process development
    B. Improving performance
    C. Decreasing the process variation
    D. Statistical analysis

Answers: 1. B   2. A   3. D   4. A   5. D   6. D   7. B
8. C   9. C   10. C

REFERENCES

Advisory Commission of Consumer Protection and Quality in the Health Care Industry. (1998). *Better Health Care for all Americans* Quality First. www.hcqualitycommission.gov/final/.

American Nurses Association. (2013). *Nursing sensitive indicators.* www.nursingworld.org/MainMenuCategories/ThePracticeofProfessionalNursing/PatientSafetyQuality/Research-Measurement/The-National-Database/Nursing-Sensitive-Indic. August 16, 2014. ators_1.

Baldrige National Quality Program. (2014). *Health care criteria for performance excellence.* Gaithersburg: MD: National Institute of Standards.

Bronson Methodist Hospital. (2007). *Baldrige application.* baldrige.nist.gov/PDF_files/Bronson_Methodist_Hospital_Application_Summary.pdf.

Clinical Dashboard Metrics. (n.d.). www.dashboardzone.com/hospital-dahsboard-clinical dashboard-metrics.

Deming, W. E. (2000a). *Out of the crisis.* Cambridge, MA: Massachusetts Institute of Technology.

Deming, W. E. (2000b). *The new economics: for industry, government, education* (2nd ed.). Cambridge, MA: MIT Press.

Donabedian, A. (1992). The role of outcomes in quality assessment and assurance. *Quality Review Bulletin, 18,* 356–360.

GE's DMAIC Approach. (2014). www.ge.com/capital/vendor/dmaic.htm.

Institute for Healthcare Improvement. (2015). *The Triple Aim.* www.ihi.org/Engage/Initiatives/TripleAim/pages/default.aspx.

Institute for Medicine. (1998). *Crossing the quality chasm: a new health system for the 21st century.* Washington, DC: National Academies Press.

Joint Commission. (2014). *National patient safety goals.* Oak Brook, IL: Author.

Joint Commission. (2015). *National Patient Safety Goals.* 2015. Oak Brook, IL. www.jointcommission.org/assets/1/6/2015_HAP_NPSG_ER.pdf.

Joint Commission. (2007). *Sentinel event policies and procedures.* www.jointcommission.org/SentinelEvents/PolicyandProcedures/.

Joosten, T., Bongers, I., & Janssen, R. (2009). Application of lean thinking to health care: Issues and observations. *International Journal of Health Care Quality, 21,* 341–347.

Juran, J. M. (1989). *Juran on leadership for quality: An executive handbook.* New York: Free Press.

Kavaler, F., & Spiegel, A. (2003). *Risk management in health care institutions: A strategic approach* (2nd ed.). Boston: Jones & Bartlett.

Miller, D. B. (Ed.). (2005). *Going lean in health care. IHI Innovation Series white paper: 2005.* Cambridge, MA: Institute for Healthcare Improvement. 5 www.ihi.org/IHI/Results/WhitePapers/GoingLeaninHealthCare.htm.

Naik, G. (2006). Hospital races to learn lessons of Ferrari crew. *The Wall Street Journal,* November 14, 2006.

Nielsen, D. M., Merry, M. D., Schyve, P. M., & Bisognano, M. (2004). Can the gurus' concepts cure health care? *Quality Progress,* Sept, 25–34

Phelps, C. E. (1997). *Health economics* (2nd ed.). Reading, MA: Addison-Wesley.

Sackett, D., Strauss, S., Richardson, W., Rosenberg, W., & Haynes, R. (2000). *Evidence-based medicine: How to practice and teach EBM* (2nd ed.). Edinburgh: Churchill Livingstone.

Womack, J., & Jones, D. (2003). *Lean thinking: Banish waste and create wealth in your corporation.* New York: Free Press.

Yoder-Wise, P. (2011). *Leading and managing in nursing.* St. Louis: Mosby.

19

Evidence-Based Practice

OBJECTIVES

- Differentiate among research, evidence-based practice (EBP), and performance improvement.
- Review the nurse's role in the implementation of evidence-based practice.
- Identify the various models of evidence-based practice (EBP).

- Identify the hierarchy of evidence.
- Discuss the critical appraisal process in evaluating evidence.
- Identify the PICOT (population, intervention, comparison, outcome, time) format of identifying a question.

OUTLINE

KEY TERMS

correlational study a study examining the relationship between, or among two or more variables in a single group; it does not examine cause and effect

descriptive study used to identify and describe variables and examine relationships that exist in a situation; provides an accurate portrayal of the phenomenon of interest

evidence-based practice conscientious use of current best practice or research evidence in making clinical decisions

nonrandomized clinical trial same as a randomized clinical trial, but patient placement in treatment or

nontreatment group depends on study variables, with not every individual having an opportunity for selection

observational study use of structured and unstructured observations to measure study variables

randomized clinical trial effects of an intervention are examined by comparing the treatment group with the nontreatment group; patients are placed in treatment or nontreatment group through random sampling

research generation of new knowledge through the rigorous study of variables

research use findings from a single study or a set of studies for the development of patient care

TREATMENT MYTHS AND TRUTHS

Two sentinel publications by the Institute of Medicine (IOM), *To Err Is Human* and *Crossing the Quality Chasm* (Institute of Medicine [IOM], 2000; 2001), drew attention to quality issues in U.S. health care. A major theme of both reports is that although the technology of health care has advanced at lightning speed, the delivery system has not advanced, causing potentially lethal situations in health care. One of the most common situations seen is the increased rate of hospital-acquired infections, and one of the proposed solutions to the improvement of care is the use of evidence-based decision making in health care.

The vision for the future of nursing in *The Future of Nursing* report (IOM, 2011) focuses on the convergence of knowledge, quality, and new functions in nursing. The recommendation that nurses lead interprofessional teams in improving delivery systems and care, brings to the fore the necessity for new competencies, beyond evidence-based practice that are requisite as nurses transform health care. These competencies focus on using knowledge in clinical decision making, and producing research evidence on interventions that promote uptake and use by individual providers and groups of providers (Stevens, 2013).

Evidence-based practice (EBP) requires a shift from the traditional paradigm of clinical practice grounded in pathophysiology and clinical experience to one of the integration of best practice and scientific evidence. This paradigm shift allows for the continuous improvement of practice and a creation of environments that stimulate innovation.

A recent survey of the state of EBP in nurses indicated that although nurses had positive attitudes toward EBP and wished to gain more knowledge and skills, they still faced significant barriers in employing it in practice (Melnyk, Fineout-Overholt, Gallagher-Ford, & Kaplan, 2012). This will prove to be a challenge if we are to meet the IOM goal of 90% of practice being informed by evidence by 2020.

As a new nurse there will be many times that you ask yourself, "Why do we do it this way?" or "There must be a better way to do this." For answers to these questions you must look to the evidence. What does the evidence tell you? What is the best practice, or what is the best way to do this? Some of our standard practices are "sacred cows," meaning they represent "the way it has always been done." For instance, does every patient admitted to your unit need their temperature taken at 7 AM? Perhaps not, but that is just the "way that we do it," or

perhaps that was the "best practice" when the policy was implemented. But what does the evidence (scientific data) tell us today? As nurses, you should remain current within your practice area, because the evidence is always changing and growing. Estabrooks (1998) and Pravikoff et al. (2005) found that knowledge sources most frequently used by nurses were school experiences and colleague experience. Assuming this is the case, a nurse with 15 years of experience may be using "evidence" that is 15 years out of date, and this experienced nurse who is mentoring new nurses may be fostering practice in the new nurse that is 15 years out of date. A colleague of this author once said that "health care was a long history of tradition unimpeded by progress"—the move to evidence-based practice is changing this.

EXAMPLES OF SOME TRADITIONAL PRACTICES NOT SUPPORTED BY EVIDENCE

Use of Oxygen in Patients with Chronic Obstructive Pulmonary Disease

The use of oxygen at levels that potentially may eliminate "hypoxic drive" in patients with chronic obstructive pulmonary disease (COPD) has long been a clinical concern (Makic et al., 2013). Statements such as "if you give oxygen, you will wipe out their drive to breathe and their carbon dioxide will increase," and "it is ok for the COPD patient to have a high $PaCO_2$ and a low PaO_2, they live there" are often repeated in clinical practice settings, in academic classrooms, and even in textbooks (Table 19-1).

Use of Large-Bore IV Needles for Blood Administration

Administration of packed red blood cells (PRBCs) is often a life-sustaining measure for patients to replace lost blood or treat symptomatic anemia (Makic et al., 2013). The size of the intravenous catheter traditionally was believed to influence the delivery of PRBCs; it was thought that smaller-bore catheters (e.g., 22-gauge needle or smaller) result in slower infusion rates and cell hemolysis. The common misperception, or sacred cow, is the belief that it is necessary to insert the largest-bore intravenous catheter possible to administer PRBCs so as to avoid destruction of cells through the administration process (Table 19-2).

TABLE 19-1   Debunking "hypoxic drive" and support for providing oxygen to patients with chronic obstructive pulmonary disease (COPD)

Evidence-based literature (Authors, year)	Provide oxygen for acute on chronic respiratory failure	Provide oxygen for chronic respiratory failure	Main points
Rudolf et al.,[38] 1977	NA	NA	Hypercapnia during oxygen therapy in acute exacerbations of chronic respiratory failure not due to "hypoxic drive" but other mechanisms
Easton et al.,[36] 1986	NA	NA	Minute ventilation may decrease in some patients in acute respiratory failure who are given oxygen; $Paco_2$ subsequently increases
Crossley et al.,[40] 1997	Yes	NA	Described response of COPD patients to high fractions of inspired oxygen after a period of rest on mechanical ventilation; provision of oxygen did not result in hypercarbia or respiratory muscle failure
Dick et al.,[35] 1997	NA	NA	Described the oxygen-induced change in ventilation and ventilatory drive in COPD; was not due to "hypoxic drive"; although hypoxic drive is a real phenomenon, it is responsible for only ~10% of the total drive to breathe
Pierson,[28] 2000	NA	Yes	Dangerous to withhold oxygen. Effects of chronic hypoxia include organ failure and a shortened life span
Singapore Ministry of Health,[30] 2006	Yes	Yes	Evidence-based recommendations for the use of oxygen in both chronic and acute on chronic COPD
West,[34] 2008	NA	NA	Describes Haldane effect and hypoxic vasoconstriction as mechanisms of increased carbon dioxide with provision of oxygen in COPD
Global Initiative for Chronic Obstructive Lung Disease,[29] 2009	Yes	Yes	Evidence-based recommendations for the use of oxygen in both chronic and acute on chronic COPD

Abbreviation: NA, not applicable.

Evaluating practice and continually questioning "why" should become a norm in every nurse's practice.

DECISION-MAKING MODEL

Evidence-based practice is a decision-making model based on the "conscientious, explicit and judicious use of current best practice in making decisions about the care of individual or groups of patients" (Sackett et al., 1996).

"This practice requires the integration of individual clinical expertise with the best available external clinical evidence from systematic research, available resources, and our patient's unique values and circumstances" (Sackett et al., 1996). This definition requires nurses to carefully and thoroughly integrate evidence into their practice. But how do they do this?

This new paradigm of evidence-based practice requires the development of a clinical inquiry approach.

TABLE 19-2   **Catheter gauge recommendations and blood product infusion based on American Association of Blood Banks practice guidelines**

Gauge of intravenous catheter	Description
22-14	Acceptable for transfusion of cellular blood components in adults (catheter size may need to be adjusted for rate of infusion)
24-22	Acceptable for transfusion of cellular blood components in infants and toddlers (may require infusion through pump or syringe)

Based on information from Roback et al.[45]

Nurses must ask themselves the following questions, and not blindly accept standard practice (Salmon, 2007):

- Why are we doing it this way?
- Is there a better way to do this?
- What is the evidence to support what we are doing?
- What practice guidelines support this practice?
- Would doing this be as effective as doing that?
- What constitutes best practice?

MODELS OF EVIDENCE-BASED PRACTICE

There are numerous models of evidence-based practice. These models are:

- The Iowa Model of Evidence-Based Practice to Promote Quality Care
- Johns Hopkins Nursing Evidence-Based Practice Model
- Stetler Model of Research Utilization
- ACE Star Model of Knowledge Transformation
- ARCC Model: Advancing Research and Clinical Practice Through Close Collaboration Model

The ACE Star Model of Knowledge Transformation is depicted as a five-point star defining the following forms of knowledge: Point 1 Discovery, representing primary research studies; Point 2 Evidence Summary, which is the synthesis of all available knowledge compiled into a single harmonious statement, such as a systematic review; Point 3 Translation into action, often referred to as evidence-based clinical practice guidelines, combining the evidential base and expertise to extend recommendations; Point 4 Integration into practice is evidence-in-action, in which practice is aligned to reflect best evidence; and Point 5 Evaluation, which is an inclusive view of the impact that the evidence-based practice has on patient health outcomes, satisfaction, efficacy and efficiency of care, and health policy (Stevens, 2013).

EVIDENCE-BASED PRACTICE

Evidence-based practice consists of five steps (Strauss, 2005):

1. Ask a searchable clinical question;
2. Find the best evidence to answer the question;
3. Appraise the evidence;
4. Apply the evidence with clinical expertise, taking the patient's wants/needs into consideration;
5. Evaluate the effectiveness and efficiency of the process.

Question Formulation

The first thing you will need to do is to formulate the question. The definition and narrowing down of the problem is very important. As nurses, we often decide on an intervention before we adequately define the problem. The first step in EBP is to identify either a problem-focused trigger or a knowledge-focused trigger that will initiate the need for change. A problem-focused trigger could be a clinical problem, or a risk management issue; knowledge triggers might be new research findings, or a new practice guideline (Dontje, 2007). Patient outcomes are a perfect starting point.

As nurses, we make numerous decisions when caring for our patients. As we make these decisions we are influenced by a number of factors (Craig & Smyth, 2002):

- Clinical expertise;
- Beliefs, attitudes;
- Routine (tradition);
- Organizational factors;
- State and federal policies;
- Regulatory factors;
- Funding;
- Time;
- Factors related to the patient;
- Clinical circumstances; and
- Preferences, beliefs, attitudes, needs.

Up-to-date, valid evidence needs to be integrated with these factors to maximize the likelihood of what we want to happen (the outcome). The more explicit the question, the easier it is to run searches through the multiple electronic databases available to nurses (CINAHL, MEDLINE, and Cochrane). For example, you are interested in determining best practice for end-of-shift reports. If you enter "end-of-shift report" into the search line, you will receive 56 references. If you narrow the search to within the past 5 years, the number of references is cut to 32. A focused question makes your "search strategy" much easier. It is very helpful for any nurse working in a hospital to develop a good relationship with the hospital librarian, who will assist you in the gathering of research evidence (Table 19-3).

Reliable Evidence

Once you have focused your question, you need to select the best evidence. Just because something has been published either in print or on the Internet, does not mean it is a valid source of evidence. You must first determine the reliability of the source. Your librarian will assist you in this. A research study on urinary catheters funded by the company that makes urinary catheters may not be the most reliable source of evidence; a study supporting their catheter is in the company's best interest. The first question in your critical appraisal of the evidence is whether or not this study is good enough to use the findings. You will be attempting to determine if the quality of the study that you are reading is good enough for you to use the results in the design of a nursing protocol. You would need to look at the research design, the sample, and the sample size. Obviously results from a study directed at children may not be appropriate in the design of a protocol addressed to adults. Also, a study with a sample size of four will not carry as much strength as will a study with a sample size of 1000. Some research designs are more powerful than others. The fact that some studies are more powerful than others has given rise to the hierarchy of evidence (Peto, 1993). The hierarchy of evidence for questions about effectiveness of an intervention follows (Polit & Beck, 2013):

Level 1
   a. Systematic review of **randomized controlled trials**
   b. Systematic review of **nonrandomized trials**
Level 2
   a. Single randomized controlled trial
   b. Single nonrandomized trial

TABLE 19-3 Resources for Forms of Knowledge in the Star Model

Form of Knowledge	Description of Resources
Point 1: Discovery	Bibliographic databases such as CINAHL—provide single research reports, in most cases, multiple reports.
Point 2: Evidence Summary	Cochrane Collaboration Database of Systematic Reviews—provides reports of rigorous systematic reviews on clinical topics. See www.cochrane.org/
Point 3: Translation into Guidelines	National Guidelines Clearinghouse—sponsored by the Agency for Healthcare Research and Quality (AHRQ), provides online access to evidence-based clinical practice guidelines. See www.guideline.gov
Point 4: Integration into Practice	AHRQ health care innovations exchange—sponsored by AHRQ, provides profiles of innovations, and tools for improving care processes, including adoption guidelines and information to contact the innovator. See http://innovations.ahrq.gov/
Point 5: Evaluation of Process and Outcome	National quality measures clearinghouse—sponsored by AHRQ, provides detailed information on quality measures and measure sets. See http://qualitymeasures.ahrq.gov/

Stevens, K. (2013) The Impact of Evidence-Based Practice in Nursing and the Next Big Ideas. *OJIN: The Online Journal of Issues in Nursing,* 18(2).

Level 3 Systematic review of **correlational/observational studies**
Level 4 Single correlational/observational study
Level 5 Systematic review of descriptive/qualitative/physiologic studies
Level 6 Single **descriptive/qualitative/physiologic study**
Level 7 Opinions of authorities, expert committees
Figure 19-1 shows an example of an evidence-based pyramid.

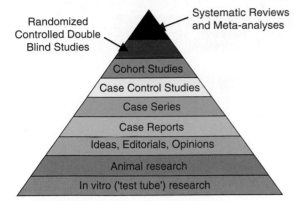

Randomized Controlled Double Blind Studies

Systematic Reviews and Meta-analyses

Cohort Studies

Case Control Studies

Case Series

Case Reports

Ideas, Editorials, Opinions

Animal research

In vitro ('test tube') research

FIGURE 19-1 Example of evidence-based pyramid.

There will be differences in the actual numbers associated with the varying levels of evidence depending on the model used. You need to become knowledgeable about the model used in your institution.

Critical Appraisal

The next question to ask in your critical appraisal is whether or not the findings are applicable to your setting. The patients used in a study will never be identical to yours, but there may be similarities. The following questions can be asked to determine applicability of the study to your practice area:

- Is it clear what the study is about?
- Is the sample/context adequately described?
- Are my patients/contexts so different that the results will not apply?
- Is the intervention available, or is the change possible in my setting?
- Do the benefits of the change for my patient/context outweigh the costs?
- Are the patients' values and preferences satisfied by change?

Part of this question will be to ask what these results mean for your patients.

POPULATION, INTERVENTION, COMPARISON INTERVENTION, OUTCOME

A framework for formulating evidence-based questions is PICOT (population, intervention, comparison intervention, outcome, time). Box 19-1 describes the focus of the population, intervention, comparison intervention, outcome (PICO) question.

BOX 19-1 Focus of the PICOT (Population, Intervention, Comparison Intervention, Outcome, Time) Question

Patient or **P**opulation	Define who or what the question is about. Tip: Describe a group of patients similar to yours.
Intervention	Describe the intervention, test, or exposure that you are interested in. An intervention is a planned course of action. An exposure is something that happens such as a fall, anxiety, exposure to house mites, etc. Tip: Describe what it is that you are considering doing or what has happened to the patient.
Comparison intervention (if any)	Describe the alternate intervention. Tip: Describe the alternative that can be compared to the intervention.
Outcomes	Define the important outcomes, beneficial or harmful. Tip: Define what you are hoping to achieve or avoid.
Time	Over what period of time will this happen?

Adapted from Craig, J., & Smyth, R. (2002). *The evidence-based manual practice manual for nurses* (p. 30). Edinburgh: Churchill Livingstone.

The last step in the implementation of any change is the monitoring of outcomes. Was the evidence-based practice change successful? And are the outcomes sustained over time?

In health care organizations, there may be many triggers that initiate the need for change. They can be data driven, resulting from performance review data, risk management data, benchmarking data, and financial data. Or they can be knowledge driven, resulting from new research findings, change in regulatory guidelines and standards, or questions from practitioners.

As a nurse manager, your role will be in the promotion and implementation of evidence-based practice in your organization. The algorithm of The Iowa Model of Evidence-Based Practice provides a visual representation of the development of evidence-based practice in a clinical facility (Figure 19-2).

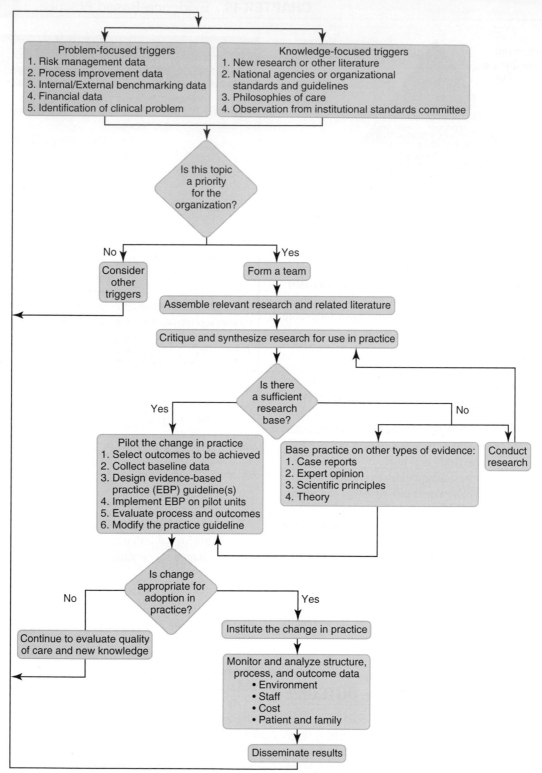

FIGURE 19-2 The Iowa Model of Evidence-Based Practice to promote quality care. (From Titler, M.G., et al. [2001]. The Iowa Model of Evidence-Based Practice to promote quality care. *Crit Care Nurs Clin of North Am, 13*[4], 497-509; reprinted from Burns, N., & Grove, S. K. [2007]. *Understanding nursing research: building an evidence-based practice,* [p. 514]. St. Louis: Saunders Elsevier.)

As a summary evidence-based practice can be used as a guide for implementing a research-based protocol. The steps in this model are to:

- Synthesize relevant research.
- Determine the sufficiency of the research base for use in practice.
- Pilot the change in practice.
- Institute the change in practice.
- Monitor outcomes (Chapter 20).

RESEARCH USE

Evidence-based practice differs from research use. Research use is the process of using research-generated knowledge to make an impact on or a change in existing practices (Burns et al., 2012). Evidence-based practice requires synthesizing research study findings to determine best research evidence. Research evidence is a synthesis of high-quality, relevant studies to form a body of empirical knowledge for the selected area of practice. The best research evidence is then integrated with clinical expertise and patient values and needs, to deliver quality, cost-effective care (Sackett et al., 2000).

RESEARCH

Research is the systematic investigation, testing, and evaluation designed to generate new knowledge or to contribute to generalizable knowledge (adapted from U.S. Department of Health and Human Services, 2014). There is now a focus on patient-centered outcomes research (PCOR). As evidence mounted on standard medical metrics (mortality and morbidity), it was noted that metrics and outcomes of particular interest to patients and families (such as quality of life) were understudied. Thus attention is now drawn to the need to produce evidence on patient-centered outcomes from the perspective of the patient.

Research is critical to the growth of any profession, and in nursing is mandatory for the continued improvements in patient care. The Iowa Model offers a visualization of how a clinical inquiry brought by a nurse may develop into a research project. In reviewing and appraising the evidence the nurse may find that there is little or no published information about the clinical inquiry. This will then lead to the development of research. Health care institutions that are centers of excellence will have infrastructures and resources available for nurses interested in pursuing research.

A first step for any nurse interested in research is to join the nursing research committee at the institution. Such research committees are part of the shared governance structures within the nursing departments (Chapter 6). A novice nurse may assist in an ongoing research project as step one, and gradually increase research responsibilities as he or she matures in professional responsibilities. Another important step is to continually ask those clinical questions that come to mind. This constant spirit of clinical inquiry is what differentiates the nurse with a passion for improving care from the nurse who sees nursing as "just a job."

The following is the Magnet template for the communication of research across the institution.

Introduction
- Research question and hypothesis
- Study rationale
- Literature review

Participants
- Nurses at the organization who are the PI (principal investigator or co-PI) involved in the study

Methods
- Study design
- Study timeline (start date/completed date)
- IRB (Institutional Review Board) approval date: full committee/expedited/exempt
- Research sample (study participants, sample size, sampling plan)
- Data collection methods

Results
- Results of data analysis (quantitative) of findings (qualitative)

Discussion
- Summary of key findings
- Analysis of findings
- Implications of the findings

SUMMARY

As a new nurse entering the profession, it is imperative that you maintain currency within your profession. Here are some strategies for using research evidence in your own practice:

- Read widely and critically: Professionally accountable nurses keep abreast of their practice by reading journals relating to their practice.
- Join a professional organization related to your specialty: Many innovations in practice and best practices are shared through professional organizations.
- Attend professional conferences and continuing education seminars.

- Participate in evidence-based projects.
- Participate in nursing research.
- Always assume that it "can be done better."
- Focus on the triple aim: delivery of effective, efficient, and patient centered care.

The IOM report (2003) stated that as a core competency nurses must employ evidence-based practice, integrate best research with clinical expertise and patient values for optimum care, and participate in learning and research activities to the extent feasible.

CLINICAL CORNER

The Staff Nurse Role in Research

I have written a short research story about the nursing research process, which I encountered as a graduate nursing student conducting nursing research at Hackensack University Medical Center. I started out with a brief nursing background about myself, which led up to my interest in the research idea and investigation.

I have been a nurse for approximately eight and a half years and have always worked at Hackensack University Medical Center. I started on the congestive heart failure unit for the first 4 years of nursing, before moving to the emergency room clinical decision unit (CDU) called the "Observation Unit" for the adult emergency room (ER). In September 2014, I transferred to the adult emergency room as a staff nurse, and currently work full-time in the adult emergency trauma department.

I gained experience working with congestive heart failure patients during the first 4 years of my nursing career. These patients were critically ill and required a multidisciplinary care approach to help them live longer with better quality of life. The treatments provided to the patients included the latest medical and surgical innovations and modalities, which required specialized training in both the aspect of medicine and nursing. As a nurse taking care of patients in acute and chronic congestive heart failure, the care was always transitioned over to the intensive care unit (ICU), in addition to receiving those patients downgraded from the ICU. This nursing experience provided me with strong critical thinking skills in a specialized and more controlled health care environment.

Approximately 4 years later, the unit in which I worked, transitioned over to an emergency room "observation" clinical decision unit (CDU). The term "observation" meant

a 24 to 48 hour hospitalization stay to determine a diagnosis, if further treatment was necessary, to complete current treatment in process, or to move forward to an "admission" status. The unit functioned like an ER overflow and the pace was rapid. The nursing dilemmas encountered in this health care environment were different than problems encountered in the congestive heart failure environment. I encountered a nursing dilemma that affected safety, quality care, and cost including the ordering of prescription medication during the patient's hospitalization, on a daily basis. For example, I would check the list of daily medications the patient was ordered, based on what the patient would take at home. I noticed that the active medication administration record (MAR) for 10:00 A.M. medications had multiple medications listed to administer. These medications were either no longer taken by the patient, or the patient stated that they have never taken that medication before or have never heard of it. Some medications were wasted or discarded once the package was opened, and some medications were consumed; the patient may state that if the doctor ordered the medication then it is all right to take it.

I also noticed that the ordering of blood pressure medications presented a medication dilemma. The once daily medications always default to 10:00 A.M., and there could be several blood pressure medications all given at the same time. The prior to admission (PTA) medication list, or home medication list was often not accurate, leading to inappropriate ordering of medication. This dilemma leads to a safety and health concern for the adult population ages 65 years and older. The administration of multiple blood pressure medications at the same time during the day may lead to dizziness, hypotension, orthostatic hypotension, and a prolonged hospital stay. Patients who are prescribed multiple antihypertensives are usually taught to take certain mediations during the day and certain medications at night or with dinner.

The majority of our patients who stayed in "observation" were 65 years and older. The hypothesis that I developed was that as older adults took more medications they experienced more symptoms. Medication plays a large part of the patient's hospitalization stay. As a nurse I observed that as more medications were ordered and given, the patient's hospitalization stay increased in length.

I began to develop some ideas about research projects and research ideas that I was interested in. Research ideas I wished to investigate included interrelated factors such as polypharmacy, quality of life, and symptom assessment in the older population, aged 65 years and older. I wanted to find out if there was some relationship among the three factors. I started to research articles on polypharmacy and quality of life, in addition to symptom assessment and quality of life. I continued to find interesting articles on the related topics and then developed my research question, which was: "What are the relationships between polypharmacy, symptom assessment, and quality of life in the older adult population ages 65 years and older?" My hypothesis states that those patients exposed to polypharmacy will have a higher symptom assessment score (based on the scoring tool for symptoms), and have a poorer quality of life (based on the quality of life questionnaire). I developed a proposal including chapters 1, 2, & 3 and made several revisions to the proposal. The proposal included a thorough literature review, definitions of variables, tools to be used, permission to use the tools, validity and reliability of the tools, consent information, and the systematic approach with rationales to the research project. Once the proposal was final, I then submitted an application through my college's international review board (IRB), William Paterson University IRB, with the approval of my mentor and thesis advisor. I received WPUNJ IRB approval within 2 weeks. After receiving an approval from my college IRB, I submitted the proposal to our hospital's Proposal Committee. Once receiving approval from our Proposal Committee, I then focused on the IRB application process at Hackensack University Medical Center. I submitted an application to the hospital's IRB via their electronic IRB portal to obtain approval to conduct the research project at the facility. Several colleagues reviewed the research proposal thoroughly and included nursing and medicine administration. This section of the research project took the most time and patience, approximately 3 to 4 months. Because my project was pharmacy related, a pharmacist had to thoroughly read through my proposal and IRB application. After multiple revisions to the proposal and IRB application, I received approval and permission to conduct the research project at Hackensack University Medical Center. I was truly ecstatic at this time.

I enrolled in an SPSS (Statistical Package for Social Sciences) class on campus, which taught me how to use the program during the data collection period. I met with my statistician on the college campus to confirm my Excel spreadsheets were set up accurately in accordance to my data collection tools. I then started my data collection in the adult observation unit at Hackensack University Medical Center. The interviews conducted took approximately 1 hour per patient. I waited until the end of my shift to start conducting interviews. After an interview was completed, I simultaneously entered the data into my computer Excel spreadsheet. The purpose for this was to avoid entering all the information at the end, which is far more time consuming. I continued data collection for approximately 5 weeks. I was gathering very interesting data. Approximately week five, I met with the statistician to confirm that my data collection was completed at this time, and that I had obtained a statistically significant result. I also met with Hackensack University Medical Center's statistician, along with several colleagues of the research team who helped guide my research project. I had several statistical methods and reports, which confirmed my data analysis was completed. I continued to write my thesis research paper on chapters 4, 5, & 6 on data analysis, data interpretation, final results, discussion, and conclusion and implications for future practice. I had to send several rough drafts to my thesis advisor for editing. After several revisions of my thesis, I was able to finalize the final copy and submit the paper to my professor. The final copy included an abstract, acknowledgment letter, table of contents, list of appendices, result charts, title page, and reference list. I submitted a final hard copy and electronic copy to my thesis advisor and nursing director of my college. I submitted my PowerPoint presentation along with original poster presentation. This research study was a pilot study and can be expanded upon with more participants. One major barrier in this research study is that I had approximately 6 weeks from IRB approval, to collect patient data including 1-hour interviews, meet with the statistician, and complete chapters 4, 5, & 6 of my thesis. The total sample size included 48 participants in the time allotted. I would have liked to gather more participants over a longer period of time.

My goal now is to build on this nursing research study foundation for my doctoral degree and publish these data in a scientific nursing journal.

Tina Vacante, MSN, RN
HackensackUMC

EVIDENCE-BASED PRACTICE

Spencer, G., et al. (2010) Determination of Analgesia Effectiveness Using the "Ice Test Method" in Adult Patients Receiving Epidural Infusions in the Post Anesthesia Care Unit. In Spencer, G. *Changes in Practice: Evidence Based Nursing Revealed.* Houston: University of Texas MD Anderson Cancer Center.

Abstract

The objectives were to identify the evidence-based project in the MD Anderson Cancer Center (MDACC) post-anesthetic care unit (PACU), and to describe the determination of analgesia effectiveness using the "Ice Test Method" in adult patients receiving epidural infusions in the PACU.

The team reviewed the literature on the "Ice Test Method." The team researched data from epidural records from January 2009. The total number of patient charts reviewed for sensory block using the ice method were 39. The documented sensory block number was 24. The undocumented sensory block was 15.

The problem identifications were difficulty determining the reliability of sensory block or dermatome level, untimely management and delay of patients' pain relief, and the level of knowledge in assessing sensory block or dermatome level.

The evidence-based population, intervention, comparison intervention, and outcome (PICO) question was "Does cold stimulation using the ice method to check the sensory block provide reliable estimation in determining the effectiveness of epidural analgesia?"

An electronic search method was undertaken using PubMed, CINAHL, and Science Direct databases. A combined search approach was undertaken to ensure that any potentially relevant literature would not be missed.

The purpose was to standardize the use of ice as a means of testing sensory block on patients with epidural analgesia, educate nurses, and further improve nursing care in the teaching of sensory block test using ice to assess the effectiveness of epidural analgesia in the immediate postoperative period, and to improve communication of patients' adequate or inadequate pain relief among interdisciplinary teams.

The findings were: seven out of the twelve studies have used multiple variables, such as analgesia medications and pinprick; hot and cold method; and alcohol swab method; therefore exclusion criteria were applied. Five of the studies supported the independent and the outcome variables; cold stimulation by using "ice method to check the sensory block" provides "reliable estimation in determining the effectiveness of epidural analgesia."

The conclusion was that the old sensation using the ice method provided valid evidence in relation to pain management and efficacy of epidural analgesia. These consist of the assessment and estimation of dermatome level, choice of local anesthesia, and spread of analgesia or density. The ice method is reliable, effective, less invasive, inexpensive, practical, and safe.

Using the ice method as an indicator to test and estimate the sensory block is perhaps the best alternative and modality in monitoring the pain in the perianesthesia setting.

The practice change was the development of "Pain Champion Nurses" in the unit level, expansion of knowledge Epidural Workshop and Program, and incorporation of sensory block assessment using the ice test as a standard practice in adult patients receiving epidural analgesia. The Epidural Workshop and Program includes didactics and hands-on training, a 3-day rotation with the Acute Pain Team of the institution, and yearly competency check-off. The Pain Champion nurses served as mentors and educators for the PACU unit and advocated for epidural analgesia.

What was learned: Proper assessment of dermatome block is vital in the safe and effective analgesia therapy. If an epidural is working safely and effectively in the immediate postoperative care, then the chances of an epidural continuing to work for the patient are increased.

Piloting and trialing the "ice method" to assess sensory block may benefit the institution as a whole. The enhanced communication between the front-line nurses and acute pain team will improve pain management, increase patient satisfaction, and promote recovery time.

■ NCLEX® EXAMINATION QUESTIONS

1. A key component of evidence-based practice is:
   A. Traditional practice
   B. Organizational commitment
   C. Patient preference
   D. Nurse ability

2. In the hierarchy of evidence, which of the following has the highest value?
   A. Single correctional studies
   B. Randomized clinical trials
   C. Case study, opinion
   D. Descriptive studies

3. The experienced nurse can do the following to use evidence-based practice in their own practice:
   A. Use textbooks from school for reference.
   B. Maintain membership in alumni organization
   C. Review professional journals.
   D. Go back to school for an advanced degree.

4. When implementing an evidence-base practice change, the all-important final step is to:
   A. Pilot the protocol.
   B. Monitor the results.
   C. Publish the study.
   D. Do a cost-benefit analysis.

5. The first step in integrating evidence into practice is to convert the clinical concern into a:
   A. Solution
   B. Question
   C. Decision
   D. Goal

6. In the PICO framework for developing the question of concern, "I" stands for:
   A. Intervention
   B. Interdisciplinary
   C. Interrelational
   D. Integrity

7. As a nurse, you have just read about a change in intervention insertion practice that sounds like it would work on your unit. Before suggesting such a change in practice, you need to:
   A. Perform a cost-benefit analysis of the new practice.
   B. Talk with the nurse manager to gain his or her opinion.
   C. Conduct a further review of the literature.
   D. Contact the nursing research committee.

8. In reviewing a study for applicability for use on your unit, you need to evaluate the study in terms of:
   A. The sponsoring agency of the study
   B. Patient context and assess whether they are similar to patients in your unit
   C. Whether the sample adequately is described
   D. Qualifications of the study authors

9. Which of the following would be a reliable source of information for a change in pediatric practice?
   A. Physician/staff discussion
   B. Editorial in *Pediatric Nursing*
   C. Growth and development charts
   D. Clinical trial results

10. An example of a knowledge trigger for an evidence-based research question is:
    A. Patient fall data
    B. Database review
    C. Benchmark information
    D. Research study

Answers: 1. C   2. B   3. C   4. B   5. B   6. A   7. C
8. B   9. D   10. D

REFERENCES

American Nurses Credentialing Center [ANCC]. (2014). *The 2014 Magnet Application Manual*. Silver Spring, MD: ANCC.

Burns, N., & Grove, S. K. (2007). *Understanding nursing research: building an evidence-based practice* (4th ed.). St. Louis: Saunders Elsevier, 515–517.

Burns, N., Grove, S., & Gray, J. (2012). *The Practice of Nursing Research* (7th Ed.). St. Louis: Saunders Elsevier.

Craig, J., & Smyth, R. (2002). *The evidence-based manual practice manual for nurses*. Edinburgh: Churchill Livingstone.

Crossley, D. J., McGuire, G. P., Barrow, P. M., & Houston, P. L. (1997). Influence of inspired oxygen concentration on dead space, respiratory drive, and $PaCO_2$ in intubated patients with chronic obstructive pulmonary disease. *Critical Care Medicine*, 25(9), 1522–1526.

Dick, C. R., Liu, Z., Sassoon, C. S., Berry, R. B., & Mahutte, C. K. (1997). O_2-induced change in ventilation and ventilatory drive in COPD. *American Journal of Respiratory Critical Care Medicine*, 155(2), 609–614.

Dontje, K. (2007). Evidence-Based Practice: Understanding the Process. *Topics in Advanced Practice Nursing*, 7(4).

Easton, P. A., Slykerman, L. J., & Anthonisen, N. R. (1986). Ventilatory response to sustained hypoxia in normal adults. *Journal of Applied Physiology, 61*, 906–911.

Estabrooks, C. (1998). Will evidence-based nursing practice make practice perfect? *Canadian Journal of Nursing Research, 30*(1), 15–36.

Global Initiative for Chronic Obstructive Lung Disease (GOLD). (2009). *Global Strategy for the Diagnosis, Management, and Prevention of Chronic Obstructive Pulmonary Disease.* Bethesda, MD: Global Initiative for Chronic Obstructive Lung Disease (GOLD).

Institute of Medicine [IOM]. (2000). *To Err is Human: Building a Safer Health Care System.* Washington, DC: National Academy Press.

Institute of Medicine [IOM]. (2001). *Crossing the Quality Chasm: a New Health System for the 21st Century.* Washington, DC: National Academy Press.

Institute of Medicine [IOM]. (2003). In A. C. Greiner, & E. Knebel (Eds.), *Health professions education: A bridge to quality.* Washington, DC: National Academies Press.

Institute of Medicine [IOM]. (2011). *The future of nursing: Leading change, advancing health [prepared by Robert Wood Johnson Foundation Committee Initiative on the Future of Nursing].* Washington, DC: National Academies Press.

Makic, M., Martin, S., Burns, S., Philbrick, D., & Rauen, C. (2013). Putting Evidence into Nursing Practice: four traditional practices not supported by the evidence. *Critical Care Nurse, 33*(2), 28–42.

Melnyk, B., & Fineout-Overholt, E. (2011). *Evidence based practice in nursing and health care: A guide to best practice* (2nd. Ed). Philadelphia, PA: Lippincott, Williams & Wilkins.

Melnyk, B. M., Fineout-Overholt, E., Gallagher-Ford, L., & Kaplan, L. (2012). The state of evidence-based practice in US nurses: critical implications for nurse leaders and educators. *Journal of Nursing Administration, 42*(9), 410–417.

Patient-Centered Outcomes Research Institute (PCORI). (2013). *Mission and vision.* www.pcori.org/about/mission-and-vision/.

Peto, R. (1993). Large scale randomized evidence; large sample trials and overview trials. *Annals of the New York Academy of Science, 703*, 314–340.

Pierson, D. J. (2000). Pathophysiology and clinical effects of chronic hypoxia. *Respiratory Care, 45*, 39–51.

Polit, D., & Beck, C. (2013). *Essentials of Nursing Research: Appraising Evidence for Nursing Practice* (9th Ed.). Philadelphia: Lippincott Williams & Wilkins.

Pravikoff, D., Tanner, A., & Pierce, S. (2005). Readiness of US nurses for evidence-based practice. *American Journal of Nursing, 105*(9), 40–51.

Roback, J. M. D., Combs, M. K., Grossman, B., & Hillyer, C. (2008). *Chapter 21, 615 The AABB Technical Manual* (16th Ed). Hoboken, NJ: Blackwell Publishing.

Rudolf, M., Banks, R. A., & Semple, S. J. (1977). Hypercapnia during oxygen therapy in acute exacerbations of chronic respiratory failure: hypothesis revisited. *Lancet, 2*, 483.

Sackett, D., Rosenberg, W., Gray, J., Haynes, R., & Richardson, W. (1996). Evidence-based medicine: what it is and what it is not. *British Medical Journal, 312*, 71–72.

Sackett, D. L., Straus, S. E., Richardson, W. C., Rosenberg, W., & Haynes, R. M. (2000). *Evidence-based medicine: how to practice and teach EBM* (2nd Ed.). New York: Churchill Livingstone.

Salmon, S. (2007). Advancing evidence-based practice. *Orthopaedic Nursing, 26*(2), 118.

Singapore Ministry of Health [SMOH]. (2006). *Chronic Obstructive Pulmonary Disease.* Singapore: Singapore Ministry of Health.

Stevens, K. (2013). The Impact of Evidence-Based Practice in Nursing and the Next Big Ideas. *OJIN: The Online Journal of Issues in Nursing, 18*(2), Manuscript 4.

Strauss, S. E. (2005). *Evidence-Based Medicine: How to Practice and Teach EBM.* New York: Churchill Livingstone.

SUNY Downstate. (2014). *Evidence-Based Medicine Tutorial.* http://library.downstate.edu/EBM2/2100.htm.

U. S. Department of Health and Human Services. (2009). *Code of Federal Regulations Title 45: Public Welfare Part 46: Protection of Human Subjects, Title 21 Food and Drugs Part 50: Protection of Human Subjects.* Washington, D.C. Author.

West, J. B. (2008). *Respiratory Physiology: The Essentials* (8th Ed.). Philadelphia: Lippincott Williams & Wilkins.

20

Monitoring Outcomes and the Use of Data for Improvement

OBJECTIVES

- Discuss the importance in using data to drive decisions.
- Interpret visual representations of performance outcomes.
- Compare levels of performance to benchmark.
- Identify the requirements for presenting improvement initiatives.

OUTLINE

KEY TERMS

benchmark comparison information that allows an organization to evaluate its own performance in relation to others.

dashboard visual representation of performance using colors to represent levels, usually green (on target) or red (below target).

graph visual representation of levels of performance

trend three data points moving in same direction

In Chapter 18 the improvement of patient care was discussed, and in the last chapter the use of evidence-based practice (EBP) was reviewed. One final and very important step in each of these processes is the continued monitoring of outcomes. But to evaluate the success of an EBP practice change, we need to know the levels of performance before the implementation of the changes and after the changes. As nurses we need to be cognizant of the outcomes of our professional practice at all times.

The Institute of Medicine (IOM) (2003) suggested a core competency of nurses as being able to: apply quality improvement; identify errors and hazards in care; understand and implement basic safety design principles, such as standardization and simplification; continually understand and measure quality of care in terms of structure, process, and outcomes in relation to patient and community needs; and design and test interventions to change processes and systems of care, with the objective of improving quality. It is the continual measuring and monitoring of quality outcomes that this chapter will address.

NURSING-SENSITIVE INDICATORS

As stated in Chapter 18, nursing-sensitive indicators reflect the structure, process, and outcomes of nursing care. The structure of nursing care is indicated by the supply of nursing staff, the skill level of the nursing staff, and the education/certification of nursing staff. Process indicators measure aspects of nursing care such as assessment, intervention, and registered nurse (RN) job satisfaction. Patient outcomes that are determined to be nursing sensitive are those that improve if there is a greater quantity or quality of nursing care (e.g., pressure ulcers, falls, and intravenous infiltrations). Some patient outcomes are more highly related to other aspects of institutional care, such as medical decisions and institutional policies (e.g., frequency of primary C-sections, cardiac failure), and are not considered "nursing-sensitive." Performance is usually represented in **dashboards** or **graphs**.

The nursing-sensitive indicators are as follows:

- Nursing hours per patient day Registered Nurses (RN) hours per patient day
  - Licensed Practical/Vocational Nurses (LPN/LVN) hours per patient day
  - Unlicensed Assistive Personnel (UAP) hours per patient day
- Nursing turnover
- Nosocomial infections
- Patient falls
- Patient falls with injury
  - Injury level
- Pressure ulcer rate
  - Community-acquired
  - Hospital-acquired
  - Unit-acquired
- Pediatric pain assessment, intervention, reassessment (AIR) cycle
- Pediatric peripheral intravenous infiltration
- Psychiatric physical/sexual assault
- RN education/certification
- RN survey
  - Job satisfaction scales
  - Practice environment scale (PES) restraints
- Staff mix
  - RN
  - LPN/LVNs
  - UAP
  - Percent agency staff

Additional Data Elements Collected:

- Patient population: adult or pediatric.
- Hospital category, e.g. teaching, nonteaching, etc.
- Type of unit (critical care, step-down, medical, surgical, combined med-surg, rehab, and psychiatric).
- Number of staffed beds designated by the hospital.

NATIONAL COMPARISON GROUPS AND REPORTS

(www.nursingworld.org/MainMenuCategories/The PracticeofProfessionalNursing/PatientSafetyQuality/

Research-Measurement/The-National-Database/Nursing-Sensitive-Indicators_1.)

The data for these nursing sensitive indicators are collected at the institution and uploaded to the National Database of Nursing Quality Indicators. There are approximately 1500 US hospitals participating in this database. The hospitals provide unit level performance data to National Database of Nursing Quality Indicators (NDNQI). The large number of participating hospitals allows for comparisons of performance across institutions, divisions, and units. A critical care unit at a large teaching hospital on the East Coast can evaluate their performance with all other critical care units in teaching hospitals. National comparison data for the indicators are grouped based on patient (adult/pediatric), and unit type: critical care, step-down, medical, surgical, combined med-surg, rehab, psychiatric, and staffed bed size. Teaching and Magnet Status is identified as it relates to participating hospitals. The quarterly reports provide the national comparison along with unit performance data trended over eight quarters. The Magnet goal is that hospitals outperform the selected benchmark for a majority of the reporting quarters. This comparison is called benchmarking; comparing performance to other like institutions. Such comparisons also allow hospitals to evaluate their performance in relation to the competition, and to the best performers.

Some of the definitions of the datasets within NDNQI are as follows:

- Patient falls: All documented falls, with or without injury, experienced by patients on a unit in a calendar month.
- Patient falls with injury: All documented patient falls with an injury level of minor or greater.
- Pressure ulcer prevalence: The total number of patients that have nosocomial (hospital-acquired) stage II or greater pressure ulcers.
- Pressure Ulcer incidence: The total number of patients that have stage II or greater pressure ulcers.
- Skill mix: Percentage of hours worked by RN, LPN, UAP, and contract staff with patient care responsibilities, by type of unit.
- Nursing care hours per patient day: The number of productive hours worked by RN nursing staff per patient day, and the number of productive hours worked by nursing staff (RN, LVN, LPN, and UAP) per patient day. (www.wsha.org/files/127/nsqi%20binder.pdf)

Let us look at pressure ulcers. Pressure ulcers cost 9.1 to -$11.6 billion per year in the U.S. Cost of individual patient care ranges from 20,900 to 151,700 dollars per pressure ulcer. Medicare estimated in 2007 that each pressure ulcer added 43,180 dollars in costs to a hospital stay. (Agency for Healthcare Research and Quality [AHRQ], 2015). Rates are calculated as follows:

- Prevalence measures the number of patients with pressure ulcers at a certain point or period in time:
  - The numerator will be the number of patients with any pressure ulcer (count for both any ulcer and Stage II or greater).
  - Just count patients, not the number of ulcers. Even if a patient has four Stage II ulcers, they are only counted once.
  - The denominator is the number of patients on your unit or in your facility during that month.
  - Divide the numerator by the denominator and multiply by 100 to get the percentage.

Example: 17 patients with any pressure ulcer ÷ 183 patients = .093 × 100 = 9.3 percent

- Incidence measures the number of patients developing new pressure ulcers during a period in time:
  - The numerator will be the number of patients who develop a new pressure ulcer (count all ulcers and those Stage II or greater) after admission.
  - Just count patients, not the number of ulcers. Even if a patient has four Stage II ulcers, they are only counted once.
  - The denominator is the number of all patients admitted during that time period.
  - Sometimes in calculating incidence rates, studies have excluded patients with an existing pressure ulcer on admission. Neither approach is necessarily better; just be consistent.
  - Divide the numerator by the denominator and multiply by 100 to get the percentage.

Example: 21 patients with a new pressure ulcer ÷ 227 patients = .093 × 100 = 9.3 percent

(www.ahrq.gov/professionals/systems/long-term-care/resources/pressure-ulcers/pressureulcertoolkit/putool5.html)

As stated above, two types of measures can be monitored: incidence and prevalence rates. Incidence rates provide the most direct evidence of the quality of your care. Therefore your quality improvement efforts should focus on incidence rates. Prevalence may reflect a single point in time, such as on the first day of each month. This is known as point prevalence. However, it can also reflect a prolonged period of time, such as an entire hospital stay. This is known as period prevalence. Both types of prevalence rates (point and period) include pressure ulcers present on admission, in addition to new ulcers that developed while

in your facility or on your unit. Therefore they can provide a useful snapshot of the pressure ulcer burden of care on the staff, but they say less about your quality of preventive care than do incidence rates. (AHRQ, 2015)

The majority of this information is presented to the staff in graph format. The frequency of reporting varies according to the information, the monitoring timeline of the organization, and the frequency of assessment. Most institutions look at financial outcomes on a daily or weekly basis. Patient satisfaction may be monitored weekly, monthly, or quarterly. The NDNQI unit based outcomes are reported on a quarterly basis, with the nurse satisfaction data reported annually.

In reviewing graphs that represent performance, the nurse needs to be able to:

1) Recognize the current level of performance;
2) Determine the relationship of the current level to the strategic goal of the organization/department;
3) Compare performance to professional comparisons; and
4) Determine if an improvement is required.

This representation of outcomes demonstrates five quarters of performance. The red line represents the chosen benchmark. For quarters one of 2012, two of 2012, three of the 12 units outperformed the benchmark. Their rates were lower than the benchmark. With pressure ulcers, the goal is fewer than the benchmark. With outcomes such as patient satisfaction, the goal is to be above the benchmark. Something happened in the fourth quarter of 2012 and the first quarter of 2013. In the fourth quarter of 2012, 7 Tower had more pressure ulcers than the benchmark. In the first quarter of 2013, all four units were higher than the benchmark. The nurses will need to identify the concerns and necessary process or evidence-based changes.

The challenge with such dashboards is that the performance levels are made available to staff quarterly, and not in "real time". This may preclude rapid process improvement. Many institutions prioritize items such as infections, patient satisfaction, and falls, and review performance on a daily level. It is not uncommon to see units bragging about levels of performance with signs such as "200 days without an infection," or "125 days without a fall" posted on the performance board. On such units, when an event occurs, a "huddle" is called, usually within 15 minutes to review the event, and to determine actions that need to be implemented immediately so that future occurrences can be prevented. However, it is important that lessons learned from the huddle are shared with the performance-improvment representatives on the unit.

A sample of a post-fall huddle follows:

Post-Fall Huddle Guidelines

Date: _____ Time of fall: _____ Time of huddle: _____ Room #: _____ SHIFT *(circle one)*: D/PM/NOC

Diagnosis: _____ Pertinent medical Hx: _____

LOCATION of FALL:

☐ Bed/ Bedside Commode   ☐ Chair   ☐ Gurney   ☐ Hallway   ☐ Room   ☐ Restroom

☐ Other: _____

BACKGROUND: Fall risk factors / risk for injury *(check all that apply)*:

☐ Altered mental status	☐ Pain or discomfort: Location	☐ Age (>85)
☐ Dizziness/lightheadedness	☐ Diagnosis r/t *(Hypoglycemia/ Seizure/Hypotension/Parkinson/Dementia)*	☐ Prior fall history
☐ Change in vital signs	☐ Bones *(Osteoporosis)*	☐ Impaired communication
☐ Medications *(Benzodiazipines, Pain meds, B/P meds, hypnotics)*	☐ Surgery *(recent/Fracture/amputee)*	☐ New infection or illness
☐ SOB	☐ Physical condition *(poor balance, weakness)(equipment)*	☐ Environmental factors
☐ Anticoagulation	☐ Sensory or neural deficit	☐ Other: _____
☐ s/p OD or intoxication	☐ ETOH use	

Information Related to Fall Event	FINDINGS
1. Was patient on fall precaution?	_____ YES _____ NO
2. Most recent fall-risk assessment score?	
3. Was patient alone at the time of fall?	_____ YES _____ NO
4. Describe in patient's own words what they were dong prior to fall.	
5. Elimination problems : (_____ urgency; _____ diarrhea, _____ incontinence)	_____ YES _____ NO
TYPE of FALL	**DESCRIPTION**
A. _____ Accidental fall	_____ Slip _____ Trip
B. _____ Anticipated physiological fall related to: _____ loss of balance _____ impaired gait or mobility _____ impaired cognition/confusion _____ impaired vision _____ functional deficits _____ disease process _____ unrealistic assessment of their ability	
C. _____ Unanticipated physiological fall *(created by condition that cannot be predicted, e.g. unexpected orthostasis, extreme hypoglycemia, stroke or heart attack.)*	
D. _____ Intentional fall: *(Patient who voluntarily alters body position to lower level).*	

NURSING OBSERVATION/ASSESSMENT	FINDINGS
Neuro checks: Glasgow Coma Scale: _____	_____ Changes in MS *(Mental Status)* _____ Headache _____ Vomiting _____ Bleeding
Did patient hit his/her head?	_____ YES _____ NO
Fall witnessed?	_____ YES _____ NO
What were the provider's findings and orders?	__ Injury __ Pain __ Functional change __ Other:

ACTION/RECOMMENDATION/PREVENTATIVE MEASURES

_____ Assistive device *(e.g. walker, cane)*	_____ Hip protectors	_____ PT/OT evaluation
_____ Bed alarm	_____ Non-skid socks	_____ Removed clutter/ equipment
_____ Close observation	_____ Moved patient *(higher visibility)*	_____ Toileting plan
_____ Behavioral management plan	_____ Pain management assessment	

Follow–up Plan: *(Free text new interventions or family to prevent further falls).*

Print and signature (RN/LVN): _____

(www.visn8.va.gov/visn8/.../fallsteam/postfallhuddle_guideline.docx)

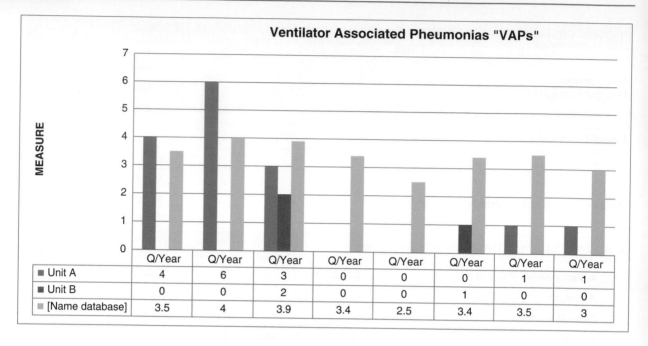

	Q/Year	Q/Year	Q/Year	Q/Year	Q/Year	Q/Year	Q/Year	Q/Year
■ Unit A	4	6	3	0	0	0	1	1
■ Unit B	0	0	2	0	0	1	0	0
▨ [Name database]	3.5	4	3.9	3.4	2.5	3.4	3.5	3

The NDNQI benchmark for ventilator associated pneumonia is compared to the actual performance of two critical units over 8 quarters. Unit A outperformed the benchmark for 6 of the 8 quarters, whereas Unit B unperformed the benchmark for 5 of the 8 quarters.

The next graph represents performance on one of the CORE measures.

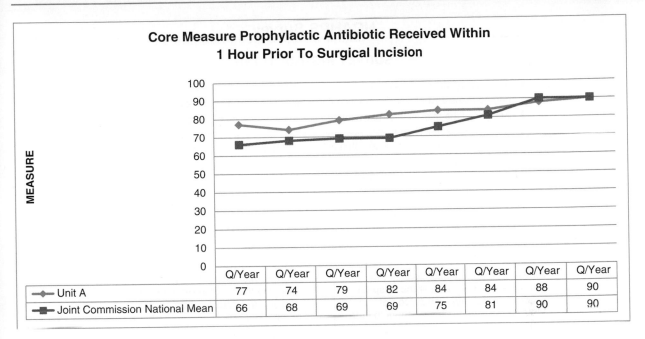

Core Measure Prophylactic Antibiotic Received Within
1 Hour Prior To Surgical Incision

	Q/Year	Q/Year	Q/Year	Q/Year	Q/Year	Q/Year	Q/Year	Q/Year
Unit A	77	74	79	82	84	84	88	90
Joint Commission National Mean	66	68	69	69	75	81	90	90

The graph demonstrates that Unit A outperformed the benchmark six of eight quarters.
When the unit results are the xsame as the benchmark, it is not considered outperforming.

This graph represents a sustained level of performance that exceeds the benchmark comparison. The hospital was above The Joint Commission national mean (the benchmark) for six of the eight quarters. When the unit results are the same as the benchmark, it is not considered outperforming.

The HCAHPS (Hospital Consumer Assessment of Healthcare Providers and Systems) survey is the first national, standardized, publicly reported survey of patients' perspectives of hospital care.

Three broad goals have shaped HCAHPS. First, the survey is designed to produce data about patients' perspectives of care that allow objective and meaningful comparisons of hospitals on topics that are important to consumers. Second, public reporting of the survey results creates new incentives for hospitals to improve quality of care. Third, public reporting serves to enhance accountability in health care by increasing transparency of the quality of hospital care (Centers for Medicare and Medicaid Services [CMS], 2015)

HCAHPS Survey

SURVEY INSTRUCTIONS

♦ You should only fill out this survey if you were the patient during the hospital stay named in the cover letter. Do not fill out this survey if you were not the patient.

♦ Answer <u>all</u> the questions by checking the box to the left of your answer.

♦ You are sometimes told to skip over some questions in this survey. When this happens you will see an arrow with a note that tells you what question to answer next, like this:

☐   Yes
☑   No   ➔ *If No, Go to Question 1*

You may notice a number on the survey. This number is used to let us know if you returned your survey so we don't have to send you reminders.
Please note: Questions 1-25 in this survey are part of a national initiative to measure the quality of care in hospitals. OMB #0938-0981

Please answer the questions in this survey about your stay at the hospital named on the cover letter. Do not include any other hospital stays in your answers.

YOUR CARE FROM NURSES

1. **During this hospital stay, how often did nurses treat you with <u>courtesy and respect</u>?**

   ¹☐ Never
   ²☐ Sometimes
   ³☐ Usually
   ⁴☐ Always

2. **During this hospital stay, how often did nurses <u>listen carefully to you</u>?**

   ¹☐ Never
   ²☐ Sometimes
   ³☐ Usually
   ⁴☐ Always

3. **During this hospital stay, how often did nurses <u>explain things</u> in a way you could understand?**

   ¹☐ Never
   ²☐ Sometimes
   ³☐ Usually
   ⁴☐ Always

4. **During this hospital stay, after you pressed the call button, how often did you get help as soon as you wanted it?**

   ¹☐ Never
   ²☐ Sometimes
   ³☐ Usually
   ⁴☐ Always
   ⁹☐ I never pressed the call button

YOUR CARE FROM DOCTORS

5. **During this hospital stay, how often did doctors treat you with <u>courtesy and respect</u>?**

   ¹☐ Never
   ²☐ Sometimes
   ³☐ Usually
   ⁴☐ Always

6. **During this hospital stay, how often did doctors <u>listen carefully to you</u>?**

   ¹☐ Never
   ²☐ Sometimes
   ³☐ Usually
   ⁴☐ Always

7. **During this hospital stay, how often did doctors <u>explain things</u> in a way you could understand?**

   ¹☐ Never
   ²☐ Sometimes
   ³☐ Usually
   ⁴☐ Always

THE HOSPITAL ENVIRONMENT

8. **During this hospital stay, how often were your room and bathroom kept clean?**

    ¹ ☐ Never
    ² ☐ Sometimes
    ³ ☐ Usually
    ⁴ ☐ Always

9. **During this hospital stay, how often was the area around your room quiet at night?**

    ¹ ☐ Never
    ² ☐ Sometimes
    ³ ☐ Usually
    ⁴ ☐ Always

YOUR EXPERIENCES IN THIS HOSPITAL

10. **During this hospital stay, did you need help from nurses or other hospital staff in getting to the bathroom or in using a bedpan?**

    ¹ ☐ Yes
    ² ☐ No ➜ **If No, Go to Question 12**

11. **How often did you get help in getting to the bathroom or in using a bedpan as soon as you wanted?**

    ¹ ☐ Never
    ² ☐ Sometimes
    ³ ☐ Usually
    ⁴ ☐ Always

12. **During this hospital stay, did you need medicine for pain?**

    ¹ ☐ Yes
    ² ☐ No ➜ **If No, Go to Question 15**

13. **During this hospital stay, how often was your pain well controlled?**

    ¹ ☐ Never
    ² ☐ Sometimes
    ³ ☐ Usually
    ⁴ ☐ Always

14. **During this hospital stay, how often did the hospital staff do everything they could to help you with your pain?**

    ¹ ☐ Never
    ² ☐ Sometimes
    ³ ☐ Usually
    ⁴ ☐ Always

15. **During this hospital stay, were you given any medicine that you had not taken before?**

    ¹ ☐ Yes
    ² ☐ No ➜ **If No, Go to Question 18**

16. **Before giving you any new medicine, how often did hospital staff tell you what the medicine was for?**

    ¹ ☐ Never
    ² ☐ Sometimes
    ³ ☐ Usually
    ⁴ ☐ Always

17. **Before giving you any new medicine, how often did hospital staff describe possible side effects in a way you could understand?**

    ¹ ☐ Never
    ² ☐ Sometimes
    ³ ☐ Usually
    ⁴ ☐ Always

WHEN YOU LEFT THE HOSPITAL

18. **After you left the hospital, did you go directly to your own home, to someone else's home, or to another health facility?**

    ¹ ☐ Own home
    ² ☐ Someone else's home
    ³ ☐ Another health facility ➜ **If Another, Go to Question 21**

19. **During this hospital stay, did doctors, nurses or other hospital staff talk with you about whether you would have the help you needed when you left the hospital?**

    ¹ ☐ Yes
    ² ☐ No

Continued

20. **During this hospital stay, did you get information in writing about what symptoms or health problems to look out for after you left the hospital?**

    ^{1}☐ Yes
    ^{2}☐ No

OVERALL RATING OF HOSPITAL

Please answer the following questions about your stay at the hospital named on the cover letter. Do not include any other hospital stays in your answers.

21. **Using any number from 0 to 10, where 0 is the worst hospital possible and 10 is the best hospital possible, what number would you use to rate this hospital during your stay?**

    ^{0}☐ 0   Worst hospital possible
    ^{1}☐ 1
    ^{2}☐ 2
    ^{3}☐ 3
    ^{4}☐ 4
    ^{5}☐ 5
    ^{6}☐ 6
    ^{7}☐ 7
    ^{8}☐ 8
    ^{9}☐ 9
    ^{10}☐ 10   Best hospital possible

22. **Would you recommend this hospital to your friends and family?**

    ^{1}☐ Definitely no
    ^{2}☐ Probably no
    ^{3}☐ Probably yes
    ^{4}☐ Definitely yes

UNDERSTANDING YOUR CARE WHEN YOU LEFT THE HOSPITAL

23. **During this hospital stay, staff took my preferences and those of my family or caregiver into account in deciding what my health care needs would be when I left.**

    ^{1}☐ Strongly disagree
    ^{2}☐ Disagree
    ^{3}☐ Agree
    ^{4}☐ Strongly agree

24. **When I left the hospital, I had a good understanding of the things I was responsible for in managing my health.**

    ^{1}☐ Strongly disagree
    ^{2}☐ Disagree
    ^{3}☐ Agree
    ^{4}☐ Strongly agree

25. **When I left the hospital, I clearly understood the purpose for taking each of my medications.**

    ^{1}☐ Strongly disagree
    ^{2}☐ Disagree
    ^{3}☐ Agree
    ^{4}☐ Strongly agree
    ^{5}☐ I was not given any medication when I left the hospital

ABOUT YOU

There are only a few remaining items left.

26. **During this hospital stay, were you admitted to this hospital through the Emergency Room?**

    ^{1}☐ Yes
    ^{2}☐ No

27. **In general, how would you rate your overall health?**

    ^{1}☐ Excellent
    ^{2}☐ Very good
    ^{3}☐ Good
    ^{4}☐ Fair
    ^{5}☐ Poor

28. **In general, how would you rate your overall <u>mental or emotional health</u>?**

    ^{1}☐ Excellent
    ^{2}☐ Very good
    ^{3}☐ Good
    ^{4}☐ Fair
    ^{5}☐ Poor

29. **What is the highest grade or level of school that you have <u>completed</u>?**

   $^1\square$ 8th grade or less

   $^2\square$ Some high school, but did not graduate

   $^3\square$ High school graduate or GED

   $^4\square$ Some college or 2-year degree

   $^5\square$ 4-year college graduate

   $^6\square$ More than 4-year college degree

30. **Are you of Spanish, Hispanic or Latino origin or descent?**

   $^1\square$ No, not Spanish/Hispanic/Latino

   $^2\square$ Yes, Puerto Rican

   $^3\square$ Yes, Mexican, Mexican American, Chicano

   $^4\square$ Yes, Cuban

   $^5\square$ Yes, other Spanish/Hispanic/Latino

31. **What is your race? Please choose one or more.**

   $^1\square$ White

   $^2\square$ Black or African American

   $^3\square$ Asian

   $^4\square$ Native Hawaiian or other Pacific Islander

   $^5\square$ American Indian or Alaska Native

32. **What language do you <u>mainly</u> speak at home?**

   $^1\square$ English

   $^2\square$ Spanish

   $^3\square$ Chinese

   $^4\square$ Russian

   $^5\square$ Vietnamese

   $^6\square$ Portuguese

   $^9\square$ Some other language (please print): _____

THANK YOU

Please return the completed survey in the postage-paid envelope.

[NAME OF SURVEY VENDOR OR SELF-ADMINISTERING HOSPITAL]

[RETURN ADDRESS OF SURVEY VENDOR OR SELF-ADMINISTERING HOSPITAL]

Questions 1-22 and 26-32 are part of the HCAHPS Survey and are works of the U.S. Government. These HCAHPS questions are in the public domain and therefore are NOT subject to U.S. copyright laws. The three Care Transitions Measure® questions (Questions 23-25) are copyright of The Care Transitions Program® (www.caretransitions.org).

Continued

Sample Initial Cover Letter for the HCAHPS Survey

[HOSPITAL LETTERHEAD]

[SAMPLED PATIENT NAME]
[ADDRESS]
[CITY, STATE ZIP]

Dear [SAMPLED PATIENT NAME]:

Our records show that you were recently a patient at [NAME OF HOSPITAL] and discharged on [DATE OF DISCHARGE]. Because you had a recent hospital stay, we are asking for your help. This survey is part of an ongoing national effort to understand how patients view their hospital experience. Hospital results will be publicly reported and made available on the Internet at www.medicare.gov/hospitalcompare. These results will help consumers make important choices about their hospital care, and will help hospitals improve the care they provide.

Questions 1-25 in the enclosed survey are part of a national initiative sponsored by the United States Department of Health and Human Services to measure the quality of care in hospitals. Your participation is voluntary and will not affect your health benefits.

We hope that you will take the time to complete the survey. Your participation is greatly appreciated. After you have completed the survey, please return it in the pre-paid envelope. Your answers may be shared with the hospital for purposes of quality improvement. [*OPTIONAL*: You may notice a number on the survey. This number is used to let us know if you returned your survey so we don't have to send you reminders.]

If you have any questions about the enclosed survey, please call the toll-free number 1-800-xxx-xxxx. Thank you for helping to improve health care for all consumers.

Sincerely,

[HOSPITAL ADMINISTRATOR]
[HOSPITAL NAME]

Note: The OMB Paperwork Reduction Act language must be included in the mailing. This language can be either on the front or back of the cover letter or questionnaire, but cannot be a separate mailing. The exact OMB Paperwork Reduction Act language is included in this appendix. Please refer to the Mail Only, and Mixed Mode sections, for specific letter guidelines.

Sample Follow-up Cover Letter for the HCAHPS Survey

[HOSPITAL LETTERHEAD]

[SAMPLED PATIENT NAME]
[ADDRESS]
[CITY, STATE ZIP]

Dear [SAMPLED PATIENT NAME]:

Our records show that you were recently a patient at [NAME OF HOSPITAL] and discharged on [DATE OF DISCHARGE]. Approximately three weeks ago we sent you a survey regarding your hospitalization. If you have already returned the survey to us, please accept our thanks and disregard this letter. However, if you have not yet completed the survey, please take a few minutes and complete it now.

Because you had a recent hospital stay, we are asking for your help. This survey is part of an ongoing national effort to understand how patients view their hospital experience. Hospital results will be publicly reported and made available on the Internet at www.medicare.gov/hospitalcompare. These results will help consumers make important choices about their hospital care, and will help hospitals improve the care they provide.

Questions 1-25 in the enclosed survey are part of a national initiative sponsored by the United States Department of Health and Human Services to measure the quality of care in hospitals. Your participation is voluntary and will not affect your health benefits. Please take a few minutes and complete the enclosed survey. After you have completed the survey, please return it in the pre-paid envelope. Your answers may be shared with the hospital for purposes of quality improvement. [*OPTIONAL*: You may notice a number on the survey. This number is used to let us know if you returned your survey so we don't have to send you reminders.]

If you have any questions about the enclosed survey, please call the toll-free number 1-800-xxx-xxxx. Thank you again for helping to improve health care for all consumers.

Sincerely,

[HOSPITAL ADMINISTRATOR]
[HOSPITAL NAME]

Note: The OMB Paperwork Reduction Act language must be included in the mailing. This language can be either on the front or back of the cover letter or questionnaire, but cannot be a separate mailing.The exact OMB Paperwork Reduction Act language is included in this appendix. Please refer to the Mail Only, and Mixed Mode sections, for specific letter guidelines.

Continued

OMB Paperwork Reduction Act Language

The OMB Paperwork Reduction Act language must be included in the survey mailing. This language can be either on the front or back of the cover letter or questionnaire, but cannot be a separate mailing. The following is the language that must be used:

English Version

"According to the Paperwork Reduction Act of 1995, no persons are required to respond to a collection of information unless it displays a valid OMB control number. The valid OMB control number for this information collection is 0938-0981. The time required to complete this information collected is estimated to average 8 minutes for questions 1-25 on the survey, including the time to review instructions, search existing data resources, gather the data needed, and complete and review the information collection. If you have any comments concerning the accuracy of the time estimate(s) or suggestions for improving this form, please write to: Centers for Medicare & Medicaid Services, 7500 Security Boulevard, C1-25-05, Baltimore, MD 21244-1850."

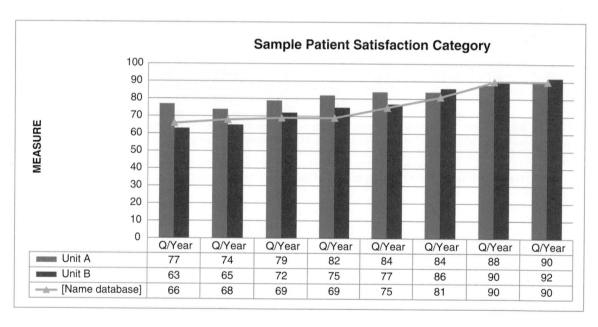

Sample Patient Satisfaction Category

	Q/Year	Q/Year	Q/Year	Q/Year	Q/Year	Q/Year	Q/Year	Q/Year
Unit A	77	74	79	82	84	84	88	90
Unit B	63	65	72	75	77	86	90	92
[Name database]	66	68	69	69	75	81	90	90

The graph demonstrates that Unit A outperformed the benchmark in six of eight quarters and that Unit B outperformed the benchmark in five of eight quarters. When the unit results are the same as the benchmark, it is not considered outperforming.

With regard to this measure of patient satisfaction, Unit A outperformed the benchmark in 6 of the 8 quarters. Unit B outperformed the benchmark for 5 of the 8 quarters.

These types of graphic representation of performance allow the staff to view **trends,** to be accountable for patient outcomes, and to continually drive performance improvement. Behind each of the above performance metrics, there are processes developed that identify targets for improvement, develop and implement plans for change, and the development and implementing plans for change and sustained high levels of performance. But there is further documentation that is needed to ascertain what actions, evidence, and research has led to the sustained improvements.

In Magnet recognized institutions, there is a template that summarizes the reporting and communication of improvements. This tool is a good template for the summarization of such efforts. (American Association of Colleges of Nursing [AACN], 2013, p. 60)

- Background/problem
  - Provide relevant background information.
  - Describe the problem that exists in the organization.
- Goal statement
  - State the goal that is the desired improvement/change/result.
  - Identify the measure selected to demonstrate the improvement/change/result (i.e., errors, incidents, indicators, satisfaction).
- Description of the intervention/initiative/activity
  - Describe the action that had an impact on the problem and resulted in the achievement of the goal.
    - Include where the intervention/initiative occurred (unit, department).
    - Include the date when the intervention/initiative occurred.
- Participants
  - List the participants involved.
  - Include name, discipline, title, and department.
- Outcomes
  - Demonstrate the achievement of the desired improvement/change/result with data displayed in a clearly labeled graph with a data table.
    - Trended data must be displayed to show change/improvement/result.
    - The selected measure must correlate with desired goal.
    - Pre-intervention/initiative data and post-intervention/initiative data must:
      - Use the same measure to demonstrate the effect of the intervention/initiative.
      - Be clearly identified with dates.
    - The intervention time frame/dates must be clearly identified on the graph.

The following clinical corner gives an example of an evidence-based improvement with the resultant graph demonstrating improvement.

SUMMARY

The continual monitoring of performance is integral to the continued excellence in the delivery of patient care. Nurses need to play an active role in the constant evaluation of the delivery of care and assume accountability for the outcomes within the organization.

CLINICAL CORNER

Investigate the use of the Kings Stool Chart when Assessing the Enterally Fed Patients

Diarrhea is defined as the passage of fluid or unformed stool. Alleviating diarrhea development and controlling its consequences can be achieved through frequent monitoring and early intervention. In the acute care setting, the incidence of diarrhea in the acute care setting varies from 2% to 95%, (Whelan, 2004). Alterations are most often made to the rate or type of feeding being infused, or changing to more expensive elemental feedings. The majority of definitions of diarrhea are subjective. Defining diarrhea among health professionals differs, basing their documentation on experience and subjective opinion (Whelan, 2004). In a retrospective chart review of 43 patients in the Medical Intensive Care Unit (MICU) and Critical Care Unit (CCU) at St. Joseph's Healthcare System, all feedings were appropriate and none were changed to elemental formula. However, there was a lack of standardized documentation at the bedside as it relates to the characteristics of stool criteria, which includes consistency, weight, and frequency.

The purpose of this evidence-based practice research pilot study was to determine if the use of standardized terminology for diarrhea, found in the Kings Stool Chart, (KSC), improve documentation of fecal output, and decrease the number of held ENT attributed to changes in bowel habits. The Registered Nurse (RN) and Patient Care Assistant (PCA) staff for the MICU/CCU were educated on benefits of feedings versus elemental intervention, the need for accurate objective guidelines for stool characteristics, and the use of the KSC. After a three month implementation period, forty-two random charts from this population were reviewed using the same audit tool. PASW (Predictive Analysis and Software, version 18, July 2009), was used for data analysis. The focus of our

Continued

CLINICAL CORNER—cont'd

research was objective documentation. Results: There was a decrease in the discontinuation of tube feeds by 10%. There was an increase in documentation of all the components of objective stool classification criteria: consistency 16%, weight 30%, and frequency 9% as compared to data collected before the use of the KSC. There was a marked increase in the identification of diarrhea by 29 % after the initiation of the KSC. However, there was a decrease in documentation of odor and color stool characteristics. Conclusion: Objective stool output documentation can be used to make an educated nutrition assessment and plan for an appropriate enteral feeding regimen. It is an invaluable tool for the interdisciplinary team of the RN and Registered Dietitian. The use of the KSC decreased discontinuing of enteral feedings by 10%, increased appropriate documentation of the three objective stool classification parameters, and increased the bedside

nurse's objectivity when identifying normal bowel changes because of enteral feedings versus diarrhea.

The Kings Stool Chart Quality Improvement Outcomes:
- Diarrhea is difficult to define, with a variation in incidence from 15% to 63%. The KSC provides documentation parameters that are clear cut, and translatable within the interdisciplinary team.
- An initial retrospective chart review of 43 patients was completed to establish a need for the KSC. Findings verified that stool documentation was not standard or objective, with a 15% occurrence of feeding disruption.
- A pilot study was completed with the KSC following staff education. A chart review found a decline in tube feed disruption by 10%.

Evidence-based objective stool output documentation can be used to make an educated nutrition assessment and plan for an appropriate enteral feeding regimen.

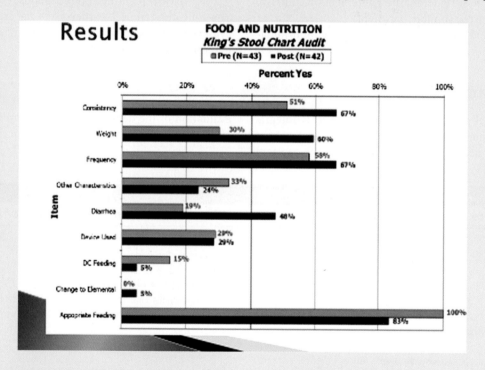

The project began in May of 2010 ending in August of 2011; after three months, forty-two random charts from this population were reviewed using the same audit tool as for the pre-implementation data.

By Kathy Faber, RN, MSN, CNL, and
Eleanor Schiavo, MS, RD

EVIDENCE-BASED PRACTICE

Wong, C., & Cummings, G. (2007). The relationship between nursing leadership and patient outcomes: a systematic review. *Journal of Nursing Management*, 6(15), 709-724.

Our aim was to describe the findings of a systematic review of studies that examine the relationship between nursing leadership practices and patient outcomes.

Background: As healthcare faces an economic downturn, stressful work environments, upcoming retirements of leaders and projected workforce shortages, implementing strategies to ensure effective leadership and optimal patient outcomes are paramount. However, a gap still exists in what is known about the association between nursing leadership and patient outcomes.

Methods: Published English-only research articles that examined leadership practices of nurses in formal leadership positions and patient outcomes were selected from eight online bibliographic databases. Quality assessments, data extraction, and analysis were completed on all included studies.

Results: A total of 20 studies satisfied our inclusion criteria and were retained. Current evidence suggests relationships between positive relational leadership styles and higher patient satisfaction, lower patient mortality, medication errors, restraint use, and hospital-acquired infections.

Conclusions: The findings document evidence of a positive relationship between relational leadership and a variety of patient outcomes, although future testing of leadership models that examine the mechanisms of influence on outcomes is warranted.

Implications for nursing management. Efforts by organizations and individuals to develop transformational and relational leadership reinforces organizational strategies to improve patient outcomes.

Evidence exists demonstrating that the nursing work environment such as staffing, has a correlation to patient mortality and adverse events in the hospital setting. Nurse leaders are responsible for ensuring proper staffing. This is challenging because of the economy and nursing workloads, to name a few.

This study was to describe findings of a systematic review of studies examining the relationship between nursing leadership and patient outcomes. Evidence was gathered from 1985 to 2012. There were a total of 20 studies reviewed. Donabedian's (1966) structure-process-outcome (SPO) framework was used. Three conceptual domains were: structure, which is concerned with organizational or setting factors; process, which is concerned with mechanisms for coordinating and facilitating patient care; and outcomes of care. Inclusion criteria for studies were the relationship between nursing leadership in all types of health care settings, and one or more patient outcomes. Leadership included: leadership styles, behaviors, competencies, direct observation of leaders, or ratings of leader behaviors made by followers.

The findings showed that there was a key relationship between relational leadership and the reduction of adverse events, specifically medication errors.

In conclusion, this study showed that there is a positive relationship between relational leadership styles, and patient satisfaction and patient outcomes.

Reference

Donabedian, A (1966). Evaluating the quality of medical care. *Mellbank Memorial Fund Quarterly, 44*(3), 166–206.

NCLEX® EXAMINATION QUESTIONS

1. Comparison information that allows organizations to evaluate their own performance in relation to others is:
   A. Benchmark
   B. Dashboard
   C. Graph
   D. Trend

2. Mechanisms related to resource identification and allocation have to be driven by internal data, and information systems that consider all domains of hospital data include:
   A. Clinical, fiscal, administrative, and patient satisfaction data
   B. Classification, financial, administrative, and patient satisfaction data
   C. Clinical, financial, social, and patient satisfaction data
   D. Clinical, financial, administrative, and patient satisfaction data

3. Nursing data fall into four domains:
   A. Patient care, provider staffing, administrative, and research
   B. Patient care, billing, administrative, and research
   C. Core values, provider staffing, administrative, and research
   D. Core values, billing, administrative, and research

4. One driving force for increasing patient satisfaction is:
   A. Clinical benefits
   B. Community benefits
   C. Classification benefits
   D. Management benefits

5. _____measures the number of patients developing new pressure ulcers during a period in time
   A. Incidence
   B. Prevalence
   C. Benchmarking
   D. Trending

6. _____measures the number of patients with pressure ulcers at a certain point or period in time.
   A. Incidence
   B. Prevalence
   C. Benchmarking
   D. Trending

7. Pressure ulcers cost $9.1 to $11.6 billion per year in the United States. The cost of individual patient care ranges from _____per year in the United States.
   A. $10,000 to $20,000
   B. $15,900 to $23,000
   C. $20,900 to $151,700
   D. $40,000 to $50,000

8. The data for nursing sensitive indicators are collected at the institution and uploaded to the National Database of Nursing Quality Indicators. There are approximately _____US hospitals participating in this database.
   A. 1000
   B. 1500
   C. 2000
   D. 2500

9. _____measure aspects of nursing care such as assessment, intervention, and Registered Nurse job satisfaction.
   A. Nursing-sensitive indicators
   B. Process indicators
   C. Core values
   D. Process improvement

10. Nursing sensitive indicators include:
    A. Nursing turnover
    B. Patient falls
    C. Nosocomial infections
    D. All of the above are correct

Answers: 1. A   2. D   3. A   4. A   5. A   6. B   7. C
8. B   9. B   10. D

REFERENCES

Agency for Healthcare Research and Quality [AHRQ]. (2015). *Pressure Ulcer Resources*. Retrieved from www.ahrq.gov/professionals/systems/long-term-care/resources/pressure-ulcers/pressureulcertoolkit/putool5.html. (January 26, 2015).

American Nurses Association [ANA]. (2014). *Nursing Sensitive Indicators*. www.nursingworld.org/MainMenuCategories/ThePracticeofProfessionalNursing/PatientSafetyQuality/Research-Measurement/The-National-Database/Nursing-Sensitive-Indicators_1.

American Nurses Credentialing Center [ANCC]. (2013). *2014 Magnet Application Manual*. Silver Spring, MD: author.

Centers for Medicare and Medicaid Services [CMS]. (2015). *HCHAPS—The Patient Perception of Care Survey*. www.cms.gov/Medicare/Quality-Initiatives-Patient-Assessment-Instruments/HospitalQualityInits/HospitalHCAHPS.html.

Cramer, E., Staggs, V., & Dunton, N. (2014). Improving the nursing work environment. *American Nurse Today*, 9(1), 55–57.

Hall, J., & Kelly, C. (2014). A partnership to enhance outcomes through quality dashboards and action planning. *American Nurse Today*, 9(1), 57–58.

Montalvo, I. (2007). The National Database of Nursing Quality Indicators™ (NDNQI®). Manuscript 2. *OJIN: The Online Journal of Issues in Nursing*, 12(3).

Northwestern Hospital Magnet Redesignation Document. 2010). ww2.nmh.org/oweb/MagnetDoc/nmh_magnet2010.htm#02_tl_transformational_leadership/tl1_narrative.htm.

VISN. (Post Falls Huddle, Palo Alto Veterans Administration Hospital. www.visn8.va.gov/visn8/.../fallsteam/postfallhuddle_guideline.docx.

Congratulations

SECTION OUTLINE

To those readers who are students, this chapter is about progression after graduation. First of all, congratulations! It is not yet time to relax, however. There is much work to be done on entry to the new role of a professional nurse. This chapter will review the process for registering and taking the licensure exam, getting your first job, the means to continue professional growth, and continuation of your nursing education.

21

New Graduates: The Immediate Future: Job Interviewing, NCLEX, and Continuing Education

OBJECTIVES

- Review the recruitment process for patient care staff.
- Identify the steps in the employment process.
- Review the importance of a résumé in the employment process.
- Differentiate between the various types of interviewing techniques used in health care.
- Differentiate between various types of questions used in the employment interview.
- Identify the role of the nurse manager in the hiring process.

- Review the process for registering for the licensing examination.
- Identify states participating in the Nurse Licensure Compact.
- Elaborate on the decision making surrounding selection of the first job.
- Identify specialty organizations in nursing.
- Review the types of certification examinations available to the nurse.
- Discuss the importance of continued education in nursing.

OUTLINE

KEY TERMS

ANCC American Nurses Credentialing Center
home state the nurse's primary state of residence
interview formal consultation to evaluate qualifications of a potential employee
NCLEX National Council Licensure Examination
NCSBN National Council of State Boards of Nursing
Nursing Licensure Compact states recognizing the license regulation of other states
party state any state that has adopted this compact

Pearson VUE company under contract with NCSBN to administer NCLEX examination
recruitment process of obtaining individuals for employment
remote state any party state other than the home state
résumé summary of an individual's past employment, education, and honors
retention preservation or maintenance of staff
specialty certification examination credential specifying the candidate's knowledge level within a specialty

THE EMPLOYMENT PROCESS

It is the responsibility of the organization to provide staffing adequate to deliver safe and competent care. The numbers of staff required will depend on the acuity of the patients, the requirements of the job, mandatory staffing law (if applicable), health department regulations, and organization policies. As positions become vacant or new ones created, the first step in the employment process is to determine the competencies required for the position. This will require a job description.

All organizations will have a template for the job description. You need to familiarize yourself with the format in your organization. An effective job description needs to minimally include: (1) title, (2) job objectives, and (3) a list of duties. The job description also includes nursing competencies and expected behaviors, and competencies as they relate to the strategic objectives of the organization. As the job description is finalized, the job is "posted" according to the organization's policies. The process of "posting" is the initial stage in the nine-stage process of recruitment (adapted from Huber, 2013).

1. Position posting;
2. Advertising;
3. Screening;
4. Interviewing;
5. Selecting;
6. Orienting;
7. Counseling/coaching/mentoring;
8. Performance evaluation; and
9. Staff development.

As a nurse manager you will play a role in each stage of this recruitment process. Your actual role in each stage of the process will depend on the organization's hierarchical structure. As a new nurse you need to be aware of the process, which you will be exposed to in your first hire.

Position Posting

Once a position becomes vacant within an organization, the facility posts the position internally for staff review and selection. Then the position is posted externally in the local newspapers and with staffing and recruiting agencies.

Advertising

Health care organizations may place ads in professional nursing journals or magazines, and/or on professional organization websites. This encourages a broad range of individuals to be exposed to the position posting.

Screening

Health care organizations use this process by reviewing applications and then determining whether or not the nurse meets the position criteria. Facilities that are equal opportunity employers must meet all federal government guidelines during the screening process. Screening for nursing positions may include criminal background checks, drug and alcohol screens, and nursing grade point averages (GPAs). Many institutions also use proficiency examinations, such as pharmacology or critical thinking examinations to screen candidates. Other institutions are now also using examinations that attempt to match the personality of the potential employee with the organizational culture.

Interviewing

Interviews are usually done in person, but they may also be conducted via telephone or teleconference. The interview may be one-on-one with the human resources representative and then with the nurse manager, or the interview may be conducted with multiple personnel at the same time.

Selecting

The nurse manager or clinical director usually makes the selection for a nursing position. If the position is a management position, the nurse manager and clinical director, and other members of the management team may select the candidate together.

THE INTERVIEW PROCESS

The most challenging aspect of the hiring process is to find the right person for the job. The job interview is the best way of determining the "fit" of the individual for the job and for your unit and organization. Remember, matching the job qualifications with the individual is only one aspect of the "right fit"; the personality and values of the individual also play a role in determination of the "right person for the job."

Before the interview process, a professional résumé is shared with individuals in the recruitment process. A **résumé** is a summary of professional and personal experiences (education, clinical experience, employment, skills, and interests) designed to introduce the candidate to potential employers. Often the résumé is the employer's first of impression of the candidate. As a new nurse manager, you will need to evaluate the résumé for "right fit."

For a résumé to be effective, it must be targeted to the job being applied for. A single "catch-all" résumé that a candidate expects to use in looking for various types of jobs is much less effective than several well-focused résumés that highlight pertinent experience or expertise. For example, if a candidate is planning to apply to both hospital-based and community-health-center–based positions, they might be better served by having two résumés, one focusing on hospital experience, and the other focusing on the community-health background. Remember, for a nurse looking for a job, the purpose of a résumé is to obtain an interview, so it must make a strong argument to the reader that you have something to offer. The purpose of the résumé to the nurse manager is for evaluation of a potential candidate's education, skills, and experience related to the open position. A résumé is different from a CV (curriculum vitae) in that a résumé is a summary of your academic and work history, whereas a CV is a more-detailed document of work history, academic experience, publications, and so on. A CV is usually used in the academic world. All nurses need to keep their résumé current; it is very frustrating to attempt to write a résumé after 5 years and try to remember everything you have accomplished! Update your résumé at least every 6 months.

RÉSUMÉ WRITING

New nurses and nurse managers and leaders all need to pay attention to their résumé. Tips for résumé writing are listed in Box 21-1.

Name and Address Section

- The name and address may be centered on the page or split on each margin.
- The name should be in a slightly larger type size than the rest of the résumé.
- The name should be in bold font.
- List a telephone number where you can be reached; list a home and/or a cell phone number, and make sure you have an answering machine or message capability so a message can be left for you (ensure that the greeting on the answering machine is appropriate for a potential employer to hear). Check your message box frequently to make sure that the box is not "full."
- Use an e-mail address that is professional and appropriate; avoid "cutesy" e-mail addresses such as Cutesypie@….
- Check e-mail and telephone messages several times a day.

BOX 21-1   Tips for Résumé Writing and Printing

- Résumés should be one page long, unless you have extensive experience in the position for which you are applying.
- Print on light blue, ivory, white, or beige paper (if you mail your résumé, the envelope must be the same color).
- Use Times Roman or similar font; do not use fancy fonts, underlining, or italics because they do not scan correctly.
- Margins should be 1 inch top, bottom, and sides.
- Use 12-point type size if possible; no smaller than 10-point type size.
- Do not use pronouns.

Objective

Be very specific, even if you have to list more than one job title. If you cannot be specific, omit this section. Make sure that this objective matches the facility to which you are applying.

Education

- List your college name, city, and state (not street address), and the years attended.
- List most recent degree first.
- List the graduation date or anticipated graduation date.
- List the degree and major or program.
- Give your grade point average (GPA) (if your overall GPA is not good, give your nursing GPA [e.g., Nursing GPA 3.5]).
- Once you have graduated, you can list your degree first and then the school and date.
- If you have graduated from a college or university, you do not need to list your high school.

Relevant Skills and Experience or Accomplishments

Use bullet format for clinical rotations, volunteer experiences, accomplishments at other jobs if relevant, computer skills, and so on. Special qualifications such as bilingual ability is important here.

Job History

- List jobs starting with the most recent and work back from there.
- List name of company, city, state (not street address), and years you worked (not months).

- Give your job title.
- Use bullets to state your accomplishments.
- Begin each bullet statement with an action verb. Use present tense for current job only; use past tense for all previous jobs.
- Do not use "responsible for" or "duties include"; list accomplishments in each job.
- If you have had jobs in the health care field or experience relevant to the job you are now seeking, give it more space on your résumé; jobs that are unrelated to what you are seeking can be given minimal space.

Professional Affiliation and Honors

- List any organizations that you were a member of as a student and/or other jobs you have had; list all honors and membership in honor societies.
- Do not put "References available on request" at the bottom of the résumé. References are always listed on a separate page that you can take with you to an interview.
- Do not list personal information (age, marital status, height, weight, social security number, etc.).

Proofread! Proofread! And Proofread Again!

Have someone else proofread your résumé. Do not rely on computer software (Jones, 2007, p. 380). Box 21-2 provides a sample résumé for a graduate nurse.

As a nurse manager evaluating this résumé, you would realize that this new nurse has computer skills, has demonstrated leadership qualities within her nursing education, and meets the basic needs of a new staff

---

BOX 21-2   Sample Résumé for a Nurse

Jane Doe, jdoe@email.com
1111 South Green Street
Anywhere, USA 00222
222-555-1212 (cell) 555-212-3333 (home)
Job Target: Long-term association with an acute care hospital acknowledged for nursing excellence

Skills
- Registered nurse highly skilled in care of the critically ill patient
- Strong ability to rapidly prioritize patient care and manage complex patient care
- Bilingual Spanish

Education and Certifications
University of State, Anywhere, USA
Bachelor of Science Degree, Nursing. GPA 3.76, 2003
Outstanding Student Award: attained for excellence in clinical area
American Association of Critical-Care Nurses: CCRN certification current to 2015
Basic Life Support Certificate and Advanced Cardiac Life Support Certificate

Professional Experience
Surgical Intensive Care Staff Nurse: June 2007 - present
Mercy Medical Center, Somewhere, NY

Continued

BOX 21-2 Sample Résumé for a Nurse—cont'd

Level II trauma center with 678 beds. 20-bed adult surgical intensive care unit

Post-cardiac, renal, and gastrointestinal surgery patient population

Cardiac Intensive Care Staff Nurse March 2005 to June 2007, Hammondton Medical Center

Community hospital with 320 beds. 10-bed cardiac intensive care. Post-cardiac intervention unit

Staff Nurse, Telemetry July 2003 to March 2005,

Hammondton Medical Center
40-bed telemetry unit

License
State of Anywhere, USA Registered Professional Nurse
Awards
Staff Nurse of the Year Hammondton Medical Center, 2006
Sigma Theta Tau, International Honor Society of Nursing.
  Chapter, inducted 2003

---

nurse. If you were looking for a nurse with extensive experience in the cardiac setting, this candidate does not meet that need.

As a new nurse developing a first professional nursing résumé, you need to access the resources available at your school of nursing. Most schools have resources to assist you in the development of a professional CV; it is in your best interest to use these services.

EFFECTIVE COVER LETTERS

All résumés need to be accompanied by a cover letter to the institution to which you are applying. The cover letter needs to be written in a professional tone. As a new nurse, this letter will set the tone for the individual reading the cover letter. For the nurse manager, this letter will let you know if this individual is someone who may be appropriate for the position. The qualities of an effective cover letter follow (Jones, 2007, p. 383):

- Brief, neat, and without errors.
- In business format.
- Name and title of person to whom the letter is addressed.
- Why you are interested, and what position you would like to apply for.
- Appointed time for taking NCLEX-RN (for a new nurse).
- Certifications that match the posted job (for an experienced nurse).
- Express appreciation for consideration and eagerness to be part of team.
- How you can be reached (telephone number).
- Use 9- by 12-inch envelope to send résumé and cover letter (first-class mail).

BOX 21-3 Example of an Effective Cover Letter

May 1, 2014
Elizabeth B. Wise, PhD, RN
Director of Nurse Recruitment and Hiring
Caring Hospital USA
Joy City, LA 70777
RE: Nursing Position on Medical-Surgical Unit
Dear Dr. Wise:
I have just graduated from Caring College and would like to apply for a new graduate nurse position on Medical-Surgical Unit II at Caring Hospital. I served there as a nurse technician while attending nursing school. I plan to take the NCLEX-RN examination in early June 2014 and will be available to start work by July 1, 2014.

Having worked as a nurse technician on Medical-Surgical Unit II for 3 years, I developed positive interpersonal and professional relationships with the team. Furthermore, I am well organized, have effective time-management skills, and am enthusiastic about the prospect of returning to the unit. I am proud to have worked at Caring Hospital for 3 years in light of its high rating and Magnet status. The mission of Caring Hospital is congruent with my values.

Thank you very much for your consideration. You may reach me any time on my cell phone at (999) 709-2525. I look forward to hearing from you to schedule an interview at your convenience.
Sincerely,
Scelitta Source

Adapted from Jones, R. A. (2007). *Nursing leadership and management: Theories, processes, and practice*. Philadelphia: F. A. Davis.

- Expect response to letter in 2 weeks.
- If not, call after 3 weeks; check with Human Resources.

Box 21-3 provides an example of an effective cover letter.

THE INTERVIEW

Credentials are often reviewed before or during the interview. These credentials usually consist of the following:

- Copy of the complete résumé.
- Copy of nursing license or a copy of notice of passing board scores.
- Two copies of a complete typed list of all references and previous managers (one copy for the human resources department, and one for the hiring manager). Be sure to include the references' complete names and titles, and current addresses and telephone numbers.
- Permission for a criminal background check. Be sure to have a list of your addresses from the previous 5 to 7 years.
- Permission for a drug and alcohol screen.
- For a new nurse, a copy of a recent cumulative grade report to show that you are a graduation candidate, and that you are not at risk for failing the licensing examination.

In many institutions, the initial interview is with the nurse recruiter. During this interview the employment process is reviewed, the salary and benefits are reviewed in a cursory manner, and the potential employee is evaluated as to what position in the organization might be appropriate. The individual is then interviewed by the nurse manager of the particular area of interest. Some nurse managers will also include staff in the interviewing process. This is a reflection of the culture of the organization.

It is important that you have prepared for the interview and do not try to "wing it." This is important for both the job candidate and the nurse manager. As the candidate, before the interview you will need to make a self-assessment of your abilities, your strong points, and your challenges. You also need to do a thorough review of the organization: What is their mission, vision, values? What is the philosophy of nursing? What is the care delivery model? Much of this information is available on the organization website. Remember you need to be able to put your best foot forward, and your self-awareness and organization awareness will greatly assist you in this endeavor. As the nurse manager, this is when the candidate assesses your abilities and judges whether or not they would like to work with you.

Styles of Interviewing

As you move forward to the interview process, you will need to have an idea of what you will ask or be asked. There are various styles of interviewing for the nurse manager, but you need to remember that the goal of the interview is to determine the capabilities of the individual, and to determine if this individual would be an asset to the unit.

The more traditional styles of interviewing ask questions that elicit standard questions from the prospective employee. Samples of such questions would be:

- How would you describe yourself?
- What specific goals have you established for your career?
- What will it take to attain your goals, and what steps have you taken toward attaining them?
- Please describe the ideal job for you.
- How would you describe yourself in terms of your ability to work as a member of a team?
- What short-term goals and objectives have you established for yourself?
- How would you evaluate your ability to deal with conflict?
- Describe what you have accomplished toward reaching a recent goal for yourself.
- Can you describe your long-range goals and objectives?
- What plans do you have for continued study? An advanced degree?
- Can you describe your long-range goals and objectives?
- Why have your chosen this health care organization?

Many institutions are moving toward a behavior-based interviewing technique. This technique allows the manager to more critically evaluate a person's capabilities based on the following questions:

- Describe a situation in which you were able to use persuasion to successfully convince someone to see things your way.
- Describe a time when you were faced with a stressful situation that demonstrated your coping skills.
- Give me a specific example of a time when you used good judgment and logic in solving a problem.
- Give me an example of a time when you set a goal, and were able to meet or achieve it.
- Give me a specific example of a time when you had to conform to a policy with which you did not agree.

- Tell me about a time when you had to go above and beyond the call of duty to get a job done.
- Tell me about a time when you had too many things to do, and you were required to prioritize your tasks.
- Give me an example of a time when you had to make a split-second decision.
- What is your typical way of dealing with conflict? Give me an example.
- Tell me about a time you were able to successfully deal with another person even when that individual may not have personally liked you (or vice versa).
- Tell me about a difficult decision you have made in the last year.
- Give me an example of a time when you tried to accomplish something and failed.
- Give me an example of when you showed initiative and took the lead.
- Tell me about a recent situation in which you had to deal with a very upset customer or co-worker.

These questions can also be customized to deal with specific patient situations.

Lawful and Unlawful Inquiries

As the manager, there are also some rules for things to avoid in the interviewing process as follows:
- Do not make promises that you cannot keep.
- Do not ask about anything that the law prohibits you from considering, in making your decision. For example, do not ask about an applicant's race or religion because you are not allowed to consider these factors in making your decision. Table 21-1 provides some ideas about how to get relevant information while staying within the bounds of the law. And do not panic if an applicant raises a delicate subject (such as disability or national origin) without any prompting from you. You cannot raise such subjects, but the applicant can.
- Respect the applicant's privacy. Although federal law does not require you to do so, many state laws and rules of etiquette do.

It is also a good strategy to ask the candidate if they have any questions of you, the interviewer. The interview is a time for both the candidate and interviewer to find the answers to any potential questions they have regarding the candidate and the organization. Box 21-4 provides guidelines for the interview process for the nurse manager.

RECRUITMENT STRATEGIES

The final stage in the recruitment process, the selection and acceptance of the candidate, often relies on many of the various recruitment activities of the organization. Many of these strategies reflect compensation, benefits, or work alternatives that are important to the nurses whom the organization is trying to recruit. Some recruitment strategies are listed in Box 21-5.

If you are the individual being interviewed, you need to know in advance, which of these recruitment strategies are important to you. If you are the nurse manager, you need to be aware of the recruitment strategies that are made available to members of your unit. Some questions that may be asked include:
- What are the specific duties of the position?
- What are the strategic objectives for this unit?
- What is the nurse-to-patient ratio?
- Is there support staff on the unit to assist nurses?
- In what ways are nurses held accountable for high qualities of practice?
- How much input do nurses have regarding systems, equipment, and the care environment? As a new nurse, what opportunities will I have to participate in shared governance?
- What particular opportunities/challenges presently exist on this unit?
- What professional development opportunities are available to nurses?
- Tell me about your culture of patient safety in this institution.
- Can you tell me how the nurses at this institution strive for excellence?
- Tell me about your commitment to the educational advancement of your nurses.

As a new nurse, you should determine the qualities of a work environment that are important to you before the interview. Review the organization's mission, philosophy, and vision to determine if it is congruent with your professional values. As a nurse manager, realize which qualities of the work environment are important to members of your staff. Although pay is an important issue, it is generally not an acceptable first or early question to ask of an interviewer. Pay information is usually available on the job posting site.

Many of these strategies play an important role in the satisfaction of the nurses and serve to assist with

TABLE 21-1 Interview Questions that May and May not be Asked

Subject	Lawful Inquiry/Areas You Can Inquire About	Unlawful Inquiry/Areas You Cannot Inquire About
Age	Are you 18 years of age or older? (to determine if the applicant is legally old enough to perform the job) If applicant is over age 21 (if jobrelated, e.g., bartender)	How old are you? Date of birth Date of high school graduation Age
Citizenship; national origin or ancestry	Are you legally authorized to work in the United States on a full-time basis? Ability to speak/write English fluently (if job related) Other languages spoken (if job related)	Are you a native-born citizen of the United States? Where are you from? Ethnic association of a surname Birthplace of applicant or applicant's parents Nationality; lineage, national origin Nationality of applicant's spouse Whether applicant is citizen of another country Applicant's native tongue/English proficiency
Disability	These [provide applicant with list of job functions] are the essential functions of the job. How would you perform them?	Do you have any physical disabilities that would prevent you from doing this job? If applicant has a disability Nature or severity of a disability Whether applicant has ever filed a workers' compensation claim Recent or past surgeries and dates Past medical problems
Drug and alcohol use	Do you currently use illegal drugs?	Have you ever been addicted to drugs?
Sex and family arrangements	If applicant has relatives already employed by the organization	Sex of applicant Number of children Marital status Spouse's occupation Childcare arrangements Health care coverage through spouse
Race	No questions acceptable	Applicant's race or color of skin Photograph to be affixed to application form
Religion	No questions acceptable	Maiden name (of married woman) Religious affiliation/availability for weekend work Religious holidays observed
Other	Convictions, if job-related Academic, vocational, or professional schooling Training received in the military Membership in any trade or professional association Job references	Number and kinds of arrests Height or weight, except if a bona fide occupational qualification Veteran status, discharge status, branch of service Contact in case of an emergency (at application or interview stage)

Modified from Development Dimensions International, Inc. (2003). *Legal considerations in selection; U.S. version.* Bridgeville, PA: Author.

BOX 21-4 Important Guidelines for the Nurse Manager Interview Process

- Prepare questions in advance on an interview guide.
- Take accurate and complete notes, without writing on the résumé or application.
- Save interview notes of all the candidates interviewed, in case of potential legal challenges.
- Use behavioral interviewing techniques in addition to skills assessments. When feasible, include an additional person in the interview process.
- Confirm that Human Resources will conduct thorough reference and background checking.
- Collaborate with Human Resources before extending an offer, promising compensation, and scheduling orientation planning.
- Human Resources will prepare an offer letter of employment for the Chief Nursing Officer's (CNO's) signature.

From Yoder-Wise, P. S., & Kowalski, K. E. (2006). *Beyond leading and managing: Nursing administration for the future* (p. 319). St. Louis: Elsevier.

BOX 21-5 Recruitment/Retention Strategies

- Flexible hours
- Competitive salaries
- Bonus pay
- Relocation pay
- Fixed shifts
- Weekend option program
- Part-time pay with bonus hours
- Flexible benefits packages
- Scholarships for Bachelor of Science in Nursing (BSN) or graduate studies
- Tuition benefit plan
- Educational loan repayment
- Registered nurse (RN) specialty internships
- Professional development opportunities
- Career opportunities
- Specialty certification reimbursement
- Low nurse-to-patient ratios (workload staffing)
- Shared governance/leadership models
- Care delivery model that promotes professional care at the bedside
- Clinical ladder/career ladder
- Free parking
- Magnet recognition
- Culture of safety: zero tolerance for incivility
- Research/evidence-based practice
- NCLEX review course
- Qualified managerial support
- Clinical support; staff educators, clinical nurse specialists
- Workforce diversity
- Interdisciplinary collaboration opportunities

From Huber, D. (2006). *Leadership and nursing care management* (p. 633). Philadelphia Elsevier.

the **retention** of nurses. With the nursing shortage, the competition for qualified staff members is at an all-time high, and the environment created with the emphasis on some of these strategies plays a vital role in the recruitment and retention of staff. Salaries vary according to locale, type of institution, the professional credentials, and past experience of the staff member.

Once the employee is hired, it is the responsibility of the organization to provide orientation, performance evaluation, training, and professional development and a professional work environment.

When the nurse has entered the professional work environment, there are policies and programs that support a safe work environment (Chapter 9). The autonomous work environment, supported by a shared governance was discussed in Chapter 6.

YOUR FIRST JOB AS A NURSE

This is a very exciting time, and the decision about the first professional position is a challenging one. John (2006) has suggested a few tips to help the new graduate get through this decision and survive the first year as a nurse:

- Go on several interviews. Try to find a job that feels "right." That is important in making the decision.

The culture of the institution; its mission, vision, and values; and the work environment are all important variables in determining if the institution is a "good fit." Evaluate your own strengths and challenges, and determine what type of work environment is important for your success.

- Get to know the new job. Gather all of the materials that you were given during the interview process. Read them and look at your job description; do they match what you want to do?
- Find out how long your orientation will be. Will you have a mentor? The first year of work is a period of tremendous learning, and it is important that you

will be supported through this process. You need to realize that you are a novice nurse, with lots to learn and experience. Be realistic about your abilities and choose a workplace based on these abilities and expectations.

- Take some time off before you begin work. You have just finished an arduous journey through your nursing education. Take some time for yourself to recover and to prepare for the next challenge in your nursing life.
- Take care of yourself. One of the major challenges in the first work year has been found to revolve around balancing work and life. Watch your diet, sleep, and exercise. Try to maintain a balance. Also, find someone you can speak to about work outside of the workplace. Have you ever noticed that when nurses get together, they all talk "shop"? You will need to talk about your experiences with someone who will understand. Keep in touch with the support group that you formed at school.
- Stay positive and motivated. Be positive every day, and avoid negative energy and negative people who will drain you.

New Nurse Residency Programs

The first year of nursing has been demonstrated, in multiple studies, to be a period of high stress, with many new nurses opting out of nursing after less than a year of practice (Halfer & Graf, 2006; Pricewaterhouse Coopers, 2007). To address this concern, new nurse residency programs have been developed to support the new nurse in the critical first year of practice. Such programs have been demonstrated to decrease the turnover of new nurses, and to increase their feelings of confidence in the first year of employment (Williams et al., 2007; Casey & Goode, 2008). Registered nurse (RN) residency programs are designed to provide new nurse graduates with new learning opportunities through mentorships within a framework that supports the advancement from beginner nurse to advanced beginner nurse role, while promoting increased competency in the RN role (Benner et al., 2010; Williams et al., 2007). They consist of a curriculum, guidance from a preceptor, support groups, and access to a facilitator (usually an experienced nurse who has advanced through a clinical ladder), who guides the residents in professional role development. They vary in length, with some lasting upwards of 1 year. Residency programs vary in length of time, pay benefits, and

guarantee of employment, so it is important to know the expectations of a residency program.

YOUR FIRST JOB INTERVIEW

At this time in the career path, it is the new nurse's responsibility to make a concerted effort in the job search. This decision should be made diligently with several factors taken into consideration. Preparation for the interview is key. Begin by listing your strengths and weaknesses. Take into consideration your student clinical evaluations from your professors. Was one of your weaknesses tardiness? If yes, you can list or discuss it as one of your weaknesses, but you can add ways in which you have made corrections to this issue. If one of your strengths was clinical group leadership, play this up during the interview process. Be prepared with a list in hand on the day of the interview. You will be asked for references, both personal and professional. Request a letter of recommendation from one of your clinical professors in a course where you did exceptionally well that will clearly point out your assets and strengths. Be prepared to answer the question, "Why do you want to work at this facility?" You may know the culture, the mission, and vision of an association if you have worked there, but if you have not, do some investigation. Evaluate the website for information about the organization, including the facility's mission and vision. Note this in answering a question that addresses why you have chosen to interview at this particular facility. If the health care organization holds Magnet status, you may say you would very much like to begin your nursing career at a facility with Magnet status. You may be asked about your short-term goals and long-term goals. For example, you may be interviewed for a 7 PM to 7 AM nursing position on the Pediatric Unit. A short-term goal might be that you may want to be working the 7 AM to 7 PM shift within 1 year. A long-term goal would be that you plan on taking the ANCC (American Nurses Credentialing Center) Pediatric Nursing Certification when you are eligible. Some institutions will ask you to analyze clinical situations and to present potential solutions.

Where to Look

Where do you look for a nursing position? There are endless ways to search for positions; the Sunday newspaper classified section, nursing journals, online at a facility's website, by word of mouth, and on in-hospital human resources job postings. Job fairs are also an excellent place to job search. The National Student Nurses Association website is one place to evaluate (www.nsna.org/).

Most hospitals have numerous components to the application process. The first contact will be through the application process on the web. That is usually followed by the interview by human resources personnel or the nurse recruiter. This interview is usually used to determine the potential "fit" between the institution and candidate. Afterwards the candidate is usually interviewed by the nurse manager and perhaps staff. Potential interview topics and questions are listed earlier in this chapter.

After the Interview

Once the interview is complete, it is very professional to send a brief message thanking the interviewer for their time and consideration for the position. The message should be handwritten on professional stationery, not a quick email. If it is the candidate's first choice for a position, they should state interest in further discussion about the position at the interviewer's convenience. This is a perfect way to begin a professional future.

PREPARING FOR LICENSURE EXAMINATION

Entry into the practice of nursing in the United States and its territories is regulated by the licensing authorities within each jurisdiction. To ensure public protection, each jurisdiction requires a candidate for licensure to pass an examination that measures the competencies needed to perform safely and effectively as a newly licensed, entry-level registered nurse. The **National Council of State Boards of Nursing (NCSBN)** develops two licensure examinations: the National Council Licensure Examination for Registered Nurses and the National Council Licensure Examination for Practical Nurses, which are used by state and territorial boards of nursing to assist in making licensure decisions.

The new nurse needs to decide where they wish to be licensed. Most graduates take the examination in the state where they intend to work. They first contact the state board of nursing in the state where they intend to work. For the current addresses and contact information on the various state boards go to the following website of the National Council of State Boards of Nursing: www.ncsbn.org/contactbon.htm

TABLE 21-2 Nurse Licensure Compact (NLC) States

Compact States	Implementation Date
Arizona	7/1/2002
Arkansas	7/1/2000
Colorado	10/1/2007
Delaware	7/1/2000
Idaho	7/1/2001
Iowa	7/1/2000
Kentucky	6/1/2007
Maine	7/1/2001
Maryland	7/1/1999
Mississippi	7/1/2001
Missouri	6/1/2010
Montana	10/1/2015
Nebraska	1/1/2001
New Hampshire	1/1/2006
New Mexico	1/1/2004
North Carolina	7/1/2000
North Dakota	1/1/2004
Rhode Island	7/1/2008
South Carolina	2/1/2006
South Dakota	1/1/2001
Tennessee	7/1/2003
Texas	1/1/2000
Utah	1/1/2000
Virginia	1/1/2005
Wisconsin	1/1/2000

If you have questions regarding NLC licensure, please contact your state board of nursing in your primary state of residence for specific requirements.
This table indicates which states have enacted the registered nurse (RN) and licensed practical nurse/vocational nurse (LPN/VN) nurse licensure compact (NLC). Please note that Illinois, Massachusetts, Minnesota, New York, and Oklahoma are pending legislation in 2016.
From Nurse Licensure Compact Administrators. (2008). *Participating states in the NLC.* www.ncsbn.org/nurse-licensure-compact.htm. Last updated March 2015.

Although many states require practicing nurses to take the examination in that state or to apply through the state board for reciprocity, the **Nurse Licensure Compact** of the National Council of State Boards of Nursing (**NCSBN**) is moving toward mutual recognition of licensure by the states. There are 24 such states, with legislation pending in four others as of this writing. Not all state boards have enacted such legislation, but a list of states participating in the Nurse Licensure Compact is given in Table 21-2.

If you move to another state and one of the states has a compact agreement, the process is listed below:

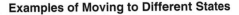

Examples of Moving to Different States

From noncompact to compact:
You must apply for licensure by endorsement in the new state of residency. Your individual state license issued by the noncompact state is not affected and will remain active if you maintain licensure and if so provided by the laws of the nonparty state.

From compact to noncompact:
You must apply for licensure by endorsement in the new state of residency. Your compact license is changed to a single-state license valid only in that state. You must notify the board of nursing that you have moved out of state.

From one compact state to another:
You can practice on the former residency license for up to 30 days. You will be required to:
- Apply for licensure by endorsement (It is recommended that nurses apply 1 to 2 months in advance of a move.).
- Pay any applicable fees.
- Complete a declaration of primary state of residency in the new home state. You will be issued a new multistate license and the former is inactivated. You must notify the board of nursing in the former residency state that you have moved out of state. Proof of residency may be required.

(www.ncsbn.org/nlc.htm)

FIGURE 21-1

After the graduate decides where to take the examination, he or she needs to begin the registration process. NCSBN maintains a website for all candidates for the NCLEX examination, which provides answers for most questions that applicants have.

This process needs to begin before graduation. The steps identified by NCSBN are listed in Box 21-6. The examination is administered by Pearson VUE; this company is contracted by NCSBN to provide test administration services.

An overview of the registration process follows:

Registration Process Overview

1. Submit an application for licensure to the board of nursing where you wish to be licensed.
2. Meet all of the board of nursing's eligibility requirements to take the NCLEX examination.
3. Register for the NCLEX examination with Pearson VUE.
4. Receive confirmation of registration from Pearson VUE.
5. The board of nursing makes the candidate eligible to take the NCLEX examination.
6. Receive authorization to test (ATT) from Pearson VUE.

If you choose to provide an e-mail address at the time you register for the NCLEX examination (whether by mail, telephone, or via the Internet), please note that all of your correspondence from Pearson VUE will arrive only by e-mail. If you do not provide an e-mail address when you register, your correspondence from Pearson VUE will arrive only through U.S. mail.

If more than 2 weeks have passed after you have submitted a registration for an NCLEX examination and received confirmation from Pearson VUE, and you have not received an ATT, please call Pearson VUE at the appropriate number listed on the inside front cover (NCSBN, 2008).

BOX 21-6   The Eight Steps of the NCLEX Examination Process

1. Apply for licensure to the board of nursing in the state or territory where you wish to be licensed. Contact the state board for the requirements.
2. Register for the NCLEX examination with Pearson VUE by mail, telephone, or via the Internet.
   A. The name with which you register must match exactly with the printed name on the identification you present at the test center
   B. If you provide an e-mail address when registering for the NCLEX examination, all subsequent correspondences from Pearson VUE will arrive only by e-mail If you do not provide an e-mail address, all correspondences will arrive only through the U.S. mail.
   C. All NCLEX examination registrations will remain open for a 365-day time period during which a board of nursing may determine your eligibility to take the NCLEX examination.
   D. There is no refund of the $200 NCLEX registration fee for any reason.
3. Receive confirmation of registration from Pearson VUE.
4. Receive eligibility from the state board of nursing you applied for licensure with.
5. Receive the Authorization to Test (ATT) from Pearson VUE.
   If more than 2 weeks have passed after you have submitted a registration for the NCLEX examination and you received a confirmation from Pearson VUE, and have not received an ATT, please call Pearson VUE.
   A. You must test within the validity dates of your ATT. These validity dates cannot be extended for any reason.
   B. The printed name on your identification must match exactly with the printed name on your ATT. If the name with which you have registered is different from the name on your identification, you must bring legal name change documentation with you to the test center on the day of your test. The only acceptable forms of legal documentation are: marriage licenses, divorce decrees, and/or court action legal name change documents. All docu-

ments must be in English, and must be the original documents.

1. Schedule an appointment to test by visiting www.pearsonvue.com/nclex or by calling Pearson VUE.
   A. To change your appointment date:
   • For examinations scheduled on Tuesday, Wednesday, Thursday, and Friday, call Pearson VUE at least 24 hours in advance of the day of the appointment.
   • For examinations scheduled on Saturday, Sunday, and Monday, call Pearson VUE no later than the Friday at least 1 full business day in advance of your appointment.
2. Present one form of acceptable identification and your ATT on the day of the examination.
   A. The only acceptable forms of identification in test centers in the United States, American Samoa, Guam, Northern Mariana Islands, and Virgin Islands are:
   • U.S. driver's license (not a temporary or learner's permit);
   • U.S. state identification; or
   • Passport.
   B. For all other test centers (international), only a passport is acceptable. All identification must be written in English, have a signature in English, be valid (not expired), and include a photograph. Candidates with identification from a country on the U.S.-embargoed countries list will not be admitted to the test.
   C. You will not be admitted to the examination without acceptable identification and your ATT. If you arrive without these materials, you forfeit your test session and must re-register; this includes re-payment of the $200 registration fee.
3. Receive your NCLEX examination results from the board of nursing you applied for licensure with within 1 month from your examination date.

For more detailed information on the NCLEX examination and registration process, consult the Candidate Bulletin by visiting www.ncsbn.org or www.pearsonvue.com/nclex.

From National Council of State Boards of Nursing (NCSBN). Used with permission.

Before the Examination

Some schools of nursing administer "readiness examinations" as a requirement for graduation. These examinations are also administered by companies that manage NCLEX review courses. Many students take such courses upon graduation as a preparation for the examination. Most of these courses are valuable preparation tools for examination candidates. They offer large test banks that allow the graduate to constantly practice and review NCLEX-type questions. Although they are an additional expense for the student, many students believe that the continued exposure to testing situations is worth the expense. Most schools of nursing will assist the student in finding appropriate courses in the area.

PROFESSIONAL GROWTH

As nurses mature in the profession, it is expected that they take a leadership role. How a nurse chooses to do this depends on their practice area. The most important thing is to maintain currency in the profession. Many states require nurses to obtain continuing education credits to renew the nursing license. Although this is a way to maintain currency, much more work is required to keep up with the rapid changes occurring on a day-to-day basis in the profession. A good way to keep up-to-date is to belong to a professional organization that represents the area of practice and interest. There are numerous organizations representing the various specialties within the profession.

Professional nursing organizations, at both the national and local chapter level, provide opportunities to connect with peers in your specialty, share best practices, and learn about new trends, education, and technical advances. There are many reasons for a nurse to join a professional organization. They include:

- Education: Science and technology change rapidly and you need to keep up with the changes that affect health care. Some of these boards even offer continuing education (CE) activities to members at reduced prices.
- Annual conventions: As a member of a professional organization, you'll get notices announcing major conventions that you may be able to attend at a discount rate. Making professional contacts is a big draw at these conventions, where you'll meet other nurses in your specialty.
- Networking: As a member of a professional association, you'll have plenty of other networking opportunities besides connecting with other health care professionals at national, state, or local conventions. For example, you'll probably have access to online chats or forums at your association's Internet site. Not only can you network with your peers and other professionals, but you can also hear how others are handling some of the same issues you face.

- Certification: Many professional organizations offer certification.
- Targeted products and resources: When you join a professional organization, you may get discounts to obtain online CE, newsletters, certification review materials, and much more. Some nursing organizations offer members discounts on auto, life, and professional liability insurance and feature special credit card offers. Many nursing organizations offer members an official journal that may contain peer-reviewed clinical articles and research relevant to the specialty.
- Career assistance: When you're searching for a new job, look to your association's career center for openings, advice, and opportunities. In fact, keep an eye on that information periodically, whether you're job searching or not, to stay in touch with the latest trends in your specialty. Review job openings for salaries and benefits so you know current earning potentials.
- The Internet: Practically all nursing associations have Internet sites you can explore. Typically, they offer general information about the association that anyone can access, in addition to member-only areas with restricted access.

(Adapted from **Greggs-McQuilkin, 2015**.)

A sample listing of professional organizations is given in Chapter 10.

When the nurse has decided on a specialty, it is highly recommended that when eligible, they sit for the certification examination in the chosen specialty field. Specialties have differing requirements for eligibility for the examination. There are advanced level examinations for nurse practitioners and clinical nurse specialists. There are also specialty examinations for specific practice areas; the ANCC certifications are listed in Chapter 10.

Other certification examinations are given by specialty organizations, such as the Certified Emergency Nurse (CEN) examination, which is administered by the Emergency Nurses Association, and the CCRN (Adult, Neonatal and Pediatric Acute/Critical Care Nursing Certification), and several other certification examinations, which are administered by The Association of Critical Care Nurses Certification Corporation.

Some institutions recognize these accomplishments through monetary awards. It is also an accreditation that would provide the nurse with "an edge" if they were to seek an advanced position in nursing.

CONTACT HOURS

Many states have passed legislation that requires a nurse to have obtained a certain number of contact hours of continuing education to renew a nursing license. When hired it is important to ask about the hospital policy on funding for continuing education, both within the facility and out of the facility. Ask whether the facility will pay a travel allowance for the nurse to attend a conference out of state. There are also contact hours offered in nursing magazines and online continuing education contact hours. It is up to the nurse to be aware of the state's licensure requirements for renewal.

RETURNING TO SCHOOL

As a nurse begins to assume a leadership role within the profession, it is time to think about advancing his or her education. Most hospitals have tuition reimbursement for nurses who return to school for an advanced degree. There has been movement in some states (New York and New Jersey) to require nurses to receive the Bachelor of Science in Nursing degree within 10 years of becoming a registered nurse. Some hospitals, especially Magnet-certified hospitals, expect their nurses to continue their education and receive an advanced degree. There are numerous studies that document better patient outcomes in facilities with nurses with advanced education (Aiken, et al., 2003; Aiken, 2004). Remember that although the new nurse has just finished their initial education, it is only the first step. Nursing is a profession that demands continued education and growth.

SUMMARY

You've finally done it! You've graduated; but this is only the first step. You will need to prepare for the NCLEX licensing examination, decide on your first job, and settle into the profession. The profession will demand that you keep up-to-date with changes in patient care, evidence, practice, and professional issues. You will need to join a professional organization, consider taking the certification examination, and return to school for an advanced degree.

CLINICAL CORNER

What I Look for in a Potential Hire

I am going to direct this to you, the potential hire, and I hope that you take this advice, freely given, to make you the hire for the job that you aspired to, and now have the background and experience necessary to apply for the position. This also goes for you, the new registered nurse (RN) graduate, because your first job is extremely important to you; the foundation that you will build your career on.

After 25 years in recruitment, and doing a job that I absolutely love, when I find that fantastic hire, it truly makes my day. Here are some tips for applicants that I hope will help make you that fantastic hire!

- A cover letter is your introduction to the recruiter. Not every recruiter feels as strongly as I do regarding an excellent cover letter, but it sure cannot hurt to do a good one and grab that recruiter's attention. For me, I want to hear your passion about being an RN, and why you would want to work at my institution. Do your homework for this letter and for the interview. It also helps to direct this to the person who will be doing the hiring. Just call the Human Resources Department to find out the name. It shows you have done that little bit extra and that can go a long way.

- Your résumé is going to tell a story of sorts regarding your education, experience, and your other accomplishments. It should begin with your current experience and other experience to follow. Make sure that your dates of employment are correct, and check again when you fill out the application that the dates match with your résumé because background checks are done before the hiring process is complete.

- Make sure a professional message is on your phone or answering machine, for you are a professional seeking employment. When you get to speak use proper grammar (as you have done in your cover letter), and communicate well, as this is a screening process for the recruiter. I cannot even count the times that I have called to set up a possible interview and have not done so because of poor communication skills; after all, an RN is going to communicate with patients, family, physicians, and everyone else connected with patient care. Effective communication is so very important in the life of a nurse or any health care employee. I listen for proper grammar, tone, and attitude in my first contact and I wish more applicants understood how very important this first voice contact is.

Continued

CLINICAL CORNER—cont'd

- You have made it to having an interview scheduled. Give yourself enough time to get to the location where the interview will take place. Take a ride there beforehand, at the same time of day your interview is scheduled, so that you have an idea of what traffic is like at that time. If your interview is on a weekday, as most are, do not take that trip on a Sunday when there is a completely different traffic pattern. Take a good look in the mirror before you leave; "dress for success" is not just a tag line. If any recruiter is being honest they will tell you that first impressions set the tone for any interview. "Dress for success" states how you feel about yourself, and how you wish to be viewed. The less skin shown the better; go light on the makeup and the perfume, and for men, the cologne. Suits give a professional appearance, and are a good and wise investment.

- Prepare for the interview by coming with questions that you might have. Remember that an interview is a conversation with the recruiter wanting to get to know you and your desire for information about the position. I think that if you keep that in mind and are honest, your interview will go well. Show your passion, why you have chosen nursing, and what you can bring to the institution you are interviewing for. Be prepared to be asked behavioral questions because they show how you have handled situations in the past, and they are a good indicator of how you will handle things in the future. This gives the recruiter excellent insight on how you will probably handle situations in the future. Body language is observed, and I watch facial expressions very closely. I want to see a face light up when talking about a patient or why you have chosen nursing; to me it shows your compassion, and I get a fairly good idea about your commitment to nursing. We can teach clinical aspects of nursing but cannot change one's personality and traits, and you will not only be caring for patients, but you will also be an ambassador for your institution, both at work and in the outside world. No one leaves my office for a second interview without my feeling that I would want them to take care of me or my family. And remember, this is your chance to convince the recruiter that you are the one for this position.

- Follow up with a cover letter to both the recruiter and to anyone else who has interviewed you. An e-mail is acceptable but a written letter or note shows that little bit extra. This follow-up shows both courtesy and professionalism, and is extremely important. It keeps you in mind. It is perfectly okay to follow up with an e-mail if you have not heard in a few weeks, but stop at one.

- I hope that these pieces of advice have and will help you to be not just the potential hire but that hire. The last thing I will leave you with is to just be yourself. Good Luck!

Joan Orseck
Nurse Recruiter
Holy Name Medical Center
Teaneck, NJ

EVIDENCE-BASED PRACTICE

Building the Case for More Highly Educated Nurses

Trio of researchers affiliated with Robert Wood Johnson Foundation's (RWJF's) interdisciplinary nursing quality research initiative (INQRI) program lead scientific efforts to show the link between nurse education levels and patient outcomes.

www.rwjf.org/en/about-rwjf/newsroom/newsroom-content/2014/04/building-the-case-for-more-highly-educated-nurses.html

Nursing is the only health profession with multiple pathways to entry-level practice.

Three leading health scientists affiliated with the RWJF are among those who have shown that pathways that lead to the bachelor's degree in nursing (BSN) and higher may improve patient outcomes.

Hospitals that employ larger numbers of BSN-prepared nurses have lower patient mortality rates, according to Linda Aiken, PhD, RN, FAAN, director of the Center for Health Outcomes and Policy Research at the University of Pennsylvania School of Nursing. In a study published in February 2014 in the *Lancet,* she found a 10% increase in the proportion of nurses with BSNs was associated with a 7% decrease in patient deaths.

In 2003, Aiken found that patients in hospitals in Pennsylvania had "a substantial survival advantage" if they were treated in hospitals with higher proportions of BSN-prepared nurses. Her study published in the *Journal of the American Medical Association,* found that a 10% increase in the number of BSN-prepared nurses reduced the likelihood of patient death by 5%.

In 2011, Aiken published a study in *Medical Care* that found that a 10% increase in the proportion of BSN-prepared nurses. Then in 2013, Aiken co-authored a study in *Health Affairs* that found that hospitals that hired more

EVIDENCE-BASED PRACTICE—cont'd

BSN-prepared nurses between 1999 and 2006 experienced greater declines in mortality than hospitals that did not add more BSN-prepared nurses.

Aiken is a research manager supporting the Future of Nursing: Campaign for Action, a joint effort of RWJF and American Association of Retired Persons (AARP) that is working to transform health care through nursing. The Institute of Medicine (IOM) recommends that 80% of the nation's nurses should hold bachelor's degrees or higher by 2020.

Patients are living longer and they are sicker. The BSN-prepared nurses are needed to care for these patients.

Yakusheva and Lindrooth have found positive correlations that if patients are cared for by a higher proportion of BSN-prepared nurses, patients were less likely to die, they stayed in the hospital for shorter periods, and they faced lower health care costs.

More employers are hiring BSN-prepared nurses.

■ NCLEX® EXAMINATION QUESTIONS

1. An effective job description includes:
   A. Title, job objectives, list of duties
   B. Title, job opportunity, list of duties
   C. Job objectives, unit, competencies needed
   D. Job objectives, unit, list of duties

2. A nurse manager is legally not allowed to ask the following question:
   A. Race
   B. When you can begin
   C. Past work history
   D. University attended

3. A nurse manager is legally allowed to ask the following question:
   A. Work history
   B. Age
   C. Number and ages of children
   D. Religion

4. A résumé is different from a curriculum vitae in that:
   A. A résumé is a summary of academic and work history.
   B. A curriculum vitae is a summary of academic and work history.
   C. A résumé is usually used in academia.
   D. A curriculum vitae is education and skills.

5. The credentials that will be evaluated when on initial interview are:
   A. Nursing license
   B. List of references
   C. Permission for drug screen
   D. All of the above

6. An effective cover letter should be sent with a résumé for all jobs you are seeking. The cover letter should include:
   A. A business format
   B. How to be reached
   C. Addressed to a specific individual
   D. All of the above are correct

7. In respect to relevant skills and experience or accomplishments, which of the following should not be included?
   A. Clinical rotations
   B. Volunteer work
   C. Awards
   D. All of the above should be listed

8. For a résumé to be effective it should be:
   A. Targeted to the position being sought
   B. Targeted to any nursing position available
   C. Hospital-based only
   D. Community-based only

9. Facilities that are equal opportunity employers must meet all _____guidelines during the screening process.
   A. Federal government
   B. Federal
   C. Government
   D. Cultural

10. Regarding position posting, once a position becomes vacant in an organization, the institution posts the position _____first.
    A. Externally
    B. Online
    C. Internally
    D. In nursing journals

Answers: 1. A 2. A 3. A 4. A 5. D 6. D 7. D 8. A 9. A 10. C

REFERENCES

Aiken, L. H. (2004). RN education: a matter of degrees. *Nursing, 34*, 50–51.

Aiken, L. H., Clarke, S. P., Cheung, R. B., Sloane, D. M., & Silber, J. H. (2003). Education levels of hospital nurses and patient mortality. *Journal of the American Medical Association, 290*, 1617–1623.

American Nurses Credentialing Center [ANCC]. (2014). *National certifications.* www.nursecredentialing.org/Magnet/Magnet-CertificationForms.

Benner, P., Sutphen, M., Leonard, V., & Day, L. (2010). *Educating nurses: A call for radical transformation.* San Francisco: Jossey-Bass.

Fink, R., Krugman, M., Casey, K., & Goode, C. (2008). The graduate nurse: Qualitative residency program outcomes. *Journal of Nursing Administration, 38*(7), 341–348.

Greggs-McQuilkin, D. (2015). Why join a professional organization? *Nursing, 35*, 19.

Huber, D. (2013). *Leadership and nursing care management.* Philadelphia: Elsevier.

John, T. (2006). Your first year as a nurse. *NSNA Imprint.*

Jones, R. A. (2007). *Nursing leadership and management: Theories, processes, and practice.* Philadelphia: F. A. Davis.

National Council of State Boards of Nursing. Nurse Licensure Compact. www.ncsbn.org/nlc.htm.

National Council of State Boards of Nursing. Application for Licensure Flowchart. www.ncsbn.org/NCLEX_Flowchart.pdf

PricewaterhouseCoopers' Health Research Institute. (2007). *What works: Healing the healthcare staffing shortage.* http://pwchealth.com/cgilocal/.

Williams, C. A., Goode, C. J., Krsek, C., Bednash, G. D., & Lynn, M. R. (2007). Postbaccalaureate nurse residency: 1-year outcomes. *Journal of Nursing Administration, 37*(7/8), 357–365.

Vice Provost for University Life at the University of Pennsylvania. (2008). *Resume guide for undergraduates.* www.vpul.upenn.edu/careerservices/nursing/resume.html#sample_resume.

Yoder-Wise, P. S., & Kowalski, K. E. (2006). *Beyond leading and managing: Nursing administration for the future.* St. Louis: Elsevier.

INDEX

Note: Page numbers followed by *b, t,* or *f* refer to boxes, tables, or figures, respectively.